Selected Papers from the 2nd Conference with International Participation "Basic Research in Endocrinology: A Modern Strategy for the Development and Technologies of Personalized Medicine"

Selected Papers from the 2nd Conference with International Participation "Basic Research in Endocrinology: A Modern Strategy for the Development and Technologies of Personalized Medicine"

Guest Editors

Yuliya I. Ragino
Oksana D. Rymar

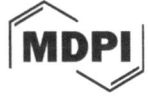

Basel • Beijing • Wuhan • Barcelona • Belgrade • Novi Sad • Cluj • Manchester

Guest Editors

Yuliya I. Ragino
Research Institute of Internal
and Preventive Medicine
Institute of Cytology and
Genetics
Siberian Branch of Russian
Academy of Sciences
Novosibirsk
Russia

Oksana D. Rymar
Research Institute of Internal
and Preventive Medicine
Institute of Cytology and
Genetics
Siberian Branch of Russian
Academy of Sciences
Novosibirsk
Russia

Editorial Office
MDPI AG
Grosspeteranlage 5
4052 Basel, Switzerland

This is a reprint of the Special Issue, published open access by the journal *Journal of Personalized Medicine* (ISSN 2075-4426), freely accessible at: www.mdpi.com/journal/jpm/special_issues/conference_endocrinology.

For citation purposes, cite each article independently as indicated on the article page online and as indicated below:

Lastname, A.A.; Lastname, B.B. Article Title. *Journal Name* **Year**, *Volume Number*, Page Range.

ISBN 978-3-7258-4018-2 (Hbk)
ISBN 978-3-7258-4017-5 (PDF)
https://doi.org/10.3390/books978-3-7258-4017-5

© 2025 by the authors. Articles in this book are Open Access and distributed under the Creative Commons Attribution (CC BY) license. The book as a whole is distributed by MDPI under the terms and conditions of the Creative Commons Attribution-NonCommercial-NoDerivs (CC BY-NC-ND) license (https://creativecommons.org/licenses/by-nc-nd/4.0/).

Contents

Preface vii

Oksana Rymar, Alla Ovsyannikova and Elena Shakhtshneider
Materials of the 2nd Conference with International Participation "Basic Research in Endocrinology: A Modern Strategy for the Development and Technologies of Personalized Medicine"
Reprinted from: *J. Pers. Med.* 2025, 15, 139, https://doi.org/10.3390/jpm15040139 1

Danil E. Kladov, Vladimir B. Berikov, Julia F. Semenova and Vadim V. Klimontov
Nocturnal Glucose Patterns with and without Hypoglycemia in People with Type 1 Diabetes Managed with Multiple Daily Insulin Injections
Reprinted from: *J. Pers. Med.* 2023, 13, 1454, https://doi.org/10.3390/jpm13101454 5

Evgeniia V. Garbuzova, Lilia V. Shcherbakova, Oksana D. Rymar, Alyona D. Khudiakova, Victoria S. Shramko and Yulia I. Ragino
Triglycerides, Obesity and Education Status Are Associated with the Risk of Developing Type 2 Diabetes in Young Adults, Cohort Study
Reprinted from: *J. Pers. Med.* 2023, 13, 1403, https://doi.org/10.3390/jpm13091403 19

Ahmad Bairqdar, Dinara Ivanoshchuk and Elena Shakhtshneider
Functionally Significant Variants in Genes Associated with Abdominal Obesity: A Review
Reprinted from: *J. Pers. Med.* 2023, 13, 460, https://doi.org/10.3390/jpm13030460 29

Dinara Ivanoshchuk, Elena Shakhtshneider, Svetlana Mikhailova, Alla Ovsyannikova, Oksana Rymar, Emil Valeeva, et al.
The Mutation Spectrum of Rare Variants in the Gene of Adenosine Triphosphate (ATP)-Binding Cassette Subfamily C Member 8 in Patients with a MODY Phenotype in Western Siberia
Reprinted from: *J. Pers. Med.* 2023, 13, 172, https://doi.org/10.3390/jpm13020172 48

Nurana Nuralieva, Marina Yukina, Leila Sozaeva, Maxim Donnikov, Liudmila Kovalenko, Ekaterina Troshina, et al.
Diagnostic Accuracy of Methods for Detection of Antibodies against Type I Interferons in Patients with Endocrine Disorders
Reprinted from: *J. Pers. Med.* 2022, 12, 1948, https://doi.org/10.3390/jpm12121948 59

Yulia G. Samoilova, Mariia V. Matveeva, Ekaterina A. Khoroshunova, Dmitry A. Kudlay, Oxana A. Oleynik and Liudmila V. Spirina
Markers for the Prediction of Probably Sarcopenia in Middle-Aged Individuals
Reprinted from: *J. Pers. Med.* 2022, 12, 1830, https://doi.org/10.3390/jpm12111830 69

Sofia Malyutina, Elena Mazurenko, Ekaterina Mazdorova, Marina Shapkina, Ekaterina Avdeeva, Svetlana Mustafina, et al.
The Profile of Glucose Lowering Therapy in Persons with Type 2 Diabetes Mellitus in an Aging Russian Population
Reprinted from: *J. Pers. Med.* 2022, 12, 1689, https://doi.org/10.3390/jpm12101689 80

Gerson Fabián Gualdrón-Bobadilla, Anggie Paola Briceño-Martínez, Víctor Caicedo-Téllez, Ginna Pérez-Reyes, Carlos Silva-Paredes, Rina Ortiz-Benavides, et al.
Stomatognathic System Changes in Obese Patients Undergoing Bariatric Surgery: A Systematic Review
Reprinted from: *J. Pers. Med.* 2022, 12, 1541, https://doi.org/10.3390/jpm12101541 93

Xavier Eugenio León Aguilera, Alexander Manzano, Daniela Pirela and Valmore Bermúdez
Probiotics and Gut Microbiota in Obesity: Myths and Realities of a New Health Revolution
Reprinted from: *J. Pers. Med.* **2022**, *12*, 1282, https://doi.org/10.3390/jpm12081282 . . . . **117**

Vladimir B. Berikov, Olga A. Kutnenko, Julia F. Semenova and Vadim V. Klimontov
Machine Learning Models for Nocturnal Hypoglycemia Prediction in Hospitalized Patients with Type 1 Diabetes
Reprinted from: *J. Pers. Med.* **2022**, *12*, 1262, https://doi.org/10.3390/jpm12081262 . . . . **129**

Preface

The 2nd all-Russia conference with international participation "Basic Research in Endocrinology: A Modern Strategy for the Development and Technologies of Personalized Medicine" was held in Novosibirsk on 24–25 November 2022. The purpose of this conference was to disseminate the latest basic and clinical findings in the fields of etiology, clinical characteristics, and modern diagnostics and treatments of endocrine disorders among various relevant specialists. The conference was intended for practicing endocrinologists, primary care physicians, medical geneticists, pediatric endocrinologists, pediatricians, and physician–scientists. The conference included plenary sessions, specialty sessions, satellite symposia, an open competition for young scientists, and the 2nd-in-Russia educational course for physicians: "Maturity Onset Diabetes of the Young (MODY): Molecular Genetic Determinants and a Personalized Approach to Patient Management."

The main topics included the epidemiology and pathogenesis of endocrine disorders; genomic research in endocrinology; biochemical characteristics of endocrine aberrations; immunology and immunogenetics in endocrinology; cellular technologies in endocrinology; metabolomic research in endocrinology; pharmacogenetics; basic pathomorphology; high-tech care of patients with endocrine disorders; iodine-deficiency-related, autoimmune, and oncological diseases of the thyroid; modern diagnostic and therapeutic strategies for diabetes mellitus; osteoporosis and osteopenias; polyendocrinopathies; an interdisciplinary approach to the diagnosis and treatment of obesity and metabolic syndrome; hypo- and hyperparathyroidism; vitamin D; neuroendocrine disorders; reproductive health; rehabilitation of patients with endocrine disorders; and health resort and spa treatments of endocrine disorders and comorbid conditions.

Scientists from Siberian cities, Moscow, St. Petersburg, and Kazan, as well as Kazakhstan, delivered presentations at the conference. The conference was organized by the Institute of Internal and Preventive Medicine, Branch of the Institute of Cytology and Genetics, Siberian Branch of the Russian Academy of Sciences (IIPM—a branch of the ICG SB RAS). The objectives and subject areas of the IIPM are basic, exploratory, and applied scientific studies in priority areas of molecular medicine and human genetics as well as safeguarding and improving human health, the development of health care and medical science, and the preparation of advanced specialists in science and medicine.

Yuliya I. Ragino and Oksana D. Rymar
Guest Editors

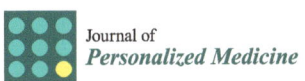

Editorial

Materials of the 2nd Conference with International Participation "Basic Research in Endocrinology: A Modern Strategy for the Development and Technologies of Personalized Medicine"

Oksana Rymar, Alla Ovsyannikova and Elena Shakhtshneider *

Research Institute of Internal and Preventive Medicine—Branch of the Institute of Cytology and Genetics, Siberian Branch of Russian Academy of Sciences, Borisa Bogatkova Str. 175/1, 630089 Novosibirsk, Russia
* Correspondence: shakhtshneyderev@bionet.nsc.ru

1. Introduction

There has been an increase in patients with diabetes mellitus (DM) all over the world, with the advent of new modern research methods (for example, molecular genetic diagnostics), non-classical types of diabetes are increasingly being identified [1,2]. These types include MODY (Maturity Onset Diabetes of the Young). One of the days of the 2nd Conference with International Participation, "Basic Research in Endocrinology: A Modern Strategy for the Development and Technologies of Personalized Medicine", was devoted to this topic. On another day, presentations were given on the most relevant topics in endocrinology, including various thyroid diseases, modern diagnosis and therapy of diabetes, neuroendocrine diseases, reproductive health, and more.

This Special Issue features several articles, the data of which were presented in the conference reports. The articles describe the results of studies on type 1 diabetes mellitus (T1DM), type 2 diabetes mellitus (T2DM), MODY, and sarcopenia, as well as reviews on obesity and type 1 interferon antibodies. The abstracts of these articles are presented below.

2. Review of Published Articles

In the article by Danil E. Kladov et al. (contribution 1), the development of nocturnal hypoglycemia depending on nocturnal glucose profiles in T1DM was described. A total of 395 patients underwent indirect glucose monitoring, during which ten clusters without hypoglycemia and six clusters with episodes of nocturnal hypoglycemia were identified. Predictors of decreased glucose were determined in clusters without hypoglycemia. The results demonstrated the diversity of nocturnal glucose profiles in patients with T1DM, which underscores the need for a differentiated approach to prescribing insulin therapy.

Evgeniya V. Garbuzova et al. (contribution 2) reported in their article the prevalence of T2DM in a cohort study of people aged 25–44 years and also identified risk factors for diabetes in this age group. The prevalence of DM was 0.82%. Patients with T2DM had a larger waist circumference; higher body mass index, systolic blood pressure, and triglyceride levels; and lower HDL levels than patients without T2DM. They were also less likely to have higher education. The risk of developing T2DM increases 6.5-fold with a BMI of ≥ 30 kg/m^2 and 5.2-fold with a triglyceride level of ≥ 1.7 mmol/L, regardless of other risk factors. In the absence of higher education, the risk of developing T2DM increases 5.6-fold. Thus, the levels of these indicators should be taken into account in young people, and when they increase, the individuals should be screened for the presence of T2DM.

In the article by Dinara Ivanoshchuk et al. (contribution 3), the genetic aspects of MODY diabetes are described in detail. One patient and his relatives were diagnosed with a pathogenic variant in the *ABCC8* gene and in the *HNF1a* gene, which makes it possible to plan the therapy for and prevention of specific complications for these patients.

Yulia G. Samoilova et al. (contribution 4) demonstrated in their article the importance of pro-inflammatory markers in the prognostic diagnosis of sarcopenia. The study included two groups: the main group consisted of 146 participants, and the control group consisted of 75 participants. A twofold increase in nitrates was detected in the main group, and a negative relationship between nitrate levels with weak grip strength and appendicular muscle mass was determined in the main group, adjusted for multiple variables. The results of this study can be used to develop a screening method for the diagnosis of sarcopenia at the outpatient stage.

In the article by Sofia Malyutina et al. (contribution 5), glucose-lowering therapy was analyzed in a random sample of the population (n = 3898, comprising both men and women aged 55–84) in Novosibirsk in 2015–2018 (HAPIEE project). Among patients with T2DM, 59% of individuals received hypoglycemic therapy, and 32% did not. Glycemic control (fasting plasma glucose < 7.0 mmol/L) was achieved in every fifth participant with T2DM (35% of those who received therapy). In terms of the frequency of use of hypoglycemic therapy, biguanides ranked first (75%), sulfonylurea derivatives ranked second (35%), insulins ranked third (12%), and inhibitors of DPP4 ranked fourth (5%). In a sample of the population aged 55–84 years, examined in 2015–2018, glycemic control was achieved in every fifth participant with T2DM and in every third participant who received therapy. The data obtained show a low percentage of achieving the target glycemia levels in elderly patients.

Vladimir B. Berikov et al. (contribution 6) developed machine learning-based models for the short-term prediction of nocturnal hypoglycemia in patients with T1DM. The models were created based on continuous glucose monitoring data, and eight parameters from this study were included. Combinations of continuous monitoring parameters and clinical data (23 parameters) were also evaluated. Basal insulin dose, duration of diabetes, proteinuria, and HbA1c were the most important clinical predictors of nocturnal hypoglycemia. Machine learning is a modern method for predicting various conditions, including hypoglycemia.

In an article by Ahmad Bairqdar et al. (contribution 7), variants of genes related to adipocyte function, as well as variants of genes associated with metabolic aberrations and concomitant disorders in visceral obesity, are considered. It is known that genetic predisposition and the influence of environmental factors contribute to the development of obesity. The article presents an extensive analysis of changes in the structure and functional activity of the genes encoding adipocytokines.

Xavier Eugenio León Aguilera et al. (contribution 8) analyzed the data on the influence of microbiota on the development of obesity. Dysbiosis was recognized as one of the many factors associated with obesity characterized by the predominance of Firmicutes, a decrease in Bifidobacterium in the intestine, and a subsequent decrease in the synthesis of short-chain fatty acids, which led to a decrease in the action of incretins and increased intestinal permeability. Bacteria, bacterial endotoxins, and toxic bacterial products enter the bloodstream, leading to systemic inflammation associated with obesity. The authors examined these relationships in detail, as well as the effects of pro- and prebiotics on them.

Nurana Nuralieva et al. (contribution 9) compared three different methods—multiplex micromatrix, cellular, and enzyme immunoassays—to detect antibodies to omega-interferon and alpha2-interferon. Only a cell-based immunoassay can determine the neutralizing activity of autoantibodies; a microarray-based immunoassay can serve as a highly specific and sensitive screening test to identify patients with positive results for antibodies to interferon 1.

In an article by Gerson Fabián Gualdrón-Bobadilla et al. (contribution 10), the changes occurring in the stomatognathic system of patients with obesity following bariatric surgery were studied. Studies published between 2010 and October 2021 in the main databases were reviewed. An analysis of changes and structures in patients with obesity and candidates for bariatric surgery showed that changes in the stomatognathic system during the preoperative period are understandable due to the availability of a wide range of information. However, information remains limited regarding the postoperative period. Therefore, further research is needed, focusing on the characteristics of the system after surgery.

3. Conclusions

This collection of articles on topical issues in endocrinology covers modern methods of diagnosis and therapy of common endocrine diseases. The articles describe the results of research on common endocrine pathologies (type 1 and type 2 diabetes mellitus) and rare diseases (MODY and sarcopenia), which is of interest not only to endocrinologists but also to doctors of other specialties.

Conflicts of Interest: The authors declare no conflicts of interest.

List of Contributions:

1. Kladov, D.E.; Berikov, V.B.; Semenova, J.F.; Klimontov, V.V. Nocturnal Glucose Patterns with and without Hypoglycemia in People with Type 1 Diabetes Managed with Multiple Daily Insulin Injections. *J. Pers. Med.* **2023**, *13*, 1454. https://doi.org/10.3390/jpm13101454.
2. Garbuzova, E.V.; Shcherbakova, L.V.; Rymar, O.D.; Khudiakova, A.D.; Shramko, V.S.; Ragino, Y.I. Triglycerides, Obesity and Education Status Are Associated with the Risk of Developing Type 2 Diabetes in Young Adults, Cohort Study. *J. Pers. Med.* **2023**, *13*, 1403. https://doi.org/10.3390/jpm13091403.
3. Ivanoshchuk, D.; Shakhtshneider, E.; Mikhailova, S.; Ovsyannikova, A.; Rymar, O.; Valeeva, E.; Orlov, P.; Voevoda, M. The Mutation Spectrum of Rare Variants in the Gene of Adenosine Triphosphate (ATP)-Binding Cassette Subfamily C Member 8 in Patients with a MODY Phenotype in Western Siberia. *J. Pers. Med.* **2023**, *13*, 172. https://doi.org/10.3390/jpm13020172.
4. Samoilova, Y.G.; Matveeva, M.V.; Khoroshunova, E.A.; Kudlay, D.A.; Oleynik, O.A.; Spirina, L.V. Markers for the Prediction of Probably Sarcopenia in Middle-Aged Individuals. *J. Pers. Med.* **2022**, *12*, 1830. https://doi.org/10.3390/jpm12111830.
5. Malyutina, S.; Mazurenko, E.; Mazdorova, E.; Shapkina, M.; Avdeeva, E.; Mustafina, S.; Simonova, G.; Ryabikov, A. The Profile of Glucose Lowering Therapy in Persons with Type 2 Diabetes Mellitus in an Aging Russian Population. *J. Pers. Med.* **2022**, *12*, 1689. https://doi.org/10.3390/jpm12101689.
6. Berikov, V.B.; Kutnenko, O.A.; Semenova, J.F.; Klimontov, V.V. Machine Learning Models for Nocturnal Hypoglycemia Prediction in Hospitalized Patients with Type 1 Diabetes. *J. Pers. Med.* **2022**, *12*, 1262. https://doi.org/10.3390/jpm12081262.
7. Bairqdar, A.; Ivanoshchuk, D.; Shakhtshneider, E. Functionally Significant Variants in Genes Associated with Abdominal Obesity: A Review. *J. Pers. Med.* **2023**, *13*, 460. https://doi.org/10.3390/jpm13030460.
8. Aguilera, X.E.L.; Manzano, A.; Pirela, D.; Bermúdez, V. Probiotics and Gut Microbiota in Obesity: Myths and Realities of a New Health Revolution. *J. Pers. Med.* **2022**, *12*, 1282. https://doi.org/10.3390/jpm12081282.
9. Nuralieva, N.; Yukina, M.; Sozaeva, L.; Donnikov, M.; Kovalenko, L.; Troshina, E.; Orlova, E.; Gryadunov, D.; Savvateeva, E.; Dedov, I. Diagnostic Accuracy of Methods for Detection of Antibodies against Type I Interferons in Patients with Endocrine Disorders. *J. Pers. Med.* **2022**, *12*, 1948. https://doi.org/10.3390/jpm12121948.

10. Gualdrón-Bobadilla, G.F.; Briceño-Martínez, A.P.; Caicedo-Téllez, V.; Pérez-Reyes, G.; Silva-Paredes, C.; Ortiz-Benavides, R.; Bernal, M.C.; Rivera-Porras, D.; Bermúdez, V. Stomatognathic System Changes in Obese Patients Undergoing Bariatric Surgery: A Systematic Review. *J. Pers. Med.* **2022**, *12*, 1541. https://doi.org/10.3390/jpm12101541.

References

1. Eizirik, D.L.; Pasquali, L.; Cnop, M. Pancreatic β-cells in type 1 and type 2 diabetes mellitus: Different pathways to failure. *Nat. Rev. Endocrinol.* **2020**, *16*, 349–362. [CrossRef] [PubMed]
2. Shestakova, M.V.; Sukhareva, O.Y. Type 2 diabetes mellitus: Is it easy to diagnose and how to choose a treatment. *Doctor RU* **2017**, *13–14*, 44–51. Available online: https://journaldoctor.ru/catalog/endokrinologiya/sakharnyy-diabet/ (accessed on 3 February 2025).

Disclaimer/Publisher's Note: The statements, opinions and data contained in all publications are solely those of the individual author(s) and contributor(s) and not of MDPI and/or the editor(s). MDPI and/or the editor(s) disclaim responsibility for any injury to people or property resulting from any ideas, methods, instructions or products referred to in the content.

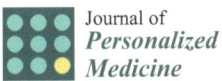

Article

Nocturnal Glucose Patterns with and without Hypoglycemia in People with Type 1 Diabetes Managed with Multiple Daily Insulin Injections

Danil E. Kladov [1,2], Vladimir B. Berikov [1,3], Julia F. Semenova [1] and Vadim V. Klimontov [1,4],*

[1] Laboratory of Endocrinology, Research Institute of Clinical and Experimental Lymphology—Branch of the Institute of Cytology and Genetics, Siberian Branch of Russian Academy of Sciences (RICEL—Branch of IC&G SB RAS), 630060 Novosibirsk, Russia; ekmxtyjr@yandex.ru (J.F.S.)
[2] Department of Mathematics and Mechanics, Novosibirsk State University, 630090 Novosibirsk, Russia
[3] Laboratory of Data Analysis, Sobolev Institute of Mathematics, Siberian Branch of Russian Academy of Sciences, 630090 Novosibirsk, Russia
[4] V. Zelman Institute of Medicine and Psychology, Novosibirsk State University, 630090 Novosibirsk, Russia
* Correspondence: klimontov@mail.ru

Abstract: Nocturnal hypoglycemia (NH) is a potentially dangerous and underestimated complication of insulin therapy. In this study, we aimed to determine which patterns of nocturnal glucose profiles are associated with NH in patients with type 1 diabetes (T1D) managed with multiple daily insulin injections. A dataset of continuous glucose monitoring (CGM) recordings obtained from 395 adult subjects with T1D was used for modeling. The clustering of CGM data was performed using a hierarchical clustering algorithm. Ten clusters without hypoglycemia and six clusters with NH episode(s) were identified. The differences among the clusters included initial and final glucose levels, glucose change during the night, and the presence of uptrends or downtrends. Post-midnight hyperglycemia was revealed in 5 out of 10 clusters without NH; in patterns with downtrends, initially elevated glucose prevented NH episodes. In clusters with initially near-normal glucose levels and downtrends, most episodes of NH were observed from midnight to 4 a.m.; if glucose was initially elevated, the episodes occurred at 2–4 a.m. or 4–6 a.m., depending on the time of the start of the downtrend. The results demonstrate the diversity of nocturnal glucose profiles in patients with T1D, which highlights the need for a differentiated approach to therapy adjustment.

Keywords: type 1 diabetes; hypoglycemia; continuous glucose monitoring; clustering; prediction

1. Introduction

According to the International Diabetes Federation Atlas Report from 2022 [1], there are 8.75 million people living with type 1 diabetes (T1D) globally, and there were an estimated 182,000 deaths due to T1D in 2022. In real-world clinical practice, glycemic control remains sub-optimal for most people with T1D [2]. Hypoglycemia is a known barrier to achieving glycemic control goals in people with diabetes. Fear of hypoglycemia is common in subjects with T1D and affects their psychosocial well-being and diabetes management [3].

In the population of people with diabetes, individuals with T1D on basal–bolus insulin therapy have the greatest risk of hypoglycemia. In a recent international study evaluating the incidence of hypoglycemia in patients with insulin-treated diabetes, hypoglycemic events were reported by 97.4% of participants with T1D, with an estimated rate of 6.86 events per patient per month [4]. A growing body of evidence indicates that hypoglycemia induces a wide range of molecular and physiological changes in targeted organs, including the cardiovascular and nervous systems [5]. In patients with T1D, severe hypoglycemia is associated with a 4–10% increase in mortality [6]. Nocturnal hypoglycemia (NH) is considered to be a particular challenge, given the difficulty in recognition, prevention, and treatment. In healthy subjects, hypoglycemia usually triggers awakening,

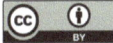

but this effect is reduced in patients with T1D [7]. An episode of NH may be a cause of sleep disturbances and morning headache, chronic fatigue, and mood changes; it is also associated with cardiac arrhythmias, resulting in "death-in-bed syndrome" [8,9]. Therefore, the prevention of NH is an important task in T1D management.

Continuous glucose monitoring (CGM) has provided new opportunities for the assessment of nocturnal glucose profiles and the detection of NH. Studies with the use of CGM showed a significantly higher prevalence of asymptomatic NH in patients with T1D than previously anticipated [10,11]. The forecasting of NH events is a difficult challenge. Previous studies indicate that both low and high glycated hemoglobin A1c (HbA1c) levels are associated with NH episodes in patients with T1D [10–13]. Additionally, glucose variability and antecedent daytime hypoglycemia turned out to be reliable predictors of NH [12,13]. Therefore, the existence of various NH patterns with different relationships with mean and pre-bedtime glucose levels and nocturnal glucose trends could be speculated.

In this study, we applied cluster analysis to CGM data to identify different patterns of interstitial glucose fluctuations at night in people with T1D managed with multiple daily insulin injections (MDIs). Clustering analysis is applied in medical research for mining knowledge and classifying patients, events, laboratory data, etc. [14]. In diabetology, cluster analysis techniques were used for the identification of diabetes subtypes [15]. In some recent studies, the clustering of CGM data was applied to different clinical tasks. Kahkoska et al. identified three dysglycemia clusters in youth with T1D based on CGM parameters measuring hypoglycemia, hyperglycemia, and glucose variability [16]. Schroder et al. applied clustering algorithms for the classification of postprandial glycemic patterns in T1D subjects under closed-loop control [17]. Tao et al. recognized four glucose clusters in patients with type 2 diabetes (T2D) based on CGM and clinical data [18]. Li et al. extracted and clustered the trend components of CGM data to assess and predict the effect of treatment on T2D [19]. In the study by Varghese et al., "time in range profile", "hypo profile", and "hyper profile" were identified from the CGM data of patients with T2D [20]. Inayama et al. categorized the CGM data of women with gestational diabetes into three clusters depending on glucose level and variability [21].

The aim of this study was to identify patterns of nocturnal glucose profiles with and without NH episodes by clustering CGM data in patients with T1D.

2. Materials and Methods

2.1. Database

We used a dataset of CGM recordings from the database of RICEL—a branch of IC&G SB RAS—a tertiary referral hospital. The recordings were obtained from 395 T1D patients, 153 men and 242 women, aged from 18 to 67 years, managed with MDIs. We applied the following set of exclusion criteria: current diabetic ketoacidosis, hyperglycemic hyperosmolar state, congestive heart failure (class IV according to NYHA), end-stage renal disease, known malignant neoplasm, acute infectious disease, and pregnancy.

CGM was performed with Medtronic Paradigm MMT-722, MiniMed Paradigm Veo (MMT-754), and Medtronic CareLink Pro™ v. 2.5.A software (Medtronic, Minneapolis, MN, USA). These systems measure the level of glucose in interstitial fluid at intervals of 5 min in the range from 2.2 to 22 mmol/L.

2.2. CGM Data Cleaning and Preprocessing

In the first step, nocturnal (0.00–6.00) segments with a length of 72 measurements were extracted from CGM records. Time intervals with a gap of three or more consecutive values, or more than 10% of all values, were excluded. We filled missing values with an average of the nearest left and right non-zero values. If the first or last value in the time series was omitted, the gaps were filled with the nearest numeric value.

In the next step, we divided all time series into two groups depending on the presence of NH. The NH was defined as an episode of interstitial glucose < 3.9 mmol/L lasting at least 15 min between 0 and 6 a.m. [22].

The final step of preprocessing was standardization, which consisted of transforming the glucose series from each patient into series with zero mean and unit variance.

After excluding recordings with missing data (about 17%) and outliers (4%), 2519 time series, including 256 with NH, were analyzed.

2.3. Clustering Procedure

By now, a number of methods for time series clustering have been proposed [23]. Taking into account the rather short length of the intervals (72 measurements for a nocturnal interval) and a large degree of glucose variability, we chose an algorithm of hierarchical clustering that allowed us to determine the structural properties of the data. The number of clusters was established empirically based on the Silhouette Score (SS) [24], visualization of solutions, and expert evaluation.

Ward's method was chosen as the criterion responsible for the merging classes [25]. Ward's minimum variance criterion minimizes the total within-cluster variance. To implement this method, at each step of the clustering algorithm, we found the pair of clusters that leads to the minimum increase in total within-cluster variance after merging. This increase is a weighted squared distance between cluster centers. The Euclidean distance was chosen as the metric responsible for the distance between time series since it penalizes more for the difference in coordinate positions. Moreover, Ward's method requires the distance between observations to be Euclidean.

2.4. Assessment of Clustering Quality

The evaluation of the cluster partitions was carried out by data visualization and the SS. Based on the definition of the SS, we tried to find the highest SS with a constraint on the number of clusters.

For analyzing the obtained solutions, the Monte Carlo method was applied. This is a numerical method of assessing the statistical reliability of the revealed clustering structure, which consists of testing statistical hypotheses. This method is usually applied in complicated tasks where standard techniques are impractical due to the lack of information on the statistical properties of data. We proposed a null hypothesis, which was that there is no cluster structure in our data; in other words, all observations in the dataset form one cluster. For testing the null hypothesis, we compared the quality of clustering on a real sample with the quality of clustering on synthetically generated samples of glucose data with the same number of records and lengths of time series. The quality was assessed with SS. Generation was made from a fixed probability distribution, provided that the null hypothesis is fulfilled. This meant that synthetically generated time series had no cluster structure.

In a study by Kirilyuk IL and Senko OV [26], clustering was considered reliable for a given number of selected clusters if the index value on the real sample turned out to be greater than the value of the quantile of the p level for artificial data (in our case, $p = 0.95$). However, the method proposed did not take into account the fact that clustering objects are time series. Since time series usually have a dependency between neighboring components, this means that many time series have autocovariance. Thus, to assess the statistical reliability of clustering structures, we used the Monte Carlo method and took into account the autocovariance of the clustered time series for the first few lags. In our work, the autocorrelation was taken into consideration for generating time series. This made it possible to make the artificial data more similar to the real data.

Probability distribution that was used for generating time series was multivariate Gaussian distribution N(E,C), where vector E is the sample mean, and C is a covariance matrix over the dataset. Autocorrelation was used as follows: first, over the entire time series, we found the sample means m_0, m_1, m_2, m_3 of the corresponding autocovariances at lags lag_0, lag_1, lag_2, and lag_3 (autocovariance at zero lag stands for the variance). Then, we constructed a covariance matrix as follows:

$$\begin{pmatrix} m_0 & m_1 & m_2 & m_3 & 0 & 0 & & & & & & \\ m_1 & m_0 & m_1 & m_2 & m_3 & 0 & & & & & & \\ m_2 & m_1 & m_0 & m_1 & m_2 & 0 & \cdots & & & 0 & & \\ m_3 & m_2 & m_1 & m_0 & m_1 & 0 & & & & & & \\ 0 & m_3 & m_2 & m_1 & m_0 & 0 & & & & & & \\ & & \vdots & & & & \ddots & & & \vdots & & \\ & & & & & & & m_0 & m_1 & m_2 & m_3 & 0 \\ & & & & & & & m_1 & m_0 & m_1 & m_2 & m_3 \\ & & 0 & & & & \cdots & m_2 & m_1 & m_0 & m_1 & m_2 \\ & & & & & & & m_3 & m_2 & m_1 & m_0 & m_1 \\ & & & & & & & 0 & m_3 & m_2 & m_1 & m_0 \end{pmatrix}$$

Finally, we generated a multivariate Gaussian vector that is a synthetic time series. Such an approach to generation best fits our time series model since it takes into account the autocorrelation of the original time series.

2.5. Calculation of Quantitative Parameters of Clusters

To characterize the clusters, we calculated the initial and final glucose levels, as well as the differences between these parameters (absolute glucose change). The initial and final glucose levels were determined as the average of the first three and the last three values in each time series. For clusters with NH, the start time of an episode of hypoglycemia was also estimated. If there were two or more episodes in an interval, we recorded the time of the first event.

2.6. Coding

We used PyCharm for coding and Jupiter Notebook (JetBrains, Prague, Czech Republic) to visualize the solutions. The programming language was Python v. 2020.3.3. The main libraries were NumPy, pandas, SciPy, sklearn, and matplotlib.

2.7. Other Statistical Procedures

The Statistica 13.0 software package (Dell, Round Rock, TX, USA) was used to assess the clinical parameters of the patients. The Kolmogorov–Smirnov test was applied to test the normality. Quantitative data are presented as medians and lower and upper quartiles; frequencies are expressed as percentages (%). *p*-Values below 0.05 were considered significant.

3. Results

3.1. Clinical Characteristics of Patients

We analyzed the results of CGM recordings from 395 patients with T1D, 153 men and 242 women, from 18 to 67 years of age (median 39 years). Diabetes duration varied from 0.5 to 55 years (median 16 years). All patients were on basal–bolus therapy with long-acting insulin analogs: glargine 100 IU/mL (n = 140), glargine 300 IU/mL (n = 135), detemir (n = 63), and degludec (n = 57). Daily insulin dose was 48 (12–132) IU/kg, or 0.7 (0.2–2.0) IU/kg. The level of HbA1c was 8.2 (7.4; 9.4)% (median (25; 75 percentile), range: 4.7–15.1%. The mean monitored glucose was 8.4 (7.3; 9.5) mmol/L; Time in Range (3.9–10 mmol/L): 68.9 (55.3; 81.7)%; Time Above Range: 30 (15.3; 42.4)%; Time Below Range: 0.6 (0.0; 1.9)%; and Coefficient of Variation 30.5 (27.2; 34.2)%.

Severe hypoglycemia in medical history was recorded in 113 (28.6%) patients. One hundred fifty individuals (38%) had impaired awareness of hypoglycemia. Other complications and diabetes-related diseases included diabetic neuropathy (n = 300, 75.9%), diabetic retinopathy (n = 218, 55.2%), chronic kidney disease (n = 216, 54.7%), peripheral artery disease (n = 72, 18.2%), arterial hypertension (n = 71, 18%), and coronary artery disease (n = 25, 6.3%). Most of the patients had a normal body mass index (BMI, 18.5–24.9 kg/m^2), 108 were overweight (BMI 25–29.9 kg/m^2), and 60 individuals had obesity (BMI ≥ 30 kg/m^2).

3.2. Glucose Clusters without NH Episodes

Ten clusters without NH were identified (Figures 1 and 2).

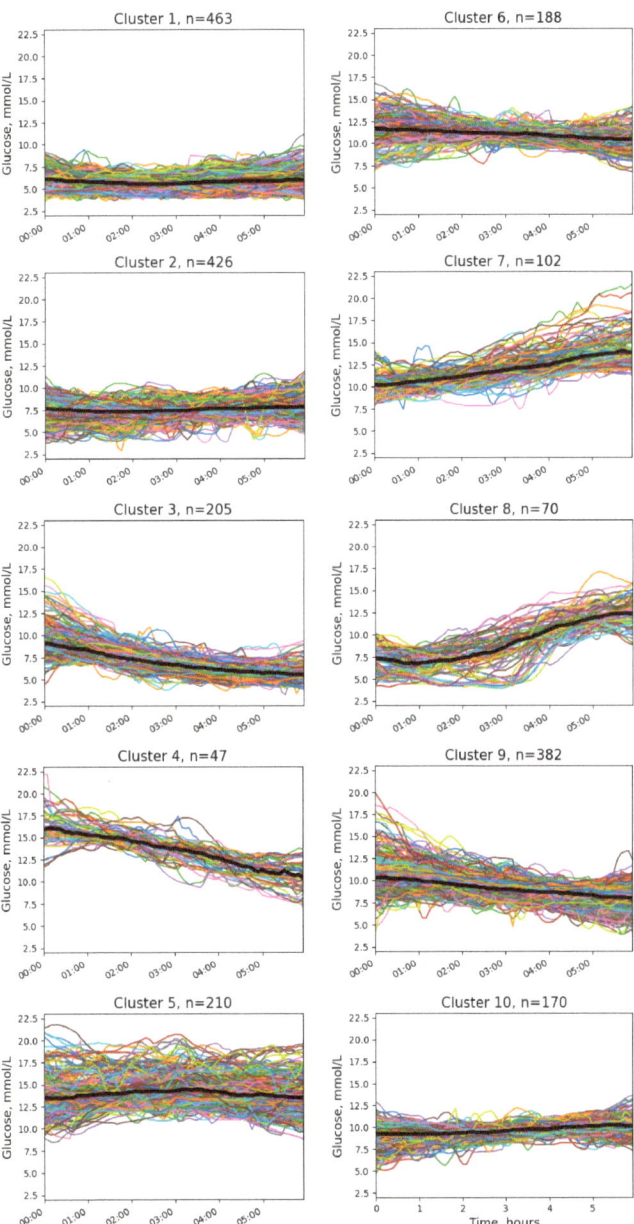

Figure 1. Clusters of nocturnal glucose without episodes of NH in patients with T1D.

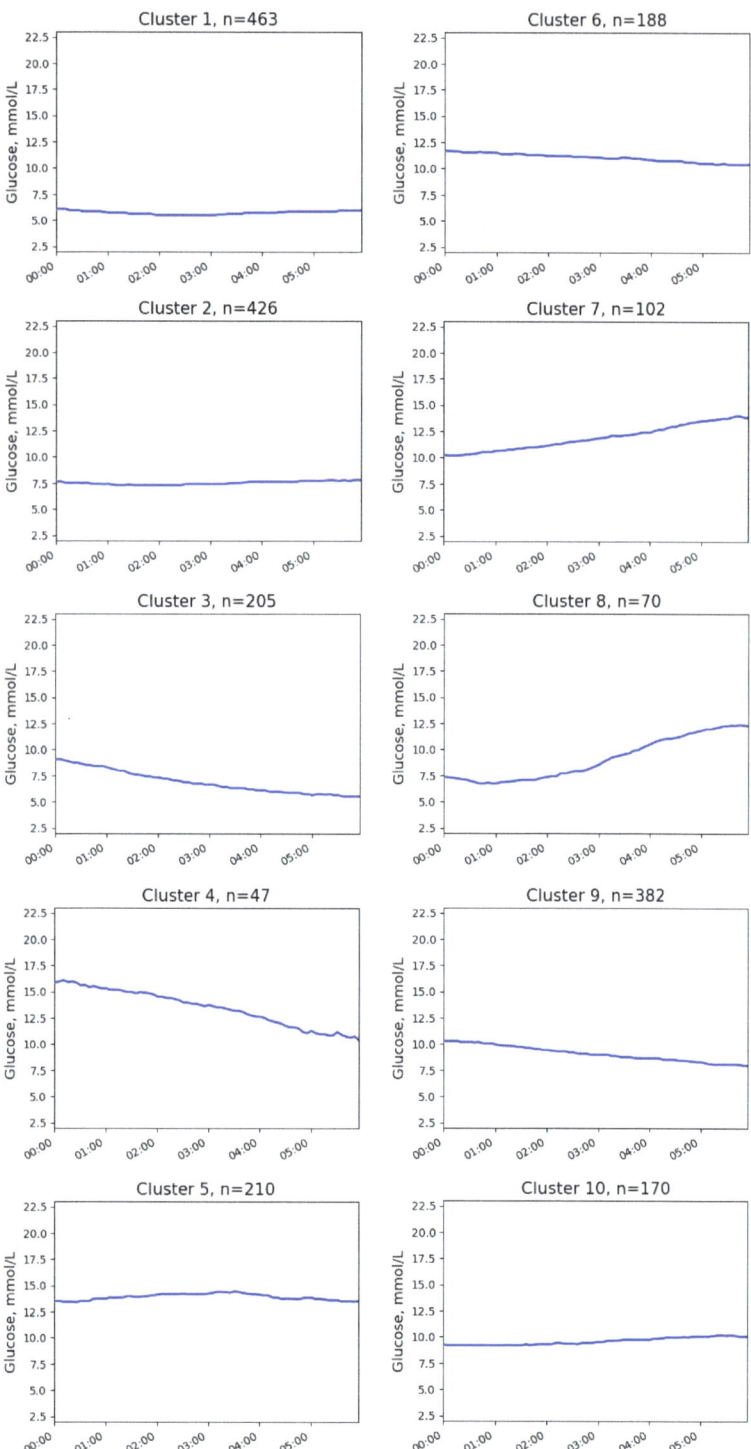

Figure 2. Medoids of glucose clusters without episodes of NH in patients with T1D.

The differences between the clusters included glucose levels at the start and at the end of the interval, absolute glucose changes, and the presence of ascending and/or descending glucose trends. The numerical parameters of the clusters are presented in Table 1.

Table 1. Parameters of glucose clusters without episodes of NH in patients with T1D.

Cluster	Parameter	Median (25; 75 Percentile)	Min–Max
1	Initial glucose, mmol/L	6.1 (5.4; 6.8)	3.8–9.0
	Final glucose, mmol/L	6.0 (5.2; 6.8)	3.9–10.8
	Glucose change, mmol/L	−0.2 (−1.1; 0.7)	−3.3–4.8
2	Initial glucose, mmol/L	7.7 (6.7; 8.4)	3.8–10.9
	Final glucose, mmol/L	7.8 (7.1; 8.8)	4.9–11.5
	Glucose change, mmol/L	0.3 (−0.8; 1.6)	−4.0–5.8
3	Initial glucose, mmol/L	9.1 (8.0; 10.4)	5.0–16.4
	Final glucose, mmol/L	5.6 (5.0; 6.2)	4.0–9.2
	Glucose change, mmol/L	−3.4 (−4.7; −2.4)	−11.9–0.5
4	Initial glucose, mmol/L	15.8 (14.9; 17.4)	11.9–21.0
	Final glucose, mmol/L	10.7 (9.4; 11.4)	7.5–13.7
	Glucose change, mmol/L	−5.6 (−7.4; −4.0)	−12.7–−1.0
5	Initial glucose, mmol/L	13.4 (12.2; 15.1)	8.7–21.6
	Final glucose, mmol/L	13.5 (12.1; 15.1)	9.0–19.5
	Glucose change, mmol/L	0.0 (−1.7; 1.6)	−7.5–7.0
6	Initial glucose, mmol/L	11.7 (10.4; 12.9)	7.3–16.7
	Final glucose, mmol/L	10.4 (9.8; 11.1)	6.9–14.1
	Glucose change, mmol/L	−1.0 (−2.6; 0.4)	−8.0–5.9
7	Initial glucose, mmol/L	10.2 (9.5; 11.1)	8.2–13.7
	Final glucose, mmol/L	14.0 (12.8; 15.3)	11.3–21.2
	Glucose change, mmol/L	3.4 (2.4; 5.4)	−0.5–12.4
8	Initial glucose, mmol/L	7.4 (5.9; 8.4)	4.2–10.0
	Final glucose, mmol/L	12.4 (11.4; 13.4)	9.0–15.9
	Glucose change, mmol/L	5.4 (3.8; 6.5)	1.8–9.9
9	Initial glucose, mmol/L	10.3 (9.3; 11.5)	5.1–19.3
	Final glucose, mmol/L	8.0 (7.3; 8.8)	4.2–13.0
	Glucose change, mmol/L	−2.2 (−3.7; −1.0)	−12.4–3.8
10	Initial glucose, mmol/L	9.2 (8.2; 10.0)	5.2–12.5
	Final glucose, mmol/L	10.1 (9.5; 10.8)	7.6–13.4
	Glucose change, mmol/L	1.2 (−0.1; 2.2)	−3.2–5.2

The most common pattern (cluster 1 in Figure 1) demonstrated a glucose profile similar to the physiological one with normal or near-normal initial glucose and stable glucose levels during the night. Cluster 2 was also characterized by stable glucose levels, but the initial and final glucose concentrations were higher.

Three clusters (clusters 3, 8, and 10) showed close to normal or slightly elevated glucose levels at the beginning of the time interval (mean levels < 10 mmol/L) but with different dynamics during the night. Cluster 3 was characterized by a decrease in glucose levels, cluster 8 had a pronounced upward trend, and the glucose level in cluster 10 was stable.

The next group of clusters was characterized by hyperglycemia (median >10 mmol/L) at the beginning of the time interval (clusters 4–7, 9). In cluster 7, glucose continued to rise during the analyzed interval (mean glucose change +3.4 mmol/L). On the contrary, clusters 4 and 9 showed marked downtrends (glucose change −5.6 and −2.2 mmol/L, respectively). The remaining clusters (5 and 6) represented stable hyperglycemia without significant changes in glucose levels (mean glucose change ≤ 1 mmol/L).

3.3. Glucose Clusters with NH

Six clusters with at least one episode of NH were identified (Figures 3 and 4). The quantitative characteristics of these clusters are presented in Table 2. No episode of severe hypoglycemia was observed.

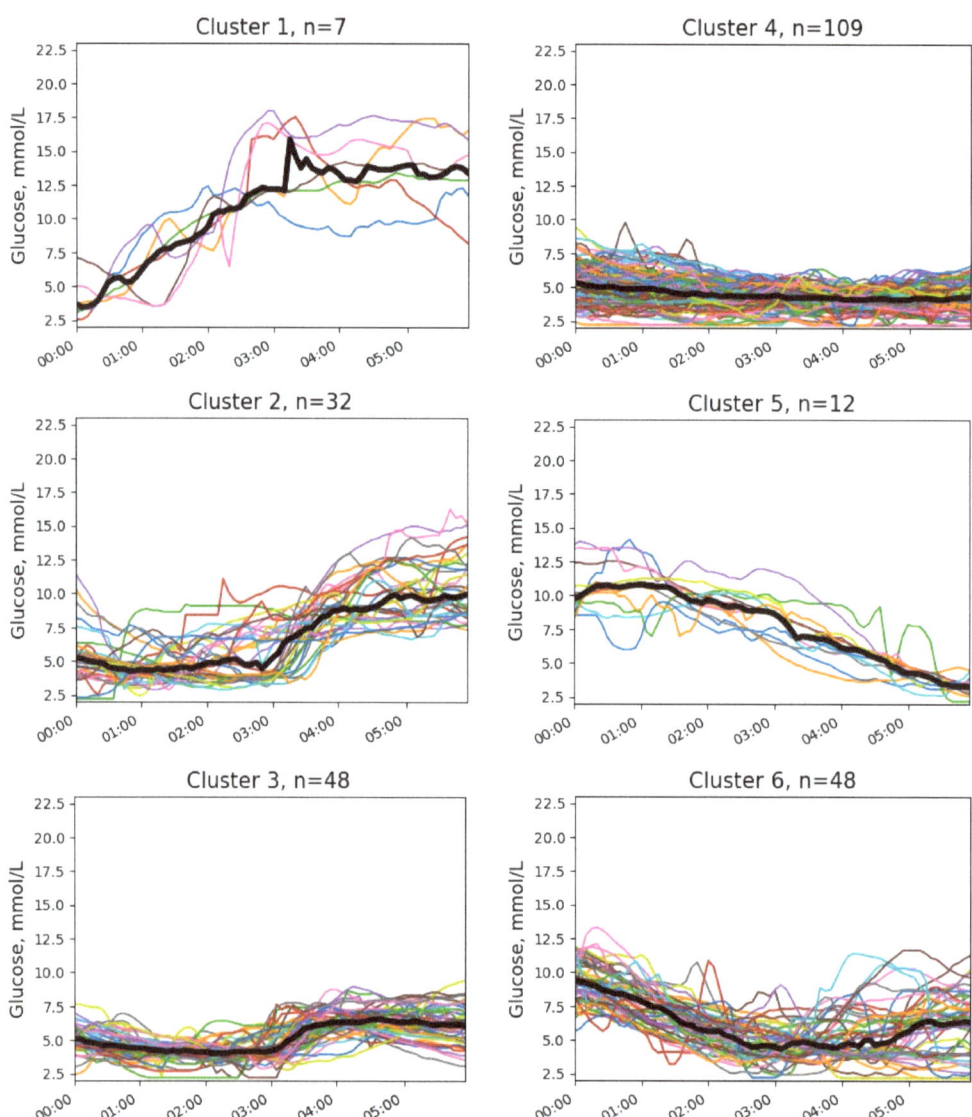

Figure 3. Glucose clusters with NH in patients with T1D.

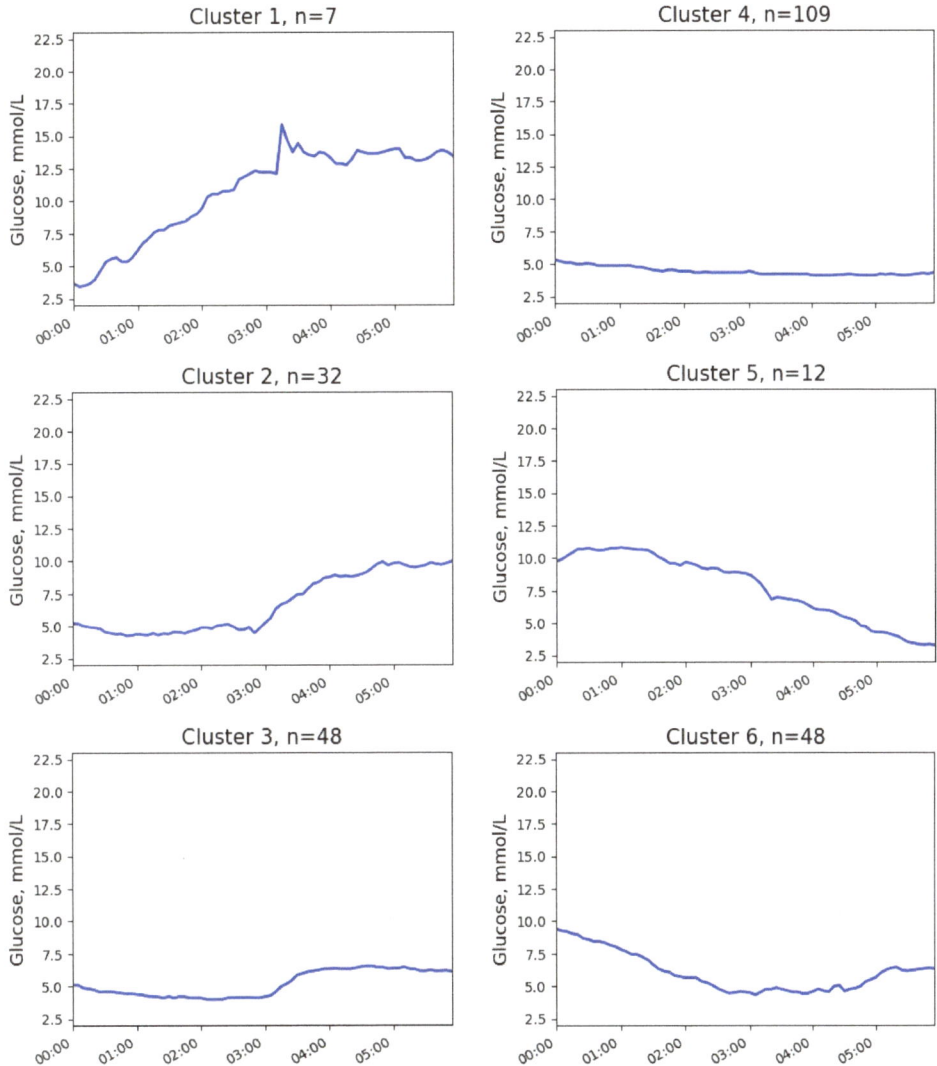

Figure 4. Medoids of the glucose clusters with NH in patients with T1D.

Most observations (clusters 2, 3, and 4) corresponded to the patterns with initially normal glucose levels (medians 5.2, 5.1, and 5.2 mmol/L, respectively) and gentle downtrends. In the most frequent pattern (cluster 4), episodes of NH typically happened between midnight and 3 a.m., the post-event uptrend was slight or even absent, and the glucose level at the end of the time interval was near the cut-off point of hypoglycemia (median 4.3 mmol/L). In cluster 3, NH was observed mainly in the first two hours after midnight, and the glucose level increased after the episode. In cluster 2, the episodes also typically occurred in the first two hours after midnight, followed by a marked increase in glucose levels, leading to hyperglycemia in the early morning.

Less commonly, NH episodes were revealed in recordings with post-midnight hyperglycemia (clusters 5 and 6). These clusters demonstrated the highest overnight glucose decline (median −6.8 and −2.8 mmol/L, respectively). In cluster 5, glucose levels began to decrease after 2 a.m., and episodes of hypoglycemia were observed at 4–6 a.m. On the contrary, in cluster 6, the downward trend was already present after midnight, and hypoglycemia occurred more often at 2–4 a.m.

In rare cases (cluster 1), NH was observed at the beginning of the time interval (0–1 a.m.). The initial glucose level was low (median 3.4 mmol/L). In addition, there was a clear uptrend during the night (+9.6 mmol/L).

Table 2. Parameters of glucose clusters with NH in patients with T1D.

Cluster	Parameter	Median (25; 75 Percentile)	Min–Max
1	Initial glucose, mmol/L	3.4 (3.2; 4.1)	2.6–7.0
	Final glucose, mmol/L	14.1 (12.7; 15.3)	8.5–16.4
	Glucose change, mmol/L	9.6 (8.3; 12.4)	5.9–12.7
	Start time of NH episode	0 (0; 0)	0–1.1
2	Initial glucose, mmol/L	5.2 (4.1; 5.8)	2.2–10.8
	Final glucose, mmol/L	9.8 (8.5; 12.2)	4.7–15.5
	Glucose change, mmol/L	4.6 (3.3; 6.6)	−2.0–11.4
	Start time of NH episode	0.8 (0.2; 1.6)	0.0–3.2
3	Initial glucose, mmol/L	5.1 (4.6; 5.6)	2.6–7.6
	Final glucose, mmol/L	6.3 (5.2; 7.2)	3.1–10.0
	Glucose change, mmol/L	1.3 (0.1; 2.6)	−2.7–5.3
	Start time of NH episode	1.3 (0.8; 2.1)	0.0–5.7
4	Initial glucose, mmol/L	5.2 (4.4; 6.1)	2.3–9.1
	Final glucose, mmol/L	4.3 (3.8; 4.9)	2.2–7.4
	Glucose change, mmol/L	−0.8 (−2.0; 0.2)	−5.3–2.3
	Start time of NH episode	2.1 (0.6; 3.9)	0.0–5.7
5	Initial glucose, mmol/L	10.0 (9.5; 10.6)	7.7–13.9
	Final glucose, mmol/L	3.4 (3.2; 3.6)	2.2–7.4
	Glucose change, mmol/L	−6.8 (−7.4; −5.3)	−5.3–2.3
	Start time of NH episode	5.2 (4.4; 5.5)	0.0–5.7
6	Initial glucose, mmol/L	9.4 (8.2; 10.6)	7.7–13.9
	Final glucose, mmol/L	6.4 (4.0; 7.9)	2.2–11.1
	Glucose change, mmol/L	−2.8 (−5.4; −0.4)	−9.1–2.7
	Start time of NH episode	2.9 (2.5; 4.0)	1.2–5.2

3.4. Clustering Quality

As mentioned above, the number of clusters was chosen based on the SS. The relationships between the SS and the number of glucose clusters are presented in Figure 5.

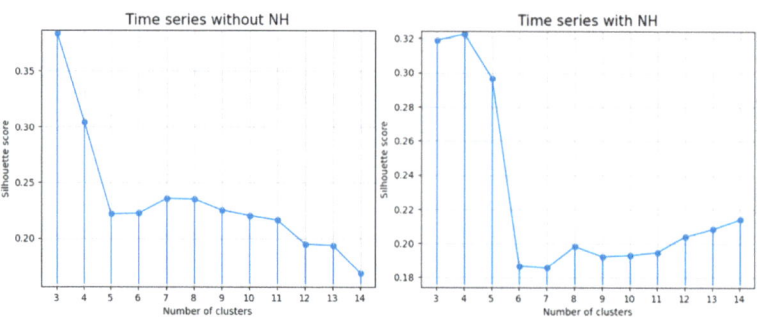

Figure 5. Relationships between the SS value and number of glucose clusters. NH, nocturnal hypoglycemia.

The index value in both cases was close to 0, but nevertheless, it was a positive indication that clusters intersect and overlap each other. The time series with NH had SS values slightly higher than those without.

The assessment of the statistical reliability of the obtained solutions showed reliable clustering at $p < 0.05$ (Figure 6).

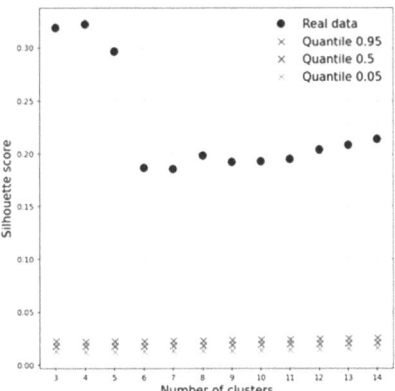

Figure 6. Dependence of the SS on the number of selected clusters.

4. Discussion

In this study, we performed a cluster analysis of CGM data from T1D patients managed with MDI to identify patterns of nocturnal glucose changes. We formed two groups of clusters depending on the presence of NH, a serious and hardly predictable event. We identified 10 glucose clusters without NH and 6 clusters with NH episodes.

In previous studies, a number of algorithms were used for cluster analysis of CGM data. In particular, hierarchical clustering [21], centroid-based clustering [17,27], non-negative matrix factorization [20], and the multilevel clustering approach [18] were tested. In this study, we applied hierarchical clustering to identify different patterns of interstitial glucose fluctuations and the Monte Carlo method to assess the statistical reliability of the obtained solutions. We also took into account the autocovariance of the initial glucose time series. Thus, our study provides further development of the cluster analysis methodology as applied to CGM data.

The obtained results indicate diversity in the patterns of nocturnal glucose profiles in T1D subjects on insulin therapy. Compared to the results of other authors [18,21], we discovered more clusters in CGM data. Although the results are clinically challenging, they may provide a rationale for a new individualized approach to diabetes management with a focus on reducing the risk of NH.

In our sample, most observations of NH belonged to three clusters with normal or near-normal glucose levels after midnight (medians 5.1–5.2 mmol/L) and delicate downtrends. Most episodes of hypoglycemia with this glucose dynamics occurred from midnight to 4 a.m. Another group of clusters was characterized by hyperglycemia at the beginning of the night. In these patterns, the timing of NH episodes depended on the start time and the rate of glucose decline. Depending on the time of the start of the downtrend, the episodes occurred between 2 and 4 a.m. or 4 and 6 a.m. These data clearly demonstrate the limited value of pre-bedtime glucose as a predictor of NH. The presence of a downtrend may be a more important risk factor than pre-bedtime glucose. In agreement, the role of glucose variability as a risk factor for NH has been established [13,28].

The rate and amplitude of the rise in glucose levels after hypoglycemia varied significantly between clusters, affecting glucose levels in the early morning. Interestingly, in the most common glucose pattern, the episodes of NH were not accompanied by a significant increase in the post-event glucose level. Impaired glucose counter-regulation as a result of the dysfunction of regulatory mechanisms and/or excessive insulin levels may be responsible for this abnormality. It should be emphasized that normal pre-bedtime and morning glucose levels do not exclude NH episodes.

Different patterns of glucose dynamics were identified in the analysis of CGM records without NH. Most of these patterns can hardly be considered optimal due to the presence of hyperglycemia and/or downward or upward glucose trends. High glucose levels at the beginning of the night without a pronounced downtrend explain the absence of NH episodes in a number of identified clusters.

Thus, the majority of the identified nocturnal glucose patterns should be considered as motivators for revision of the treatment. Identification of the pattern of glucose fluctuations may be the basis for treatment adjustment. The presence of NH in patients with initially low glucose values or a pronounced downtrend mostly indicates an overdose of basal insulin. Hyperglycemia and/or an overnight uptrend without hypoglycemia indicate the opposite. Clusters with high pre-bedtime glucose and a pronounced downtrend are a particular problem. As a first step, the causes of high pre-bedtime glucose levels should be identified and eliminated. The persistence of a downward trend in glucose levels that is not corrected by reducing the dose of basal insulin may be an indication that a change of insulin is required. Second-generation insulin analogs (glargine 300 U/mL and degludec) provide a more stable glucose profile and may have advantages over first-generation ones in reducing the incidence of NH in patients with T1D [29–31]. Switching to subcutaneous continuous insulin infusion with sensor-augmented pumps or closed-loop control systems may be another option for patients with an increased risk of NH [32–34].

Single-site data and a relatively small sample size are the obvious limitations of our study. Nevertheless, this is the first study identifying nocturnal glucose patterns in T1D patients depending on NH. The results provide the rationale for the classification of NH depending on the time of the event, preceding glucose dynamics, and pre-bedtime and early morning glucose. Identifying a nocturnal glucose profile could be considered to be a promising approach to achieving safer and individualized diabetes care. Future research should address clinical factors that contribute to different nocturnal glucose profiles in subjects with T1D.

5. Conclusions

In this study, we performed a hierarchical cluster analysis of nocturnal CGM recordings in patients with T1D depending on the presence of NH episodes. Ten clusters without NH and six clusters with NH were identified. The results clearly show a variety of nocturnal glucose patterns with and without NH and provide the rationale for the classification of NH depending on the time of the event, preceding glucose dynamics, and pre-bedtime and early morning glucose levels. Obviously, a wide range of nocturnal glucose dynamics requires a differentiated therapeutic approach. Identifying a nocturnal glucose profile could be considered a promising approach to achieving safer and individualized diabetes care.

Author Contributions: Conceptualization, V.B.B. and V.V.K.; methodology, D.E.K. and V.B.B.; software, validation, and formal analysis, D.E.K. and V.B.B.; investigation, D.E.K., V.B.B., J.F.S. and V.V.K.; data curation, D.E.K. and J.F.S.; writing—original draft preparation, D.E.K. and V.V.K.; writing—review and editing, V.V.K.; supervision, project administration, and funding acquisition, V.V.K. All authors have read and agreed to the published version of the manuscript.

Funding: This research was funded by the Russian Science Foundation, grant number 20-15-00057-П.

Institutional Review Board Statement: This study was conducted in accordance with the Declaration of Helsinki and approved by the Ethics Committee of RICEL—a branch of IC&G SB RAS (protocol N. 158, date of approval 1 June 2020).

Informed Consent Statement: Written informed consent was obtained from all subjects involved in the study.

Data Availability Statement: The source data are available from the corresponding author upon request.

Conflicts of Interest: The authors declare no conflict of interest. The funder had no role in the design of the study; in the collection, analysis, or interpretation of data; in the writing of the manuscript, or in the decision to publish the results.

Abbreviations

BMI	body mass index
CGM	continuous glucose monitoring
HbA1c	glycated hemoglobin A1c
NH	nocturnal hypoglycemia
SS	Silhouette Score
T1D	type 1 diabetes
T2D	type 2 diabetes

References

1. Type 1 Diabetes Estimates in Children and Adults. IDF Atlas Reports 2022. Available online: https://diabetesatlas.org/idfawp/resource-files/2022/12/IDF-T1D-Index-Report.pdf (accessed on 18 September 2023).
2. Prigge, R.; McKnight, J.A.; Wild, S.H.; Haynes, A.; Jones, T.W.; Davis, E.A.; Rami-Merhar, B.; Fritsch, M.; Prchla, C.; Lavens, A.; et al. International comparison of glycaemic control in people with type 1 diabetes: An update and extension. *Diabet. Med.* **2022**, *39*, e14766. [CrossRef] [PubMed]
3. Peter, M.E.; Rioles, N.; Liu, J.; Chapman, K.; Wolf, W.A.; Nguyen, H.; Basina, M.; Akturk, H.K.; Ebekozien, O.; Perez-Nieves, M.; et al. Prevalence of fear of hypoglycemia in adults with type 1 diabetes using a newly developed screener and clinician's perspective on its implementation. *BMJ Open Diabetes Res. Care* **2023**, *11*, e003394. [CrossRef] [PubMed]
4. Emral, R.; Pathan, F.; Cortés, C.A.Y.; El-Hefnawy, M.H.; Goh, S.Y.; Gómez, A.M.; Murphy, A.; Abusnana, S.; Rudijanto, A.; Jain, A.; et al. Self-reported hypoglycemia in insulin-treated patients with diabetes: Results from an international survey on 7289 patients from nine countries. *Diabetes Res. Clin. Pract.* **2017**, *134*, 17–28. [CrossRef] [PubMed]
5. Saik, O.V.; Klimontov, V.V. Hypoglycemia, Vascular Disease and Cognitive Dysfunction in Diabetes: Insights from Text Mining-Based Reconstruction and Bioinformatics Analysis of the Gene Networks. *Int. J. Mol. Sci.* **2021**, *22*, 12419. [CrossRef]
6. Nakhleh, A.; Shehadeh, N. Hypoglycemia in diabetes: An update on pathophysiology, treatment, and prevention. *World J. Diabetes* **2021**, *12*, 2036–2049. [CrossRef]
7. Schultes, B.; Jauch-Chara, K.; Gais, S.; Hallschmid, M.; Reiprich, E.; Kern, W.; Oltmanns, K.M.; Peters, A.; Fehm, H.L.; Born, J. Defective awakening response to nocturnal hypoglycemia in patients with type 1 diabetes mellitus. *PLoS Med.* **2007**, *4*, e69. [CrossRef]
8. Seaquist, E.R.; Anderson, J.; Childs, B.; Cryer, P.; Dagogo-Jack, S.; Fish, L.; Heller, S.R.; Rodriguez, H.; Rosenzweig, J.; Vigersky, R. Hypoglycemia and diabetes: A report of a workgroup of the American Diabetes Association and the Endocrine Society. *Diabetes Care* **2013**, *36*, 1384–1395. [CrossRef]
9. Siamashvili, M.; Davis, H.A.; Davis, S.N. Nocturnal hypoglycemia in type 1 and type 2 diabetes: An update on prevalence, prevention, pathophysiology and patient awareness. *Expert Rev. Endocrinol. Metab.* **2021**, *16*, 281–293. [CrossRef]
10. Juvenile Diabetes Research Foundation Continuous Glucose Monitoring Study Group. Prolonged nocturnal hypoglycemia is common during 12 months of continuous glucose monitoring in children and adults with type 1 diabetes. *Diabetes Care* **2010**, *33*, 1004–1008. [CrossRef]
11. Henriksen, M.M.; Andersen, H.U.; Thorsteinsson, B.; Pedersen-Bjergaard, U. Asymptomatic hypoglycaemia in Type 1 diabetes: Incidence and risk factors. *Diabet. Med.* **2019**, *36*, 62–69. [CrossRef]
12. Guelho, D.; Paiva, I.; Batista, C.; Barros, L.; Carrilho, F. A1c, glucose variability and hypoglycemia risk in patients with type 1 diabetes. *Minerva Endocrinol.* **2014**, *39*, 127–133.
13. Wilson, D.M.; Calhoun, P.M.; Maahs, D.M.; Chase, H.P.; Messer, L.; Buckingham, B.A.; Aye, T.; Clinton, P.K.; Hramiak, I.; Kollman, C.; et al. In Home Closed Loop Study Group. Factors associated with nocturnal hypoglycemia in at-risk adolescents and young adults with type 1 diabetes. *Diabetes Technol. Ther.* **2015**, *17*, 385–391. [CrossRef]
14. McLachlan, G.J. Cluster analysis and related techniques in medical research. *Stat. Methods Med. Res.* **1992**, *1*, 27–48. [CrossRef]
15. Sarría-Santamera, A.; Orazumbekova, B.; Maulenkul, T.; Gaipov, A.; Atageldiyeva, K. The Identification of Diabetes Mellitus Subtypes Applying Cluster Analysis Techniques: A Systematic Review. *Int. J. Environ. Res. Public Health* **2020**, *17*, 9523. [CrossRef]
16. Kahkoska, A.R.; Adair, L.A.; Aiello, A.E.; Burger, K.S.; Buse, J.B.; Crandell, J.; Maahs, D.M.; Nguyen, C.T.; Kosorok, M.R.; Mayer-Davis, E.J. Identification of clinically relevant dysglycemia phenotypes based on continuous glucose monitoring data from youth with type 1 diabetes and elevated hemoglobin A1c. *Pediatr. Diabetes* **2019**, *20*, 556–566. [CrossRef]
17. Schroder, C.; Diez, J.L.; Laguna, A.J.; Bondia, J.; Tarin, C. Classification of postprandial glycemic patterns in type 1 diabetes subjects under closed-loop control: An in silico study. *Annu. Int. Conf. IEEE Eng. Med. Biol. Soc.* **2019**, *2019*, 5443–5446. [CrossRef]

18. Tao, R.; Yu, X.; Lu, J.; Shen, Y.; Lu, W.; Zhu, W.; Bao, Y.; Li, H.; Zhou, J. Multilevel clustering approach driven by continuous glucose monitoring data for further classification of type 2 diabetes. *BMJ Open Diabetes Res. Care* **2021**, *9*, e001869. [CrossRef]
19. Li, L.; Sun, J.; Ruan, L.; Song, Q. Time-Series Analysis of Continuous Glucose Monitoring Data to Predict Treatment Efficacy in Patients with T2DM. *J. Clin. Endocrinol. Metab.* **2021**, *106*, 2187–2197. [CrossRef]
20. Varghese, J.S.; Ho, J.C.; Anjana, R.M.; Pradeepa, R.; Patel, S.A.; Jebarani, S.; Baskar, V.; Narayan, K.M.V.; Mohan, V. Profiles of Intraday Glucose in Type 2 Diabetes and Their Association with Complications: An Analysis of Continuous Glucose Monitoring Data. *Diabetes Technol. Ther.* **2021**, *23*, 555–564. [CrossRef]
21. Inayama, Y.; Yamanoi, K.; Shitanaka, S.; Ogura, J.; Ohara, T.; Sakai, M.; Suzuki, H.; Kishimoto, I.; Tsunenari, T.; Suginami, K. A novel classification of glucose profile in pregnancy based on continuous glucose monitoring data. *J. Obstet. Gynaecol. Res.* **2021**, *47*, 1281–1291. [CrossRef]
22. Danne, T.; Nimri, R.; Battelino, T.; Bergenstal, R.M.; Close, K.L.; DeVries, J.H.; Garg, S.; Heinemann, L.; Hirsch, I.; Amiel, S.A.; et al. International Consensus on Use of Continuous Glucose Monitoring. *Diabetes Care* **2017**, *40*, 1631–1640. [CrossRef] [PubMed]
23. Cassisi, C.; Montaldo, P.; Aliotta, M.; Cannata, A.; Pulvirenti, A. Similarity Measures and Dimensionality Reduction Techniques for Time Series Data Mining. In *Advances in Data Mining Knowledge Discovery and Applications*; Karahoca, A., Ed.; InTech: Rijeka, Croatia, 2012; pp. 71–96. [CrossRef]
24. Rousseeuw, P. Silhouettes: A Graphical Aid to the Interpretation and Validation of Cluster Analysis. *J. Comput. Appl. Math.* **1987**, *20*, 53–65. [CrossRef]
25. Ward, J.H. Hierarchical grouping to optimize an objective function. *J. Am. Stat. Assoc.* **1963**, *58*, 236–244. [CrossRef]
26. Kirilyuk, I.L.; Senko, O.V. Assessing the validity of clustering of panel data by Monte Carlo methods (using as example the data of the Russian regional economy). *Comput. Res. Model.* **2020**, *12*, e1501–e1513. [CrossRef]
27. Ono, M.; Katsuki, T.; Makino, M.; Haida, K.; Suzuki, A. Interpretation Method for Continuous Glucose Monitoring with Subsequence Time-Series Clustering. *Stud. Health Technol. Inform.* **2020**, *270*, 277–281. [CrossRef]
28. Klimontov, V.V.; Myakina, N.E. Glucose variability indices predict the episodes of nocturnal hypoglycemia in elderly type 2 diabetic patients treated with insulin. *Diabetes Metab. Syndr.* **2017**, *11*, 119–124. [CrossRef]
29. Owens, D.R.; Bailey, T.S.; Fanelli, C.G.; Yale, J.F.; Bolli, G.B. Clinical relevance of pharmacokinetic and pharmacodynamic profiles of insulin degludec (100, 200 U/mL) and insulin glargine (100, 300 U/mL)–a review of evidence and clinical interpretation. *Diabetes Metab.* **2019**, *45*, 330–340. [CrossRef]
30. Díez-Fernández, A.; Cavero-Redondo, I.; Moreno-Fernández, J.; Pozuelo-Carrascosa, D.P.; Garrido-Miguel, M.; Martínez-Vizcaíno, V. Effectiveness of insulin glargine U-300 versus insulin glargine U-100 on nocturnal hypoglycemia and glycemic control in type 1 and type 2 diabetes: A systematic review and meta-analysis. *Acta Diabetol.* **2019**, *56*, 355–364. [CrossRef]
31. Brøsen, J.M.B.; Agesen, R.M.; Alibegovic, A.C.; Ullits Andersen, H.; Beck-Nielsen, H.; Gustenhoff, P.; Krarup Hansen, T.; Hedetoft, C.G.R.; Jensen, T.J.; Stolberg, C.R.; et al. Continuous Glucose Monitoring-Recorded Hypoglycemia with Insulin Degludec or Insulin Glargine U100 in People with Type 1 Diabetes Prone to Nocturnal Severe Hypoglycemia. *Diabetes Technol. Ther.* **2022**, *24*, 643–654. [CrossRef]
32. Forlenza, G.P.; Li, Z.; Buckingham, B.A.; Pinsker, J.E.; Cengiz, E.; Wadwa, R.P.; Ekhlaspour, L.; Church, M.M.; Weinzimer, S.A.; Jost, E.; et al. Predictive Low-Glucose Suspend Reduces Hypoglycemia in Adults, Adolescents, and Children With Type 1 Diabetes in an At-Home Randomized Crossover Study: Results of the PROLOG Trial. *Diabetes Care* **2018**, *41*, 2155–2161. [CrossRef]
33. Chen, E.; King, F.; Kohn, M.A.; Spanakis, E.K.; Breton, M.; Klonoff, D.C. A Review of Predictive Low Glucose Suspend and Its Effectiveness in Preventing Nocturnal Hypoglycemia. *Diabetes Technol. Ther.* **2019**, *21*, 602–609. [CrossRef] [PubMed]
34. Brown, S.A.; Beck, R.W.; Raghinaru, D.; Buckingham, B.A.; Laffel, L.M.; Wadwa, R.P.; Kudva, Y.C.; Levy, C.J.; Pinsker, J.E.; Dassau, E.; et al. iDCL Trial Research Group. Glycemic Outcomes of Use of CLC Versus PLGS in Type 1 Diabetes: A Randomized Controlled Trial. *Diabetes Care* **2020**, *43*, 1822–1828. [CrossRef] [PubMed]

Disclaimer/Publisher's Note: The statements, opinions and data contained in all publications are solely those of the individual author(s) and contributor(s) and not of MDPI and/or the editor(s). MDPI and/or the editor(s) disclaim responsibility for any injury to people or property resulting from any ideas, methods, instructions or products referred to in the content.

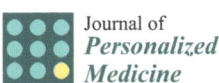

Article

Triglycerides, Obesity and Education Status Are Associated with the Risk of Developing Type 2 Diabetes in Young Adults, Cohort Study

Evgeniia V. Garbuzova, Lilia V. Shcherbakova, Oksana D. Rymar, Alyona D. Khudiakova, Victoria S. Shramko and Yulia I. Ragino *

Research Institute of Internal and Preventive Medicine—Branch of the Institute of Cytology and Genetics, Siberian Branch of Russian Academy of Sciences (IIPM—Branch of IC&G SB RAS), 630089 Novosibirsk, Russia; stryukova.j@mail.ru (E.V.G.); 9584792@mail.ru (L.V.S.); orymar23@gmail.com (O.D.R.); alene.elene@gmail.com (A.D.K.); nosova@211.ru (V.S.S.)
* Correspondence: ragino@mail.ru; Tel.: +7-(913)-376-73-42

Abstract: Background: It is important to determine the influence of traditional risk factors on the development of type 2 diabetes mellitus (T2DM) in young adults. Goal of the research: To study the incidence of T2DM and factors that increase the risk of its occurrence during the observation of a cohort of young adults. Materials and methods: 1341 people aged 25–44 were included in the study from 2013 to 2017, of whom 622 were men (46.4%). The examination included anamnesis, anthropometric data, and a blood test. Cases of developed T2DM were identified by comparing the Diabetes Mellitus Register, medical records of patients, and the database of examined individuals from 2019 to 2023. T2DM Results: In the examined population, 11 participants (0.82%) developed T2DM. The prevalence of T2DM was 0.96% in men and 0.69% in women. Patients with T2DM had a higher waist circumference, BMI, SBP, TG, and lower HDL than patients without T2DM, and were also less likely to have a higher education. The risk of developing T2DM increases 6.5 times at a BMI of ≥ 30 kg/m^2, and 5.2 times at a TG level of ≥ 1.7 mmol/L, regardless of other risk factors. In the absence of a higher education, the risk of developing T2DM is increased by 5.6 times. Conclusion: In young people, high triglyceride levels, obesity, and a low level of education are associated with the risk of developing type 2 diabetes, regardless of other factors.

Keywords: cohort study; persons 25–44 years old; type 2 diabetes mellitus; obesity; hypertriglyceridemia; educational status

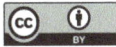

1. Introduction

Type 2 diabetes mellitus (T2DM) is a disease with a rapidly growing prevalence worldwide that is largely associated with obesity and a sedentary lifestyle [1]. The prevalence of established T2DM in Russia is 3.2% [2]. At the age of 25–44 years, according to the NATION study, the prevalence of T2DM is 1.5%. By age subgroups, the prevalence of T2DM is: at the age of 25–29 years, 1.14%; at the age of 30–34 years, 0.82%; at the age of 35–39 years, 1.64%; and at the age of 40–44 years, 2.75% [3]. At the same time, the proportion of participants with prediabetes and T2DM increased with increasing body mass index (BMI).

The global trend of increasing T2DM prevalence, including among all patients with DM [4], is also confirmed by data from Russian studies [5,6]. Global and Russian trends also predict an epidemic of type 2 diabetes among people of young working age. The influence of lifestyle and weight loss on the risk of developing T2DM may vary for different people depending on age and body composition [7]. At the same time, given the increasing prevalence of obesity in the Russian Federation at a young age [3,8], it becomes important to determine its influence as well as the influence of other traditional risk factors on the development of T2DM in young adults for personalized prevention.

The aim of this study was to study the incidence of type 2 diabetes mellitus and factors that increase the risk of its occurrence during the observation of a cohort of young adults aged 25–44 years.

2. Materials and Methods

The study design was a prospective cohort study. Based on the IIPM—Branch of IC&G SB RAS, a survey of the population of Novosibirsk from 2013 to 2017 was conducted. The study was approved by the local ethics committee of IIPM—Branch of IC&G SB RAS (Proto-col No. 6/2013 of 25 June 2013).

The Territorial Compulsory Health Insurance Fund's base, which consists of residents of one of Novosibirsk's districts between the ages of 25 and 44, was utilized to create the sample. Using a random number generator, a sample of 2500 people was selected at random to reflect the population. Since invitations to young age groups are the least likely to be accepted, step-by-step incentive approaches, such as invites sent via mail, phone calls, and media messages were employed. At the screening, 1512 individuals were assessed; those with any known form of diabetes, women who were pregnant, and individuals who had fatal events occur during follow-up were removed. 1341 individuals were included in the final analysis, including 622 men (46.4%) and 719 women (53.6%) (Figure 1). The respondents' average age was 37.08 [31.75; 41.75]. Informed consent of all was obtained for the examination and processing of personal data.

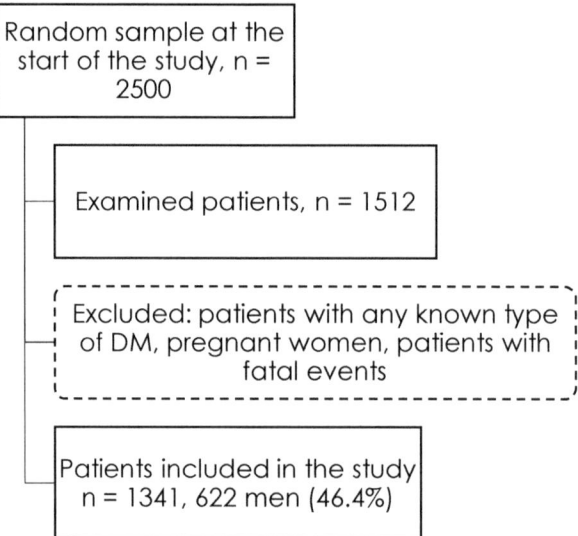

Figure 1. Flow chart of the study population according to inclusion and exclusion criteria.

The endpoint in the form of cases of developed T2DM were identified by comparing the Diabetes Mellitus Register, medical records of patients, and the database of examined individuals from 2019 to 2023. A group of medical professionals with training in standardized epidemiological screening techniques performed the screening. The survey program contained a number of components, such as demographic and social data, a smoking habits survey, a socioeconomic survey, Rose's cardiological questionnaire, anthropometry, 2-fold blood pressure measurement, spirometry, ECG recording with transcription in accordance with the Minnesota Code, and others.

Educational level was divided into 3 groups: higher education, secondary and specialized secondary education, and primary and incomplete secondary education. All groups were included in the analysis, and the final analysis included higher education against all other types of education. Waist circumference (WC) was measured with a centimeter tape placed horizontally in the center between the sacral iliac bone and the lower edge of the costal arch [9,10]. Body mass (kg) divided by the square of height (m^2) is the formula used to calculate the body mass index (BMI) [10]. Elevated BMI was considered >30 kg/m^2. Physical activity was considered sufficient if more than 3 h of physical activity per week [10].

After a 5 min break, blood pressure was checked twice with a 2 min gap on the right hand while seated and registered as the average of the two readings using an Omron M5-I automated tonometer. Systolic blood pressure (SBP) of more than 140 mmHg and/or diastolic blood pressure (DBP) of more than 90 mmHg were classified as arterial hypertension (AH) [10].

Smokers were defined as those who smoked at least one cigarette each day.

On an empty stomach, 12 h after eating, a single blood sample was taken from the ulnar vein. On a KoneLab 30i automatic biochemical analyzer (Finland), blood parameters for lipid profile (total cholesterol (TCH), low-density lipoprotein cholesterol (HDL-C), triglycerides (TG), lilow-density lipoprotein cholesterol (LDL-C)), glucose, albumin, urea, and creatinine were analyzed using an enzyme-based approach. The formula used to convert serum glucose into plasma glucose was plasma glucose (mmol/L) = −0.137 + 1.047 × serum glucose (mmol/L) [10]. The levels of low-density lipoprotein cholesterol were calculated using the Friedwald formula (TCH − (TG/5) − HDL-C). Decreased blood levels of HDL-C were estimated to be less than 1 mmol/L for men and less than 1.2 mmol/L for women, while elevated blood levels of TG were estimated to be more than 1.7 mmol/L, and elevated blood levels of LDL-C were estimated to be 3 mmol/L [10]. The calculation of GFR was carried out according to the formula CKD-EPI (Chronic Kidney Disease Epidemiology Collaboration), taking into account race, gender, age, and serum creatinine level.

The SPSS software tool (version 13.0) was used to statistically process the results. The Kolmogorov-Smirnov criterion was used to examine the distribution. Continuous variables have non-normal distributions; hence, the data are presented as Me [25; 75], where Me is the median and 25 and 75 are the first and third quartiles, respectively. For categorical indicators, the data are presented as absolute and relative values, n (%). To compare two independent samples, the nonparametric Mann-Whitney U-test was employed. To compare the fractions, Pearson's chi-squared test was employed. Multivariate models of logistic regression analysis were performed to identify independent prognostic predictors of the development of diabetes mellitus. The critical significance level of the null hypothesis (p) was assumed to be 0.05.

The work was supported by the grant of the Russian Science Foundation No. 21-15-00022 (statistical processing, collection of endpoints). The funding organization played no role in the development of the study, data collection, analysis, interpretation of data or writing of the manuscript.

3. Results

In the examined population, 11 cases (0.82%) of T2DM developed during the cohort observation. The prevalence of T2DM in men was 0.96%, and in women it was 0.69%. During the first stage of our study, the clinical and anamnestic data of patients with and without T2DM were analyzed. Patients with developed diabetes mellitus, compared to patients without T2DM, had a waist circumference 1.2 times higher (101.00 (90.00; 122.00) vs. 85.00 (76.0; 95.40]), $p < 0.001$, a BMI 1.3 times higher (32.37 (29.78; 39.44) vs. 25.01 (22.04; 28.70), $p < 0.001$, an SBP 1.1 times higher (132.50 (121.50; 140.00) vs. 119.00 (110.00; 129.00), $p = 0.033$), a TG 1.9 times higher (1.75 (1.22; 2.89) vs. 0.94 (0.68; 1.38), $p = 0.003$), and an HDL-C 1.3 times lower (1.03 (10.90; 1.16) vs. 1.29 (1.08; 1.52). $p = 0.001$), and were also less likely to have a higher education. There were no differences in age, sex, smoking status, level of physical activity, civil partnership status, employment, DBP, presence of AH, LDL-C, TCH, Creatinine, glomerular filtration rate (GFR), Albumin, Urea, and Glucose levels between patients with and without T2DM. The characteristics of the examined patients are presented in Table 1.

Table 1. Characteristics of the studied sample of 25–44-year-old participants in Novosibirsk.

Parameters	Patients with Developed T2DM n = 11	Patients without T2DM n = 1330	p
Age	39 (31; 44)	37 (31; 41)	0.253
Men (n, %)	6 (54.5%)	616 (46.3%)	0.763
Women (n, %)	5 (45.5%)	714 (53.7%)	
Physical activity less than 3 h/week (n, %)	9 (81.8%)	882 (66.6%)	0.355
Smoking (n, %)	5 (45.5%)	438 (33.1%)	0.386
Married (n, %)	7 (63.6%)	953 (71.9%)	0.515
Employed (n, %)	7 (63.6%)	1108 (83.6%)	0.076
Higher education (n, %)	2 (18.2%)	833 (62.9%)	0.003
WC, sm	101.00 (90.00; 122.00)	85.00 (76.0; 95,40)	<0.001
SBP, mm Hg	132.50 (121.50; 140.00)	119.00 (110.00; 129.00)	0.033
DBP, mm Hg	84.50 (76.00; 96.00)	78.00 (71.00; 86.00)	0.095
Presence of AH	4 (36.4%)	237 (17.9%)	0.120
BMI, kg/m^2	32.37 (29.78; 39.44)	25.01 (22.04; 28.70)	<0.001
≤25 kg/m^2	0	663 (49.9%)	
25–29.9 kg/m^2	3 (27.3%)	425 (32.0%)	<0.001
≥30 kg/m^2	8 (72.7%)	240 (18.1%)	<0.001
TG, mmol/L	1.75 (1.22; 2.89)	0.94 (0.68; 1.38)	0.003
TG ≥ 1.7 mmol/L (n, %)	7 (63.6%)	216 (16.3%)	0.001
HDL-C, mmol/L	1.03 (10.90; 1.16)	1.29 (1.08; 1.52)	0.001
HDL < 1 mmol/L for men and <1.2 mmol/L for women (n, %)	7 (63.6%)	389 (29.4%)	0.020
LDL-C, mmol/L	2.85 (2.17; 3.77)	3.13 (2.53; 3.69)	0.370
LDL-C ≥ 3 mmol/L (n, %)	4 (36.4%)	739 (55.9%)	0.231
TCH, mmol/L	5.22 (3.85; 5.68)	4.96 (4.34; 5.63)	0.715
TCH ≥ 5 mmol/L (n, %)	6 (54.5%)	646 (48.9%)	0.769
Creatinine, umol/L	72.00 (65.00; 81.50)	74.00 (67.00; 82.00)	0.701
GFR $_{CKD-EPI}$, mL/min/1.73 m^2	1 (10.0%)	220 (23.6%)	0.467
GFR $_{CKD-EPI}$ < 90 mL/min/1.73 m^2 (n, %)	106.38 (94.98; 110.323)	101.47 (90.66; 110.21)	0.505
Albumin, g/L	41.65 (38.65; 43.93)	42.70 (40.80; 44.60)	0.267
Urea, mmol/L	3.95 (3.05; 5.63)	4.30 (3.70; 5.20)	0.534
Glucose, mmol/L	5.83 (5.31; 6.98)	5.73 (5.31; 6.04)	0.251
Glucose ≥ 6.1, mmol/L	4 (36.4%)	292 (22.1%)	0.257

Note: AH—arterial hypertension, BMI—body mass index, DBP—diastolic blood pressure, HDL-C—high-density lipoprotein cholesterol, LDL-C–low-density lipoprotein) cholesterol, SBP—systolic blood pressure, TCH—total cholesterol, TG—triglycerides, WC—waist circumference.

To study the associations of cardiometabolic parameters with the risk of developing diabetes mellitus, a logistic regression analysis was performed (Table 2). The analysis showed that the risk of developing diabetes mellitus is associated with an increase in SBP (by 35.7% per 10 mm Hg), TG (by 47.5% per 1 mmol/L and by 9 times at a level of TG greater than 1.7 mmol/L), WC (by 8.6% per 1 cm and by 13 times in the presence of abdominal obesity (AO)), BMI (by 20% per 1 kg/m^2), and a decrease in HDL-C (by 45 times per 1 mmol/L and by 4.4 times at a level of HDL-C less than 1.1 mmol/L for men and <1.2 mmol/L for women), as well as with other types of education, except higher education.

Table 2. One-factor logistic regression analysis of the association of cardiometabolic risk factors with the development of diabetes mellitus adjusted for gender and age.

Indicators	Logistic Regression Analysis			p
	OR	95% Confidence Interval (CI)		
		Lower Bound	Upper Bound	
BMI, per 1 kg/m^2	1.200	1.119	1.287	<0.001
SBP, per 10 mm Hg	1.357	1.010	1.842	0.050
TG, per 1 mmol/L	1.475	1.079	2.017	0.015
TG ≥ 1.7 mmol/L vs. TG < 1.7 mmol/L	9.013	2.491	32.614	0.001
HDL-C, per 1 mmol/L	0.022	0.002	0.293	0.004
HDL-C < 1 mmol/L for men (vs. ≥1 mmol/L) and <1.2 mmol/L for women (vs. ≥1.2 mmol/L)	4.413	1.271	15.322	0.019
WC, by 1 cm	1.086	1.049	1.123	<0.001
AO (WC ≥ 80 cm vs. WC < 80 cm for women and ≥94 cm vs. WC < 94 cm for men)	12.967	1.634	102.927	0.015
Level of education, higher education vs. other types of education	7.014	1.484	33.151	0.014

Note: AO—abdominal obesity, BMI—body mass index, HDL-C—high-density lipoprotein cholesterol, SBP—systolic blood pressure, TG—triglycerides, WC—waist circumference.

The next stage was the construction of models for multivariate logistic regression analysis (Table 3). Model 1 included gender, age, TG level, and the presence of AO (determined by WC); in Model 2, the presence of AO was replaced by BMI. Models 3 and 4 additionally include education status.

Table 3. Multivariate logistic regression analysis of the association of cardiometabolic risk factors with the development of diabetes mellitus.

Analyzed Factors	Model 1		Model 2		Model 3		Model 4	
	OR (95% CI)	p	OR (95% CI)	p	OR (95% CI)	p	OR (95% CI)	p
Gender, male vs. female	1.083 (0.308–3.811)	0.901	0.992 (0.265–3.711)	0.990	0.884 (0.226–3.454)	0.860	1.353 (0.367–4.986)	0.650
Age, per 1 year	1.029 (0.922–1.149)	0.606	1.053 (0.938–1.183)	0.381	1.043 (0.925–1.176)	0.493	1.018 (0.912–1.137)	0.747
TG ≥ 1.7 mmol/L vs. TG < 1.7 mmol/L	5.314 (1.424–19.833)	0.013	5.119 (1.345–19.477)	0.017	5.365 (1.371–20.995)	0.016	5.220 (1.348–20.217)	0.017
Availability of AO vs. absence of AO	7.893 (0.945–65.914)	0.056	-	-	-	-	-	-
BMI, per 1 kg/m^2	-	-	1.184 (1.098–1.277)	<0.001	1.183 (1.083–1.293)	<0.001	-	-
BMI ≥ 30 kg/m^2 vs. BMI < 30 kg/m^2	-	-	-	-	-	-	6.461 (1.600–26.098)	0.009
Level of education, all types of education except higher vs. higher education	-	-	-	-	5.172 (1.027–26.035)	0.046	5.649 (1.178–27.094)	0.030

Note: AO—abdominal obesity, BMI—body mass index, TG—triglycerides, WC—waist circumference.

The multivariate logistic regression analysis showed that TG, BMI, and education status were associated with the risk of developing T2DM. In Model 4, the risk of developing T2DM increases 6.5 times at a BMI of ≥30 kg/m^2, as well as 5.2 times at a TG level of

≥1.7 mmol/L, regardless of other cardiometabolic risk factors. Additionally, in the absence of a higher education, the risk of developing T2DM increases 5.6 times.

4. Discussion

The main purpose of this study was to study the influence of various cardiometabolic and social factors on the risk of developing T2DM. After conducting a study on a sample of young participants in Novosibirsk, we found that high triglyceride levels, a high body mass index, and a low level of education were associated with the risk of developing T2DM, independent of other cardiometabolic risk factors. In general, our data are consistent with previous studies. The prevalence of T2DM in young adults in Novosibirsk was studied earlier and amounted to 2.2% [11], which is consistent with the all-Russian data of the NATION study. According to the results of this study, 0.82% of people in the study developed T2DM (taking into account the fact that patients with a history of T2DM were excluded from the analysis).

Chronic diseases like diabetes and obesity are becoming more prevalent everywhere [12]. Body mass index, as well as diabetes and insulin resistance are closely related. NEFA, glycerol, hormones, cytokines, proinflammatory chemicals, and other compounds that are involved in the development of insulin resistance are present in higher amounts in obese people. Insulin resistance with impairment of β-cell function leads to the development of diabetes [13]. According to the NATION study, the number of participants with prediabetes and T2DM increased as BMI increased. In the group with a BMI of less than 25 kg/m^2, the prevalence of T2DM was 1.1%. In the group with a BMI of more than 25 and less than 30 kg/m^2, the prevalence of T2DM was 3.9%, and among obese people, the prevalence of T2DM was 12.0%. The data obtained show that T2DM is more common in obese people than in people with a normal body mass ($p < 0.001$) [3]. In China, in a cross-sectional study of 5860 people, the chance of having T2DM in people with abdominal obesity was 1.55 times higher (95% CI 1.08–2.24) [14]. At the same time, in studies that included high-risk overweight and obese populations, weight loss was an important factor in preventing diabetes or delaying its development; a greater benefit was usually observed with greater weight loss [15,16]. In a cohort study of individuals aged 56.1 years (range 50–65), obesity and an unfavorable lifestyle were associated with a higher risk of developing T2DM, regardless of genetic predisposition. Even among people with a healthy lifestyle, obesity was associated with a more than 8-fold risk of developing T2DM compared to people with normal weight in the same lifestyle group [17]. In the study, all patients with T2DM had a BMI of more than 25 kg/m^2, while a BMI of more than 30 kg/m^2 is associated with a 6-fold risk of developing T2DM in young patients, which underscores the importance of early prevention in the form of recommendations for weight loss at any age. BMI does not accurately reflect the adipose tissue distribution throughout the body, and it is unable to distinguish between fat mass and muscle mass. Visceral adipose tissues seem to play a significant role in the emergence of metabolic problems linked to obesity [18,19]. The distribution of adipose tissue is a well-documented and major factor linked to the development of insulin resistance, and WC, which is an index of body fat distribution, could be used as a criterion for evaluating abdominal obesity [20]. Along with BMI, WC can be used to assess the distribution of adipose tissue in young adults. In our study, an increase in WC was associated with an increase in the risk of 2DM in a single-factor analysis; however, BMI turned out to be more significant in multivariate analysis models. Our result was consistent with some earlier studies which revealed that the TG level might be an influential factor for T2DM in young men [21] and women [22]. The results of an 8-year prospective observation of the middle-aged and elderly Chinese population (61.49 ± 13.85 at the time of inclusion) showed that triglycerides are an independent predictor of the development of T2DM. Compared with the group with a normal level of TG, the risk coefficients for developing T2DM in the borderline (TG 1.7–2.25 mmol/L) and high (TG ≥ 2.26 mmol/L) TG groups were 1.30 (95% CI 1.04–1.62) and 1.54 (95% CI 1.24–1.90), respectively. Survival analysis has shown that higher levels of TG can predict an earlier onset of T2DM [23]. In another Chinese study of 7329 people over 45 years of age, hypertriglyceridemia also increased the risk of developing T2DM by 1.9 times (95% CI 1.49–2.46) [24]. In a prospective 5-year follow-up of 5085 younger patients without T2DM, 42.8 ± 9.0 years old, every 10 mg/dL increase in triglyceride levels significantly increased the risk of developing T2DM by 4%. This relationship persisted even when the triglyceride level remained within the generally accepted norm (<150 mg/dL (<1.7 mmol/L), $p < 0.001$) [25]. In our study, the risk of T2DM was 5.2 times higher in patients with a TG level of more than 1.7 mmol/L in young adults. T2DM can be caused by a variety of things, both hereditary and acquired, but the exact mechanism is yet unknown. As an endocrine organ, adipose tissue can affect the metabolism of glucose and lipids. TGs are the most prevalent lipid in adipose tissue [26]. The free fatty acid (FFA) metabolic pathways can be mentioned as the probable mechanism connecting TG to T2DM. Because adipose tissue with an excessive amount of FFA, resistin, TNF-α, interleukin-6, and other substances might result in insulin resistance [27]. Furthermore, raising the level of FFA produced by TGs can increase insulin resistance [28].

The level of education was also previously studied in the context of the risk of developing T2DM: 17.2% of the cases of diabetes in men and 20.1% of the cases in women were associated with a lower level of education in Sweden in all age groups; diabetes mellitus was more common in the group with a low level of education in groups older than 70 years [29]. In a population of 53,159 Danish men and women aged 50–64 years with a follow-up period of 14.7 years, differences in the incidence of T2DM were estimated depending on the level of education per 100,000 person-years. Compared with a high level of education, a low level of education was associated with 454 (95% CI 398–510) additional cases of T2DM, and an average level of education was associated with 316 (CI 268–363) additional cases [30]. At the same time, the authors believe that different susceptibilities to being overweight or having obesity are important mechanisms in the relationship between education and the incidence of T2DM. Previous studies have shown that from 8% [31] to 64% [32] of the relationship between the level of education and type 2 diabetes can be explained by different exposures to being overweight or having obesity [33]. In another Danish study, which included 83,759 and 91,083 participants aged 30–65 years, from a cohort of patients with T2DM and cardiovascular diseases, respectively, a low level of education was positively associated with a higher risk of developing T2DM (OR 1.24, 95% CI 1.04–1.48) [34]. Education establishes an individual's non-material resources, such as knowledge, skills, and self-efficacy, which lowers obstacles and enables people to be more receptive to health messages and convert those messages into healthy behaviors. Additionally, people with a lower level of education are less physically active, smoke more, and consume fewer fruits and vegetables than people with a high level of education [30], which may have an indirect effect on the development of T2DM, but was not separately evaluated in this study. The analysis of our data provides very important additional data on the risk factors for developing T2DM in a young population. The results show that despite the fact that people with obesity and dyslipidemia may benefit from lifestyle changes, their high risk of developing T2DM may persist depending on their initial level of education.

Gender and age in the conducted study did not affect the risk of developing T2DM; perhaps this is due to the initially young age of the population and the insufficient follow-up period for these variables to have an impact.

This study's strengths include the large sample size and extended follow-up. We were able to account for numerous potential confounders because of the inclusion of numerous comprehensive clinical and biochemical examinations. After reading various references, our research is one of the few in Russia and the first in Novosibirsk evaluating risk factors for the development of T2DM in young adults.

This study has several limitations. First, this study was a single-center investigation, and the enrolled participants were primarily residing in the city. Further investigations should be conducted as multi-center studies that include various areas. Second, limitations of the study include lack of access to information regarding family history of diabetes mellitus, age of diagnosis, and lack of information about gestational diabetes. There was also no information about glucose levels during the observation period, which does not allow to exclude latent T2DM. Also, the estimate of the effect of educational level on type 2 diabetes may be inflated due to unmeasured confounding factors from early life, such as family socioeconomic position, family history of T2DM and fetal/neonatal factors.

5. Conclusions

In young people, high triglyceride levels, obesity, and a low level of education are associated with the risk of developing type 2 diabetes, regardless of other factors. These data can be taken into account when developing personalized preventive measures for different age groups.

Author Contributions: Conceptualization, Y.I.R. and O.D.R.; methodology, O.D.R. and L.V.S.; software, L.V.S.; validation, Y.I.R. and O.D.R.; formal analysis, L.V.S.; investigation, O.D.R., E.V.G., V.S.S. and A.D.K.; resources, O.D.R.; data curation, L.V.S.; writing—original draft preparation, E.V.G. and A.D.K.; writing—review and editing, O.D.R., L.V.S., E.V.G. and A.D.K.; visualization, E.V.G.; supervision, Y.I.R. and O.D.R.; project administration, Y.I.R.; funding acquisition, Y.I.R. All authors have read and agreed to the published version of the manuscript.

Funding: The work supported the grant of the Russian Science Foundation No. 21-15-00022.

Institutional Review Board Statement: The study was conducted in accordance with the Declaration of Helsinki. The study was approved by the local ethics committee of IIPM—Branch of IC&G SB RAS (Protocol No. 6/2013 of 25 June 2013).

Informed Consent Statement: Informed consent was obtained from all subjects involved in the study.

Data Availability Statement: Not applicable.

Acknowledgments: The team of authors expresses gratitude to Sazonova O.V. for her help in identifying new cases of diabetes mellitus.

Conflicts of Interest: The authors declare no conflict of interest.

References

1. Global Burden of Disease Study 2013 Collaborators; Vos, T.; Allen, C.; Arora, M.; Barber, R.M.; Bhutta, Z.A.; Brown, A.; Liang, X.; Kawashima, T.; Coggeshall, M.; et al. Global, regional, and national incidence, prevalence, and years lived with disability for 301 acute and chronic diseases and injuries in 188 countries, 1990–2013: A systematic analysis for the Global Burden of Disease Study 2013. *Lancet* **2015**, *386*, 743–800. [CrossRef] [PubMed]
2. Dedov, I.I.; Shestakova, M.V.; Suntsov, Y.I.; Peterkova, V.A.; Galstyan, G.R.; Mayorov, A.Y.; Kuraeva, T.L.; Sukhareva, O.Y.E. Federal targeted programme 'Prevention and Management of Socially Significant Diseases (2007–2012)': Results of the 'Diabetes mellitus' sub-programme. *Diabetes Mellit.* **2013**, *16*, 1–48. [CrossRef]
3. Dedov, I.I.; Shestakova, M.V.; Galstyan, G.R. The prevalence of type 2 diabetes mellitus in the adult population of Russia (NA-TION study). *Diabetes Mellit.* **2016**, *19*, 104–112. [CrossRef]
4. International Diabetes Federation (IDF). *IDF Diabetes Atlas*, 8th ed.; International Diabetes Fedration: Brussels, Belgium, 2017; ISBN 978-2-930229-87-4.
5. Dedov, I.I.; Shestakova, M.V.; Vikulova, O.K.; Zheleznyakova, A.V.; Isakov, M. Epidemiological characteristics of diabetes mellitus in the Russian Federation: Clinical and statistical analysis according to the Federal diabetes register data of 01.01.2021. *Diabetes Mellit.* **2021**, *24*, 204–221. [CrossRef]
6. Dedov, I.I.; Shestakova, M.V.; Vikulova, O.K.; Zheleznyakova, A.V.; Isakov, M.A. Diabetes mellitus in Russian Federation: Prevalence, morbidity, mortality, parameters of glycaemic control and structure of glucose lowering therapy according to the Federal Diabetes Register, status 2017. *Diabetes Mellit.* **2018**, *21*, 144–159. [CrossRef]
7. Al-Sofiani, M.E.; Ganji, S.S.; Kalyani, R.R. Body composition changes in diabetes and aging. *J. Diabetes Its Complicat.* **2019**, *33*, 451–459. [CrossRef] [PubMed]
8. Kelly, T.; Yang, W.; Chen, C.-S.; Reynolds, K.; He, J. Global burden of obesity in 2005 and projections to 2030. *Int. J. Obes.* **2008**, *32*, 1431–1437. [CrossRef]
9. Alberti, K.G.M.M.; Eckel, R.H.; Grundy, S.M.; Zimmet, P.Z.; Cleeman, J.I.; Donato, K.A.; Fruchart, J.C.; James, W.P.T.; Loria, C.M.; Smith, S.C., Jr. Harmonizing the metabolic syndrome: A joint interim statement of the international diabetes federation task force on epidemiology and prevention; National heart, lung, and blood institute; American heart association; World heart federation; International Atherosclerosis Society; and International Association for the Study of Obesity. *Circulation* **2009**, *120*, 1640–1645. [CrossRef]

10. Mach, F.; Baigent, C.; Catapano, A.L.; Koskinas, K.C.; Casula, M.; Badimon, L.; Chapman, M.J.; De Backer, G.G.; Delgado, V.; Ference, B.A.; et al. 2019 ESC/EAS Guidelines for the management of dyslipidaemias: Lipid modification to reduce cardiovascular risk. *Eur. Heart J.* **2020**, *41*, 111–188. [CrossRef]
11. Mustafina, S.V.; Rymar, O.D.; Malyutina, S.K.; Denisova, D.V.; Shcherbakova, L.V.; Voevoda, M.I. Prevalence of diabetes in the adult population of Novosibirsk. *Diabetes Mellit.* **2017**, *20*, 329–334. [CrossRef]
12. Wild, S.; Roglic, G.; Green, A.; Sicree, R.; King, H. Global prevalence of diabetes: Estimates for the year 2000 and projections for 2030. Diabetes Care. *Diabetes Care* **2004**, *27*, 1047–1053. [CrossRef]
13. Algoblan, A.; Alalfi, M.; Khan, M.Z. Mechanism linking diabetes mellitus and obesity. *Diabetes Metab. Syndr. Obes.* **2014**, *7*, 587–591. [CrossRef] [PubMed]
14. Lu, Y.; Yang, H.; Xu, Z.; Tang, X. Association between Different Obesity Patterns and the Risk of Developing Type 2 Diabetes Mellitus Among Adults in Eastern China: A Cross-Sectional Study. *Diabetes Metab. Syndr. Obes.* **2021**, *14*, 2631–2639. [CrossRef] [PubMed]
15. Hamman, R.F.; Wing, R.R.; Edelstein, S.L.; Lachin, J.M.; Bray, G.A.; Delahanty, L.; Hoskin, M.; Kriska, A.M.; Mayer-Davis, E.J.; Pi-Sunyer, X.; et al. Effect of Weight Loss with Lifestyle Intervention on Risk of Diabetes. *Diabetes Care* **2006**, *29*, 2102–2107. [CrossRef]
16. Lachin, J.M.; Christophi, C.A.; Edelstein, S.L.; Ehrmann, D.A.; Hamman, R.F.; Kahn, S.E.; Knowler, W.C.; Nathan, D.M.; on behalf of the DPP Research Group. Factors Associated with Diabetes Onset during Metformin versus Placebo Therapy in the Diabetes Prevention Program. *Diabetes* **2007**, *56*, 1153–1159. [CrossRef]
17. Schnurr, T.M.; Jakupović, H.; Carrasquilla, G.D.; Ängquist, L.; Grarup, N.; Sørensen, T.I.A.; Tjønneland, A.; Overvad, K.; Pedersen, O.; Hansen, T.; et al. Obesity, unfavourable lifestyle and genetic risk of type 2 diabetes: A case-cohort study. *Diabetologia* **2020**, *63*, 1324–1332. [CrossRef] [PubMed]
18. Neeland, I.J.; Turer, A.T.; Ayers, C.R.; Berry, J.D.; Rohatgi, A.; Das, S.R.; Khera, A.; Vega, G.L.; McGuire, D.K.; Grundy, S.M.; et al. Body Fat Distribution and Incident Cardiovascular Disease in Obese Adults. *J. Am. Coll. Cardiol.* **2015**, *65*, 2150–2151. [CrossRef]
19. Hayashi, T.; Boyko, E.J.; McNeely, M.J.; Leonetti, D.L.; Kahn, S.E.; Fujimoto, W.Y. Visceral Adiposity, Not Abdominal Subcutaneous Fat Area, Is Associated with an Increase in Future Insulin Resistance in Japanese Americans. *Diabetes* **2008**, *57*, 1269–1275. [CrossRef]
20. Chen, M.E.; Chandramouli, A.G.; Considine, R.V.; Hannon, T.S.; Mather, K.J. Comparison of β-Cell Function Between Overweight/Obese Adults and Adolescents Across the Spectrum of Glycemia. *Diabetes Care* **2017**, *41*, 318–325. [CrossRef]
21. Norhammar, A.; Schenck-Gustafsson, K. Type 2 diabetes and cardiovascular disease in women. *Diabetologia* **2012**, *56*, 1–9. [CrossRef]
22. Tirosh, A.; Shai, I.; Bitzur, R.; Kochba, I.; Tekes-Manova, D.; Israeli, E.; Shochat, T.; Rudich, A. Changes in Triglyceride Levels over Time and Risk of Type 2 Diabetes in Young Men. *Diabetes Care* **2008**, *31*, 2032–2037. [CrossRef]
23. Zhao, J.; Zhang, Y.; Wei, F.; Song, J.; Cao, Z.; Chen, C.; Zhang, K.; Feng, S.; Wang, Y.; Li, W.-D. Triglyceride is an independent predictor of type 2 diabetes among middle-aged and older adults: A prospective study with 8-year follow-ups in two cohorts. *J. Transl. Med.* **2019**, *17*, 403. [CrossRef] [PubMed]
24. Peng, J.; Zhao, F.; Yang, X.; Pan, X.; Xin, J.; Wu, M.; Peng, Y.G. Association between dyslipidemia and risk of type 2 diabetes mellitus in middle-aged and older Chinese adults: A secondary analysis of a nationwide cohort. *BMJ Open* **2021**, *11*, e042821. [CrossRef] [PubMed]
25. Beshara, A.; Cohen, E.; Goldberg, E.; Lilos, P.; Garty, M.; Krause, I. Triglyceride levels and risk of type 2 diabetes mellitus: A longitudinal large study. *J. Investig. Med.* **2016**, *64*, 383–387. [CrossRef] [PubMed]
26. Scherer, P.E. Adipose Tissue: From lipid storage compartment to endocrine organ. *Diabetes* **2006**, *55*, 1537–1545. [CrossRef] [PubMed]
27. Boden, G. Obesity and Free Fatty Acids. *Endocrinol. Metab. Clin. N. Am.* **2008**, *37*, 635–646. [CrossRef]
28. Boden, G.; Chen, X.; Ruiz, J.; White, J.V.; Rossetti, L. Mechanisms of fatty acid-induced inhibition of glucose uptake. *J. Clin. Investig.* **1994**, *93*, 2438–2446. [CrossRef] [PubMed]
29. E Agardh, E.; Sidorchuk, A.; Hallqvist, J.; Ljung, R.; Peterson, S.; Moradi, T.; Allebeck, P. Burden of type 2 diabetes attributed to lower educational levels in Sweden. *Popul. Health Metr.* **2011**, *9*, 60. [CrossRef]
30. Mathisen, J.; Jensen, A.K.G.; Andersen, I.; Andersen, G.S.; Hvidtfeldt, U.A.; Rod, N.H. Education and incident type 2 diabetes: Quantifying the impact of differential exposure and susceptibility to being overweight or obese. *Diabetologia* **2020**, *63*, 1764–1774. [CrossRef]
31. Demakakos, P.; Marmot, M.; Steptoe, A. Socioeconomic position and the incidence of type 2 diabetes: The ELSA study. *Eur. J. Epidemiol.* **2012**, *27*, 367–378. [CrossRef]
32. Sacerdote, C.; Ricceri, F.; Rolandsson, O.; Baldi, I.; Chirlaque, M.D.; Feskens, E.; Bendinelli, B.; Ardanaz, E.; Arriola, L.; Balkau, B.; et al. Lower educational level is a predictor of incident type 2 diabetes in Euro-pean countries: The EPIC-InterAct study. *Int. J. Epidemiol.* **2012**, *41*, 1162–1173. [CrossRef] [PubMed]

33. Smith, P.M.; Smith, B.T.; Mustard, C.A.; Lu, H.; Glazier, R.H. Estimating the direct and indirect pathways between education and diabetes incidence among Canadian men and women: A mediation analysis. *Ann. Epidemiol.* **2013**, *23*, 143–149. [CrossRef] [PubMed]
34. Duan, M.-J.F.; Zhu, Y.; Dekker, L.H.; Mierau, J.O.; Corpeleijn, E.; Bakker, S.J.; Navis, G. Effects of Education and Income on Incident Type 2 Diabetes and Cardiovascular Diseases: A Dutch Prospective Study. *J. Gen. Intern. Med.* **2022**, *37*, 3907–3916. [CrossRef] [PubMed]

Disclaimer/Publisher's Note: The statements, opinions and data contained in all publications are solely those of the individual author(s) and contributor(s) and not of MDPI and/or the editor(s). MDPI and/or the editor(s) disclaim responsibility for any injury to people or property resulting from any ideas, methods, instructions or products referred to in the content.

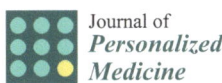

Review

Functionally Significant Variants in Genes Associated with Abdominal Obesity: A Review

Ahmad Bairqdar [1], Dinara Ivanoshchuk [1,2] and Elena Shakhtshneider [1,2,*]

[1] Federal Research Center Institute of Cytology and Genetics, Siberian Branch of Russian Academy of Sciences, Prospekt Akad. Lavrentyeva 10, Novosibirsk 630090, Russia
[2] Institute of Internal and Preventive Medicine—Branch of Institute of Cytology and Genetics, Siberian Branch of Russian Academy of Sciences, Bogatkova Str. 175/1, Novosibirsk 630004, Russia
* Correspondence: shakhtshneyderev@bionet.nsc.ru

Abstract: The high prevalence of obesity and of its associated diseases is a major problem worldwide. Genetic predisposition and the influence of environmental factors contribute to the development of obesity. Changes in the structure and functional activity of genes encoding adipocytokines are involved in the predisposition to weight gain and obesity. In this review, variants in genes associated with adipocyte function are examined, as are variants in genes associated with metabolic aberrations and the accompanying disorders in visceral obesity.

Keywords: adipocyte; obesity; gene

1. Introduction

High prevalence of obesity and of its associated diseases is a major problem worldwide [1]. Genetic predisposition and an influence of environmental factors that contribute to the development of obesity represent a set of causes of excess body weight [2–6]. Hereditary factors involved in the development of obesity lead to the formation of syndromic, monogenic, and polygenic types of obesity [7].

Monogenic obesity is a pathology caused by a mutation in a single gene. Monogenic obesity is extremely rare and is characterized by early onset, development in childhood, and extreme values of body weight [8,9]. Monogenic types of obesity are caused by a mutation in one of genes *LEP*, *LEPR*, *POMC*, *PCSK1*, and *MC4R*, which encode proteins of the leptin–melanocortin system. This system is key for the regulation of eating behavior and energy metabolism [10]. The leptin–melanocortin system is activated by leptin, which is secreted by adipocytes but exerts its action via leptin receptor, thereby leading to the activation of pro-opiomelanocortin. Under the influence of an enzyme called prohormone convertase 1, adrenocorticotropic hormone and α-melanocyte-stimulating hormone are generated from proopiomelanocortin; α-melanocyte-stimulating hormone in turn activates receptor MC4R, which launches satiety signaling [8]. Environmental factors have little effect on the development of nonsyndromic monogenic obesity but may be crucial for treatment. Physical activity, socioeconomic status, and diet type may influence obesity severity in these patients [11].

Syndromic obesity is obesity that develops in chromosomal and other genetic syndromes (e.g., Prader–Willi, fragile X, Bardet–Biedl, Cohen, and Albright) and is accompanied by a set of congenital aberrations [11].

Polygenic obesity is caused simultaneously by many genes and their interactions both with each other and with the external environment. Polygenic obesity is widespread in many populations [12]. In research on polygenic etiology of obesity by means of genome-wide association studies, 127 loci associated with obesity have been found in the human genome [7]. This number constantly changes as new studies come out regarding the polygenic etiology of obesity as a complex multifactorial disease [13]. Although polygenic

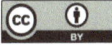

Citation: Bairqdar, A.; Ivanoshchuk, D.; Shakhtshneider, E. Functionally Significant Variants in Genes Associated with Abdominal Obesity: A Review. *J. Pers. Med.* **2023**, *13*, 460. https://doi.org/10.3390/jpm13030460

Academic Editor: Konstantinos Tsarouhas

Received: 15 December 2022
Revised: 23 February 2023
Accepted: 26 February 2023
Published: 1 March 2023

Copyright: © 2023 by the authors. Licensee MDPI, Basel, Switzerland. This article is an open access article distributed under the terms and conditions of the Creative Commons Attribution (CC BY) license (https://creativecommons.org/licenses/by/4.0/).

obesity is the most common type of obesity and is the most responsive to clinical interventions, it is the least investigated owing to its sensitivity to environmental factors and because of its variation among ethnic groups [14].

Obesity is associated with various pathological metabolic changes in the human body: impaired glucose tolerance, insulin resistance, dyslipidemia, nonalcoholic fatty liver disease, and hypertension [15–19]. Visceral adiposity may have a negative effect on longevity [20]. From the point of view of the development of metabolic disorders in obesity, it is important to study visceral adipose tissue and its role as a hormonally active structure [21]. Adipocytes of visceral adipose tissue secrete a set of biomolecules: adipocytokines, which are signaling and regulatory peptides that regulate various metabolic processes [22–24]. In Whites with a BMI ≥ 25.0 kg/m^2 and in Asians with a BMI ≥ 23.0 kg/m^2, waist circumference (WC) measurement is recommended as a simple and informative method for diagnosing abdominal obesity. Values of WC ≥ 80 cm in women and WC ≥ 94 cm in men are said to correspond to abdominal obesity and increased risk of cardiovascular events [25,26]. This method does not apply to pregnant and lactating women.

Changes in the structure and function of genes encoding adipocytokines are involved in the predisposition to weight gain and obesity [7,27,28]. In this review, selected genes associated with adipocyte function are examined, as are variants in genes associated with metabolic aberrations that contribute to visceral obesity (Table 1).

Table 1. Genes examined in this review that are associated with secretory activity of visceral adipocytes.

Gene	Genes Associated with the Secretory Activity of Visceral Adipocytes	References
ADIPOQ	This gene is expressed in adipose tissue exclusively. Mutations in this gene are associated with adiponectin deficiency.	[29]
ADRB3	This receptor is located mainly in adipose tissue and is involved in the regulation of lipolysis and thermogenesis. Obesity-related and body weight–related disorders correlate with polymorphisms in this gene.	[30]
APLN, APLNR	Apelin is secreted by adipose tissue. Apelin and its receptor are widespread in the human body and take part in many physiological processes, such as glucose and lipid metabolism, homeostasis, endocrine responses to stress, and angiogenesis.	[31]
CCL2, CCL7	Chemokines CCL2 and CL7 have been implicated in the pathogenesis of several disorders, including obesity.	[32]
FTO	This gene shows a strong association with the BMI, obesity risk, and T2DM.	[33]
GCG	The glucagon (GCG) family of peptide hormones plays a role in central control of feeding behavior.	[34]
GLP1R	The hormone called glucagon-like peptide 1 (GLP-1) plays an important part in the signaling cascades resulting in insulin secretion.	[35]
GHRL	This gene encodes ghrelin-obestatin preproprotein, which is cleaved thus yielding two peptides: ghrelin and obestatin. Ghrelin regulates multiple phenomena, including hunger and pancreatic glucose-stimulated insulin secretion. Obestatin has multiple metabolic functions, including regulation of adipocyte function and glucose metabolism.	[36]
GIP	This gene encodes an incretin hormone. This protein is important for glucose homeostasis because it is a potent stimulator of insulin secretion from pancreatic β-cells after food ingestion and nutrient absorption.	[37]
INS	This gene codes for insulin: a peptide hormone that plays a vital role in the regulation of carbohydrate and lipid metabolism.	[38]
LEP	This gene encodes a protein that is secreted by white adipocytes into the circulation and performs a major function in the modulation of energy homeostasis. Circulating leptin binds to leptin receptor in the brain, thereby triggering downstream signaling pathways that inhibit feeding and promote energy expenditure. Mutations in this gene and in its regulatory regions induce severe obesity.	[39]
NAMPT	This gene encodes a protein that participates in many important biological processes, including metabolism, stress responses, and aging. Levels of NAMPT in adipose tissue are rather high.	[40,41]

Table 1. Cont.

Gene	Genes Associated with the Secretory Activity of Visceral Adipocytes	References
PPY	This hormone acts as a regulator of pancreatic and gastrointestinal functions and may be important for the modulation of food intake.	[42]
PYY	Rare variations in this gene may increase susceptibility to obesity.	[42]
RBP4	Vitamin A can affect obesity progression and the development of obesity-related diseases including insulin resistance, T2DM, hepatic steatosis, steatohepatitis, and cardiovascular diseases.	[43]
RETN	This gene codes for a protein called resistin. Resistin is secreted by adipocytes and may be the hormone potentially linking obesity to T2DM.	[44,45]
SCT	Secretin activates brown adipose tissue, reduces central responses to appetizing food, and delays the motivation to refeed after a meal.	[46]
UCP2	This gene is expressed in many tissues, and the highest expression is seen in skeletal muscle. The product of this gene plays certain roles in unregulated thermogenesis, obesity, and diabetes mellitus.	[47]

In this review, we analyzed the PubMed database [48] by means of the following search string: "abdominal obesity" [Title/Abstract] AND "single nucleotide polymorphism" [Title/Abstract]. We found 177 full-text articles for the period 2002–2022. Only 20 of the 177 articles (11.3%) contained information on polymorphic variants of genes associated with abdominal obesity. These 20 articles were included in the review.

At the next stage, we performed an additional search in PubMed for articles containing information about single-nucleotide polymorphisms in genes associated with adipocyte secretory activity: *ADIPOQ, ADRB3, APLN, APLNR, CCL2, CCL7, FTO, GCG, GLP1R, GHRL, GIP, INS, LEP, NAMPT, PPY, PYY, RBP4, RETN, SCT,* and *UCP2*. At this stage, we included 175 full-text articles in the review (Figure 1).

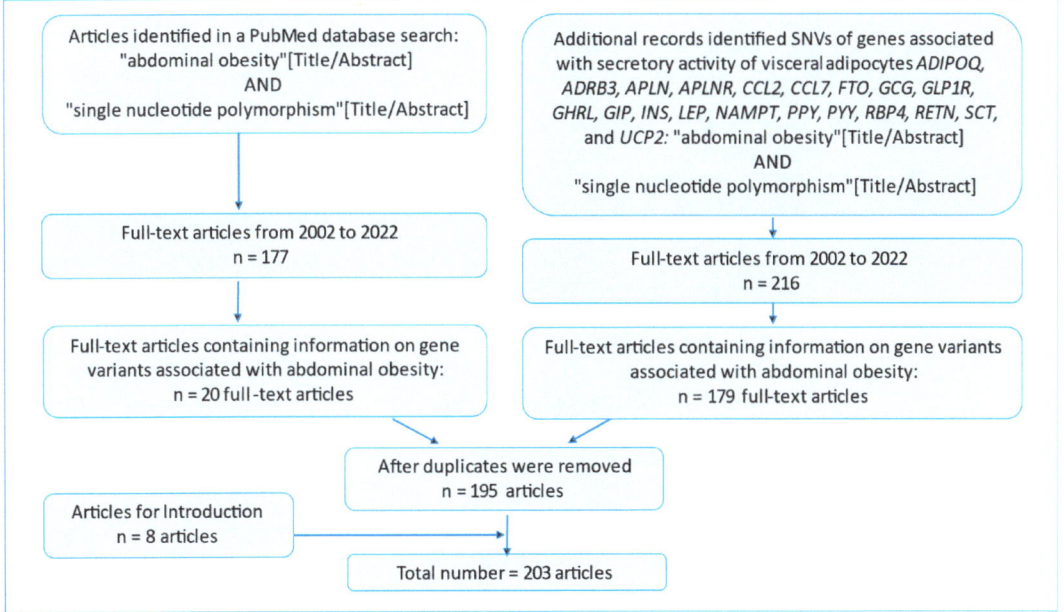

Figure 1. A flowchart of the initial publications in PubMed.

We included an additional 8 full-text articles in Introduction. In this review, the total number of articles is 203.

Variants in the genes examined in our review participate in the development of polygenic obesity.

2. Results

2.1. ADIPOQ

The *ADIPOQ* gene encodes the protein adiponectin, which shares similarities with collagens X and VIII and complement factor C1q. The gene is expressed predominantly in adipose tissue, and the encoded protein circulates as various isoforms in blood plasma. Adiponectin participates in the regulation of many metabolic and hormonal processes, including carbohydrate and lipid metabolism, and has anti-inflammatory effects. Adiponectin interacts with two types of receptors: AdipoR1 and AdipoR2 [49]. Mutations in this gene can lead to adiponectin deficiency [50]. Adiponectin levels inversely correlate with both total body weight and visceral fat mass [51].

The *ADIPOQ* gene has many variants that result in low adiponectin levels, which correlate with obesity: the rs1391272583 variant in a Brazilian population [52], rs17366568 in a Malaysian population [53], rs266729 in a young Nigerian population [54], variants rs266729, rs16861205, rs1501299, rs3821799, and rs6773957 in a Finnish population [55], and variants rs17846866 and rs1501299 in the Indian population of Gujarat [56]. Other variants in this gene have been associated with type 2 diabetes mellitus (T2DM): rs62625753 and rs17366743 in a French white population [57], rs185847354 in a Japanese population [58], and rs2241766, rs2082940, and rs266729 in a Finnish population [55]. The *ADIPOQ* rs266729-G allele affects body fatness in response to dietary monounsaturated fatty acids [59].

2.2. ADRB3

This gene encodes a receptor that belongs to the β-adrenergic receptor family. The activity of the gene is regulated by catecholamines. ADRB3 is expressed mostly in adipose tissue and is responsible for the modulation of lipolysis and thermogenesis [60]. Lipolysis-produced free fatty acids via upregulation of *ADRB3* accelerate transcription of the *UCP1* gene and raise the activity of the UCP1 protein [61].

Several variants of the *ADRB3* gene are associated with the development of obesity and T2DM. One of the first studied variants in this gene, rs4994, has been found to correlate with severe cases of obesity and insulin resistance in a Japanese population [62]. Subsequently, the rs4994 variant has been investigated in many populations and has shown an association with the risk of childhood and adolescent obesity and being overweight [63]. The correlation of rs4994 (*ADRB3* gene) with obesity may be mediated by the impact of this polymorphism on adipokines. Carriers of its C allele have anomalous blood levels of adipokines and lipids [64]. Variants rs72655364 and rs72655365 of this gene correlate with T2DM in a Chinese population [65].

2.3. APLN and APLNR

The *APLN* gene codes for a preproprotein that is subsequently cleaved and activated in the endoplasmic reticulum. The protein apelin is secreted as a peptide hormone that binds to apelin receptors located in various organs. Apelin plays an important part in the regulation of many biological functions, including insulin secretion [66].

The rs2281068 variant (*APLN* gene) is associated with T2DM in the Chinese Han population [67], whereas the rs3115757 variant correlates with obesity among women in a Chinese population [68]. The receptor (encoded by the *APLNR* gene) to which apelin binds is expressed in the spleen, brain, placenta, and adipose tissues [69].

Studies on *APLNR* gene variants have not detected any associations with diabetes mellitus or obesity [70]. Some variants in the *APLNR* gene correlate with the risk of hypertension [71].

2.4. CCL2 and CCL7

Genes *CCL2* and *CCL7* are members of the CC subfamily of the chemokine superfamily, which plays a crucial role in immunomodulatory and inflammatory processes. The two genes are located side by side on chromosome 17 [72].

The serum concentration of CCL2 correlates with insulin resistance and a high body–mass index (BMI) [73]. In a Mexican population, the G allele of variant rs1024611 is associated with lower serum insulin levels, a lower BMI, lower adipose-tissue volume, and higher adiponectin levels than is the A allele [74]. The G allele of variant rs1024611 is less common among women with gestational diabetes mellitus, whereas its GG genotype is associated with a lower BMI among women with gestational diabetes mellitus [75].

CCL7 is overexpressed in the adipose tissue of obese people [76]. This upregulation is induced by elevated expression of interferon regulatory factor 5 in adipose tissue [77].

2.5. FTO

The *FTO* gene codes for a protein that plays an important part in the development of obesity and T2DM [78]. The *FTO* gene was one of the first identified loci correlating with obesity in genome-wide association studies [7]. This gene is widely expressed within the human body, with the highest expression in the brain. Several reports from different populations indicate an association of some variants of *FTO* with obesity in children and adults [79]. Two of the earliest genome-wide association studies in this field showed a correlation of *FTO* variants with early onset of obesity in a German population [80] and with T2DM in a Finnish population [81]. The rs1421085 variant of *FTO* is associated with impaired differentiation of adipocytes. The *FTO* SNP rs1421085 disrupts the binding site of repressor ARID5B [33]. The *FTO* SNP rs1558902 correlates with the BMI [82,83]. *FTO* variants implicated in obesity have been found in diverse populations: rs1421085, rs8050136, and rs9939609 in an Indian population [84], rs9939609 in a Russian population [85], rs9939609, rs1121980, and rs1558902 in a Japanese population [86,87], and rs9939609 in a Saudi Arabian population [88]. Rs9939609 is associated of with the risk of central obesity in Chinese children [89]. Rs9939609 has shown a significant correlation with male visceral obesity in an Indonesian population [90]. Increased abdominal fatness is associated with the AA genotype of a common SNP of *FTO* (rs9939609, T/A) when measured as waist circumference and intra-abdominal adipose tissue [91]. On the other hand, the rs9939609 polymorphism of this gene correlates with fat accumulation in the whole body without being associated with abdominal fat accumulation in Turkish adults [92]. Rs9939609 is in the same linkage region as rs8050136 (r2 = 1) [93]. A rare variant—rs140101381 (R80W)—is associated with early onset of obesity [27]. The T allele at the rs3751812 locus has been implicated in increased waist circumference in Asian-Indian populations [94]. Rs7185735 is associated with an increase in subcutaneous adipose tissue and a decrease in the visceral adipose tissue/subcutaneous adipose tissue ratio and correlates with the childhood BMI [95,96]. *FTO* rs9936385 is responsible for significant differences in the BMI between adults ≤50 years of age and adults aged >50 years [97].

2.6. GCG and GLP1R

The *GCG* gene encodes glucagon, a hormone that regulates blood glucose levels. GCG is expressed mainly in pancreatic α-cells in the islets of Langerhans and in the small intestine. As a consequence of a post-translational modification in α-cells of the pancreas, glucagon is generated, and in the small intestine, a post-translational modification results in the production of glucagon-like peptides 1 and 2, oxyntomodulin, and glicentin. Glicentin is a 69 amino acid peptide, which contains the entire sequences of oxyntomodulin (and hence glucagon) and glicentin-related pancreatic peptide [98].

GCG variants related to T2DM and obesity have been identified. In a Danish population, carriers of the homozygous GG genotype of rs4664447 have lower plasma glucose-stimulated insulin levels [99]. The rs12104705 variant correlates with general and abdominal obesity [34].

The *GLP1R* gene encodes a transmembrane receptor for glucagon-like peptide 1 [100]. The receptor is internalized by binding to GLP1 or its analogs, and activation of this receptor results in insulin secretion [35].

In 2004, an association of rs367543060 of the *GLP1R* gene with both impaired insulin secretion and aberrant insulin sensitivity was identified for the first time in patients with T2DM [101]. Variants rs2268641 and rs6923761 in this gene correlate with a high BMI [102,103]. Carriers of the AA genotype of rs6923761 have a higher risk of obesity and higher glucose levels [104]. Variant rs10305492 in a European population [105] and rs3765467 and rs10305492 in a Chinese population [106] have been implicated in metabolic syndrome and a higher risk of T2DM. Interaction between various factors, including the single-nucleotide polymorphisms (SNPs) that alter signaling, transport, and receptor activity, is key to the design of next-generation personalized agonists of GLP1R [107].

2.7. GHRL

The *GHRL* gene (ghrelin and obestatin prepropeptide) encodes a preprotein that is later cleaved thereby yielding ghrelin and obestatin, which are expressed and secreted primarily in the stomach and much less often in the small intestine. The peptide ghrelin binds to its receptor (GHSR) in the hypothalamus and drives growth hormone secretion [108]. Ghrelin modulates many metabolic pathways and performs a crucial function in the reward system via the mesolimbic pathway [109]. Higher prevalence of variants rs34911341 and rs696217 has been found among obese people than in the general population [110,111].

Subsequent research has uncovered an association of various other *GHRL* variants with obesity: rs4684677 in a general-population cohort of European origin [112]; rs35682 and rs35683 in a white American population [113], and rs696217 in a Japanese population [114]; in addition, rs35681 correlates with the development of obesity in polycystic ovary syndrome [115].

Some variants in the *GHRL* gene are associated with disorders of carbohydrate metabolism. Rs27647 correlates with lower insulin levels in the oral glucose tolerance test (at 2 h after the glucose challenge) [112]. One of ghrelin's effects related to weight changes is an alteration of eating behavior; for example, variants rs696217 and rs2075356 have been implicated in bulimia nervosa [116].

2.8. GIP

The *GIP* gene (gastric inhibitory polypeptide) is located on chromosome 17 and encodes an incretin hormone that regulates insulin secretion and ensures blood glucose homeostasis [117].

Three SNPs (rs3895874, rs3848460, and rs937301) have been analyzed in the 5′ region of the human *GIP* gene. Functional studies have revealed that in the promoter region of GIP, rare alleles of these three SNPs [haplotype GIP(−1920A)] correspond to significantly lower transcriptional activity than do the common alleles of these SNPs [haplotype GIP(−1920G)] [118]. Rs9904288, which is located at the 3′ end of *GIP*, is significantly associated with visceral fat area [119].

2.9. INS

The *INS* gene codes for the hormone insulin, which is responsible for the modulation of carbohydrate and lipid metabolism. The gene is located on chromosome 11 [120]. Insulin synthesis in pancreatic β-cells starts with preproinsulin [121]. During transport to the endoplasmic reticulum, the signal peptide located at the N terminus is cleaved off, then the remaining polypeptide is folded with the formation of disulfide bridges between the α and β chains, after which proinsulin is transported to the Golgi apparatus, where it is packaged into vesicles. Proinsulin is cleaved in vesicles and loses its C-peptide, which is subsequently secreted along with insulin molecules in equal amounts [122,123].

Some mutations in the insulin gene can lead to specific subtypes of diabetes, such as mutant *INS* gene–induced diabetes of youth (MIDY), maturity onset diabetes of the young

(MODY), or neonatal diabetes [124,125]. Variants A24D, F48C, and R89C (*INS* gene), which are implicated in the development of neonatal diabetes, result in inefficient processing of proinsulin [126]. Rare variants R6H and R46Q have been described in familial cases of maturity onset diabetes of the young [127]. The A24D variant is associated with inefficient cleavage of preproinsulin [124], whereas the V92L variant weakens the affinity of insulin for insulin receptor [125], and both lead to mutant *INS* gene–induced diabetes of youth.

2.10. LEP

The leptin gene encodes a protein that is expressed by white adipocytes and secreted into the blood. Leptin plays an important role in the regulation of energy homeostasis and body weight control [128]. Leptin circulating in the blood binds to leptin receptor and has a central effect and peripheral effect. In the brain, leptin activates appetite-regulating signaling pathways that cause a decrease in food intake. The influence of metabolic stressors on leptin secretion has become a major focus of research on feeding behaviors [129]. The identification of central actions of leptin during signaling through its specific LepRls in neurons of neuroendocrine and hippocampal circuits has revealed complex integrated central control of body energy (expenditure vs. storage) and sophisticated self-defense of the brain, thus shedding light on how leptin modulates satiety and compulsion [130]. Reductions in energy reserves and in leptin production appear to cause a compensatory change in the reward system and the secretion of orexigenic and anorexigenic neuropeptides [131,132].

Leptin also regulates bone mass and the secretion of hypothalamic–pituitary–adrenal hormones. At the periphery, leptin accelerates basal metabolism and modulates the function of pancreatic β-cells and insulin secretion. In intestines, leptin activates protein kinase C and reduces glucose absorption [133]. Leptin levels also correlate with the waist-to-hip ratio and BMI. Leptin levels are higher in individuals with obesity compared to those without obesity [134].

Mutations in this gene may be the cause of severe obesity [133]. Mutations in the LEP gene have also been associated with the development of T2DM [128].

Mutations in the leptin gene leading to leptin deficiency are some of the causes of monogenic obesity with such symptoms as impaired satiety, hyperphagia, early onset of obesity, and many metabolic and immunological disorders [135]. These autosomal recessive pathogenic mutations are well studied and differ from the LEP variants that do not lead to monogenic obesity but may be a risk factor of obesity and other metabolic disorders.

In a study on common variants in the leptin gene, researchers showed an association of the AA genotype of the rs7799039 variant with the development of obesity in the population of South India [136]. The A allele of rs2167270 significantly correlates with an elevated risk of prediabetes in Jordan and in the population of South India [137–139]. Rs6966536 (allele G) of the LEP gene has been implicated in the development of obesity in a South African population [140].

Among African Americans, two SNPs of the LEP gene (rs4731427 and rs17151919) have been associated with weight, BMI, and WC. Among whites, rs2167270 and rs17151913 (in this gene) correlate with weight, whereas in women, rs28954369 is associated with weight, BMI, and WC [141]. In a study by Yaghootkar et al., missense variant Val94Met (rs17151919) was found to occur only among people of African descent, and its association with lower concentrations of leptin was specific to this origin [142].

Despite abundant research on leptin, the mechanisms of action of variants on the expression and stability of leptin or on its interaction with its receptor are still being investigated. A study by Hagglund et al. offers an explanation that includes the following mechanisms: (1) weaker affinity of leptin for its receptor, (2) blockade of leptin receptor, (3) destabilization of leptin, and (4) improper coagulation/aggregation of leptin [143].

2.11. NAMPT

This gene encodes an enzyme that catalyzes the condensation of nicotinamide with 5-phosphoribosyl-1-pyrophosphate. The gene is located on chromosome 7 [144]. The enzyme is secreted into extracellular space, and its secreted form is known as visfatin. The latter acts as a cytokine and adipokine [145].

Many *NAMPT* variants have been identified that correlate with changes in its metabolic function and adipokine activity. The T allele of the −948G/T variant is associated with lower fasting insulin levels [146] and higher levels of high-density lipoprotein cholesterol [147]. *NAMPT* variants rs10487818 and rs3801266 correlate with changes in body weight [148,149]. The rs3801267 variant has shown an association with a lower BMI in a Chinese population [150]. Rs34861192 and rs13237989 (*NAMPT*) affect insulin levels and the glycemic index [151]. The aforementioned variants cause either higher or lower serum levels of visfatin, which in turn leads to alterations of insulin and blood glucose levels [152].

2.12. PYY and PPY

Genes *PPY* and *PYY* code for two peptides from the neuropeptide family: pancreatic polypeptide (PP) and peptide YY (PYY). Both genes are located on chromosome 17 [153,154].

Neuropeptides typically affect the gut–brain axis by regulating appetite and energy homeostasis. The peptides of this family act through five receptors called "Y-receptors": Y1, Y2, Y4, Y5, and Y6. These receptors differ in their tissue distribution, function, and selectivity of binding to various neuropeptides. Peptide PYY acts on the arcuate nucleus of the hypothalamus, where the Y-receptors are located that have strong affinity for PYY [155]. Gene variants in *PYY* are associated with changes in body weight and with obesity. Variants rs11684664, rs162430, and rs1058046 have been implicated in the development of obesity in various reports [156–158].

Peptide PPY is synthesized in the pancreas as a 94-amino-acid polypeptide; then, it is cleaved into 2 peptides, with only the 36-amino-acid PPY fragment being active [153]. The secreted peptide performs a function similar to that of PYY but has stronger affinity for receptor Y4. The PPY peptide is secreted by very rare γ-cells in pancreatic islets [159]. According to one research article, the GG genotype of variant rs231472 in the *PPY* gene correlates with the risk of obesity in children in Korea [160].

2.13. RBP4

The *RBP4* gene is located on chromosome 10 and codes for a protein that binds retinol and helps to transport it from the skin to peripheral tissues. The protein is expressed mostly in the liver (and at lower levels in adipose tissues). Retinol bound to RBP4 is then imported into the cell by STRA6, which serves as a receptor of the RBP4–retinol complex [161].

RBP4 was first described as an adipokine in 2005 [162]. Variants rs34571439 and rs3758539 are associated with decreased insulin secretion in whites [163]. The rs34571439 variant (*RBP4* gene) has been implicated in hypertriglyceridemia [164] and childhood obesity [165]. Variant rs7091052 is associated with the risk of gestational diabetes mellitus [166].

2.14. RETN

This gene encodes a protein called resistin. The resistin gene is located on chromosome 19 [167]. Resistin has a pleiotropic role in inflammation, in the biology of stress, and in the pathogenesis of obesity [168].

Variants in the *RETN* gene correlate with signs of metabolic syndrome. Investigation has revealed an association of variant rs1862513 with the risk of obesity and T2DM [169,170]. Other variants (rs3745367, rs1423096, and rs10401670) of this gene have been associated with some parameters of metabolic syndrome in various populations [171–173].

Differences in serum resistin levels may be related to alterations of methylation patterns in the RETN promoter region [174]. Variants in coding regions of RETN have a greater impact on this protein's stability [175].

2.15. SCT

The *SCT* gene is located on chromosome 11 and codes for hormone secretin. Secretin stimulates bile and bicarbonate secretion in the duodenum, pancreas, and bile ducts [176].

Secretin expression activates brown adipose tissue, reduces central responses to appetizing food, and delays motivation for eating again after a meal [177,178].

2.16. UCP2

The *UCP2* gene is in the same cluster as the *UCP3* gene and is situated on chromosome 11 [179]. It is thought to take part in unregulated thermogenesis, obesity, and diabetes mellitus [180]. Variant rs659366 is associated with the risk of obesity [85,181–184], whereas variant rs660339 correlates with the risk of obesity in a specific population: Indonesians [185–187].

Modern molecular genetic and biochemical technologies are key to solving such fundamental problems as the formation of overweightness and obesity, thereby making it possible to identify genes and their products participating in the pathogenesis of obesity, to investigate the molecular mechanisms of relevant pathological processes, and to determine molecular biological heterogeneity of pathological phenotypes [7,188].

In addition to the determination of the BMI and WC, a Body Shape Index (ABSI) is used to diagnose obesity. ABSI takes into account body height, weight, and WC. ABSI has independent genetic associations [189,190]. ABSI can more precisely quantify abdominal obesity in metabolic syndrome [191]. Other indicators may also help to diagnose abdominal obesity, but all of them maintain a significant correlation with the BMI [192]. The association of polymorphisms of genes with ABSI may be an interesting research topic for clarifying functional significance of SNPs.

An effective method of early diagnosis and prevention of obesity is the identification of genetic markers of predisposition to this pathology and research on their characteristics in various populations [193]. Most results presented in the review have been obtained in case-control studies. This method complements data from genome-wide association studies [194–196]. Table 2 shows the main variants that are associated with metabolic disorders and located in the genes presented in this review.

Table 2. Single-nucleotide variants associated with metabolic disorders.

Gene	dbSNP ID	Nucleotide Changes	Type of Variation/Amino Acid Changes	Minor Allele Frequency (GnomAD)	ClinVar Variation ID/LOVD Database ID	Associated Metabolic Disorder
ADIPOQ	rs62625753	+268 G > A	Missense Variant G > S	0.004625	708724	allele A is associated with T2DM risk
ADIPOQ	rs266729	C > G	2KB Upstream Variant	G = 0.09786	-	allele C is associated with T2DM risk
ADIPOQ	rs17366743	+331 T > C	Missense Variant Y > H	0.030445	-	allele C is associated with T2DM risk
FTO	rs9939609	46-23525 T > A	Intron Variant	0.41025	-	allele A is associated with obesity
FTO	rs1421085	46-43098 T > C	Intron Variant	0.419704	214481	allele C is associated with obesity
GCG	rs4664447	254 + 672 A > T	Intron Variant	C = 0.00792 G = 0.00000	-	GG genotype is associated with insulin level abnormalities
GHRL	rs34911341	152 G > A	Missense Variant R > Q	0.007960	20100/ 00293181	allele A is associated with metabolic syndrome
GHRL	rs696217	214 C > A	Missense Variant L > M	0.080526	20101	allele T is associated with metabolic syndrome and obesity
GHRL	rs4684677	269 A > T	Missense Variant Q > L	0.06097	20102	allele A is associated with obesity

Table 2. Cont.

Gene	dbSNP ID	Nucleotide Changes	Type of Variation/Amino Acid Changes	Minor Allele Frequency (GnomAD)	ClinVar Variation ID/LOVD Database ID	Associated Metabolic Disorder
GLP1R	rs2268641	1224 + 1751 C > T	Intron Variant	0.39129	-	Associated with BMI
GLP1R	rs6923761	502 G > A	Missense Variant G > S	0.324795	-/00208599	GG genotype is associated with higher BMI and CV risks
GLP1R	rs10305492	946G > A	Missense Variant A > T	0.015874	-	allele A is associated with T2DM risk
NAMPT	rs9770242	C > A	2KB Upstream Variant	C = 0.23919	-	allele C is associated with lower fasting plasma glucose and insulin levels
NAMPT	rs1319501	T > C	2KB Upstream Variant	C = 0.23662 A = 0.00001	-	allele C is associated with lower fasting plasma glucose and insulin levels
NAMPT	rs10487818	448-303 T > A	Intron Variant	0.01841	-/00028958	allele T is associated with protection against obesity
PYY	rs11684664	C > T		A = 0.0000 T = 0.00038		allele T is associated with obesity-related phenotypes in women only
PYY	rs162430	270-61 C > T	Intron Variant	0.105072	-	allele A is associated with childhood obesity
RBP4	rs34571439	A > C	500B Downstream Variant	0.186457	-	allele C is associated with reduced insulin secretion
RBP4	rs3758539	C > T	2KBUpstream Variant	0.16303	-	allele T is associated with reduced insulin secretion
RETN	rs3745367	118 + 181 G > A	Intron Variant	0.248110	-	allele A is associated with obesity
UCP2	rs659366	C > T	2KB Upstream Variant	0.370248	22904	allele T is associated with higher BMI
UCP2	rs660339	164 C > T	Missense Variant A > V	0.402632	136143	allele A is associated with obesity

Based on the analysis of functional significance of the variants, a scale of an individual's genetic risk of obesity may be constructed. The creation of such a scale is an important task for modern endocrinology. The complexity of this task is due to population specificity of (i) prevalence rates of obesity, (ii) characteristics of climatic and social living conditions, and (iii) genetic factors. When a scale of individual genetic risk is created, it is important to take into account the ethnicity of the patients included in the research. For example, according to many studies, the same scale of individual genetic risk detects an association with cardiovascular events in one population and does not in another [197,198]. At present, there are not many published studies on the development of an ethnospecific scale of individual genetic risk of obesity. Most of these studies have been conducted on white cohorts, and the results may not be applicable to other populations. In research projects examining the association between a scale of individual genetic risk and diseases, Cox's proportional hazards model and logistic regression analysis are used. Correlations between a genetic risk scale and anthropometric and biochemical parameters are assessed via linear regression. ROC (receiver operating characteristic), the area under the ROC curve (i.e., C-statistic), NRI, and integrated discrimination improvement are metrics of the quality of a scale of individual genetic risk as compared to traditional risk factors [199].

The risk of obesity, as assessed by the genetic risk scale, can be modified, for example, by a therapy aimed at weight loss and alleviation of comorbidities. It is now recognized that our everyday exercise and nutrition choices have long-term consequences for our brain function [200–203]. Early detection of a genetic risk may help to improve quality of life and life expectancy and to reduce economic costs of treatment.

3. Conclusions

It is necessary to study each population, both in terms of the nature of the variation of genes predisposing to diseases associated with excess body weight and in terms of specific features of their phenotypic manifestation. High-throughput sequencing technologies allow investigators to obtain new information about the variation of the structure of genes in groups from the general population and in clinical groups of overweight and obese individuals.

Author Contributions: A.B.: writing—original draft; D.I.: writing—original draft; E.S.: conceptualization, writing—original draft, funding acquisition, and participation in the discussion. All authors have read and agreed to the published version of the manuscript.

Funding: The work was carried out within the framework of Russian Science Foundation grant No. 21-15-00022.

Institutional Review Board Statement: Not applicable.

Informed Consent Statement: Not applicable.

Data Availability Statement: Not applicable.

Acknowledgments: We would like to thank Nikolay Shevchuk by the English editing. We thank the reviewers for their useful comments that helped to significantly improve our paper.

Conflicts of Interest: The authors declare that they have no conflict of interest.

References

1. Caballero, B. Humans against Obesity: Who Will Win? *Adv. Nutr.* **2019**, *10* (Suppl. S1), S4–S9. [CrossRef]
2. Lin, X.; Li, H. Obesity: Epidemiology, Pathophysiology, and Therapeutics. *Front. Endocrinol.* **2021**, *12*, 706978. [CrossRef]
3. Ling, C.; Rönn, T. Epigenetics in Human Obesity and Type 2 Diabetes. *Cell Metab.* **2019**, *9*, 1028–1044. [CrossRef] [PubMed]
4. Herrera, B.M.; Lindgren, C.M. The genetics of obesity. *Curr. Diab. Rep.* **2010**, *10*, 498–505. [CrossRef]
5. Vettori, A.; Pompucci, G.; Paolini, B.; Del Ciondolo, I.; Bressan, S.; Dundar, M.; Kenanoğlu, S.; Unfer, V.; Bertelli, M.; Geneob Project. Genetic background, nutrition and obesity: A review. *Eur. Rev. Med. Pharmacol. Sci.* **2019**, *23*, 1751–1761. [CrossRef]
6. Hurtado, A.M.D.; Acosta, A. Precision Medicine and Obesity. *Gastroenterol. Clin. N. Am.* **2021**, *50*, 127–139. [CrossRef] [PubMed]
7. Singh, R.K.; Kumar, P.; Mahalingam, K. Molecular Genetics of Human Obesity: A Comprehensive Review. *C R Biol.* **2017**, *340*, 87–108. [CrossRef] [PubMed]
8. Hebebrand, J.; Hinney, A.; Knoll, N.; Volckmar, A.L.; Scherag, A. Molecular genetic aspects of weight regulation. *Dtsch. Arztebl. Int.* **2013**, *110*, 338–344. [CrossRef] [PubMed]
9. Muñoz, C.; Garcia-Vargas, G.G.; Morales, R.P. Monogenic, Polygenic and Multifactorial Obesity in Children: Genetic and Environmental Factor. *Austin J. Nutr. Metab.* **2017**, *4*, 1052.
10. Littleton, S.H.; Berkowitz, R.I.; Grant, S.F.A. Genetic Determinants of Childhood Obesity. *Mol. Diagn. Ther.* **2020**, *24*, 653–663. [CrossRef] [PubMed]
11. Mahmoud, R.; Kimonis, V.; Butler, M.G. Genetics of Obesity in Humans: A Clinical Review. *Int. J. Mol. Sci.* **2022**, *23*, 11005. [CrossRef] [PubMed]
12. GBD 2015 Obesity Collaborators. Health effects of overweight and obesity in 195 countries over 25 years. *N. Engl. J. Med.* **2017**, *377*, 13–27. [CrossRef] [PubMed]
13. Loos, R.J.F.; Yeo, G.S.H. The Genetics of Obesity: From Discovery to Biology. *Nat. Rev. Genet.* **2022**, *23*, 120–133. [CrossRef] [PubMed]
14. Heianza, Y.; Qi, L. Gene-Diet Interaction and Precision Nutrition in Obesity. *Int. J. Mol. Sci.* **2017**, *18*, 787. [CrossRef]

15. Litwin, M.; Kułaga, Z. Obesity, metabolic syndrome, and primary hypertension. *Pediatr. Nephrol.* **2021**, *36*, 825–837. [CrossRef]
16. Ahmed, B.; Sultana, R.; Greene, M.W. Adipose tissue and insulin resistance in obese. *Biomed. Pharmacother.* **2021**, *137*, 111315. [CrossRef]
17. Brunner, K.T.; Henneberg, C.J.; Wilechansky, R.M.; Long, M.T. Nonalcoholic Fatty Liver Disease and Obesity Treatment. *Curr. Obes. Rep.* **2019**, *8*, 220–228. [CrossRef]
18. Milić, S.; Lulić, D.; Štimac, D. Non-alcoholic fatty liver disease and obesity: Biochemical, metabolic and clinical presentations. *World J. Gastroenterol.* **2014**, *20*, 9330–9337. [CrossRef]
19. Zhang, T.; Chen, J.; Tang, X.; Luo, Q.; Xu, D.; Yu, B. Interaction between adipocytes and high-density lipoprotein:new insights into the mechanism of obesity-induced dyslipidemia and atherosclerosis. *Lipids Health Dis.* **2019**, *18*, 223. [CrossRef]
20. Yan, B.; Yang, J.; Zhao, B.; Wu, Y.; Bai, L.; Ma, X. Causal Effect of Visceral Adipose Tissue Accumulation on the Human Longevity: A Mendelian Randomization Study. *Front Endocrinol.* **2021**, *1*, 722187. [CrossRef]
21. Cao, H. Adipocytokines in obesity and metabolic disease. *J. Endocrinol.* **2014**, *220*, 47–59. [CrossRef] [PubMed]
22. Maximus, P.S.; Al Achkar, Z.; Hamid, P.F.; Hasnain, S.S.; Peralta, C.A. Adipocytokines: Are they the Theory of Everything? *Cytokine* **2020**, *133*, 155144. [CrossRef]
23. Zorena, K.; Jachimowicz-Duda, O.; Ślęzak, D.; Robakowska, M.; Mrugacz, M. Adipokines and Obesity. Potential Link to Metabolic Disorders and Chronic Complications. *Int. J. Mol. Sci.* **2020**, *21*, 3570. [CrossRef] [PubMed]
24. Wen, W.; Kato, N.; Hwang, J.Y.; Guo, X.; Tabara, Y.; Li, H.; Dorajoo, R.; Yang, X.; Tsai, F.J.; Li, S. Genome-wide association studies in East Asians identify new loci for waist-hip ratio and waist circumference. *Sci. Rep.* **2016**, *20*, 17958. [CrossRef] [PubMed]
25. Dedov, I.I.; Shestakova, M.V.; Melnichenko, G.A.; Mazurina, N.V.; Andreeva, E.N.; Bondarenko, I.Z.; Gusova, Z.R.; Dzgoeva, F.K.; Eliseev, M.S.; Ershova, E.V.; et al. Interdisciplinary Clinical Practice Guidelines "Management of obesity and its comorbidities". *Obes. Metab.* **2021**, *18*, 5–99. [CrossRef]
26. Yumuk, V.; Tsigos, C.; Fried, M.; Schindler, K.; Busetto, L.; Micic, D.; Toplak, H. Obesity Management Task Force of the European Association for the Study of Obesity. European Guidelines for Obesity Management in Adults. *Obes. Facts* **2015**, *8*, 402–424. [CrossRef]
27. Serra-Juhé, C.; Martos-Moreno, G.; De Pieri, F.B.; Flores, R.; Chowen, J.A.; Pérez-Jurado, L.A.; Argente, J. Heterozygous rare genetic variants in non-syndromic early-onset obesity. *Int. J. Obes.* **2020**, *44*, 830–841. [CrossRef]
28. Ghoshal, K.; Chatterjee, T.; Chowdhury, S.; Sengupta, S.; Bhattacharyya, M. Adiponectin Genetic Variant and Expression Coupled with Lipid Peroxidation Reveal New Signatures in Diabetic Dyslipidemia. *Biochem. Genet.* **2021**, *59*, 781–798. [CrossRef]
29. Iwabu, M.; Okada-Iwabu, M.; Yamauchi, T.; Kadowaki, T. Adiponectin/AdipoR Research and Its Implications for Lifestyle-Related Diseases. *Front. Cardiovasc. Med.* **2019**, *6*, 116. [CrossRef]
30. Luo, Z.; Zhang, T.; Wang, S.; He, Y.; Ye, Q.; Cao, W. The Trp64Arg Polymorphism in B3 Adrenergic Receptor (ADRB3) Gene Is Associated with Adipokines and Plasma Lipids: A Systematic Review, Meta-Analysis, and Meta-Regression. *Lipids Health Dis.* **2020**, *19*, 99. [CrossRef]
31. Li, C.; Cheng, H.; Adhikari, B.K.; Wang, S.; Yang, N.; Liu, W.; Sun, J.; Wang, Y. The Role of Apelin-APJ System in Diabetes and Obesity. *Front. Endocrinol.* **2022**, *13*, 820002. [CrossRef]
32. Ignacio, R.M.; Gibbs, C.R.; Lee, E.S.; Son, D.S. Differential Chemokine Signature between Human Preadipocytes and Adipocytes. *Immune Netw.* **2016**, *16*, 189–194. [CrossRef] [PubMed]
33. Claussnitzer, M.; Dankel, S.N.; Kim, K.-H.; Quon, G.; Meuleman, W.; Haugen, C.; Glunk, V.; Sousa, I.S.; Beaudry, J.L.; Puviindran, V.; et al. FTO Obesity Variant Circuitry and Adipocyte Browning in Humans. *N. Engl. J. Med.* **2015**, *373*, 895–907. [CrossRef] [PubMed]
34. Zhang, L.; Zhang, M.; Wang, J.J.; Wang, C.J.; Ren, Y.C.; Wang, B.Y.; Zhang, H.Y.; Yang, X.Y.; Zhao, Y.; Han, C.Y.; et al. Association of TCF7L2 and GCG Gene Variants with Insulin Secretion, Insulin Resistance, and Obesity in New-Onset Diabetes. *Biomed. Environ. Sci.* **2016**, *29*, 814–817. [CrossRef] [PubMed]
35. Mayendraraj, A.; Rosenkilde, M.M.; Gasbjerg, L.S. GLP-1 and GIP Receptor Signaling in Beta Cells—A Review of Receptor Interactions and Co-Stimulation. *Peptides* **2022**, *151*, 170749. [CrossRef] [PubMed]
36. Landgren, S.; Simms, J.; Thelle, D.S.; Strandhagen, E.; Bartlett, S.E.; Engel, J.A.; Jerlhag, E. The Ghrelin Signalling System Is Involved in the Consumption of Sweets. *PLoS ONE* **2011**, *6*, e18170. [CrossRef]
37. Nauck, M.A.; Quast, D.R.; Wefers, J.; Pfeiffer, A.F.H. The evolving story of incretins (GIP and GLP-1) in metabolic and cardiovascular disease: A pathophysiological update. *Diabetes Obes. Metab.* **2021**, *23* (Suppl. S3), 5–29. [CrossRef] [PubMed]
38. Støy, J.; Edghill, E.L.; Flanagan, S.E.; Ye, H.; Paz, V.P.; Pluzhnikov, A.; Below, J.E.; Hayes, M.G.; Cox, N.J.; Lipkind, G.M.; et al. Insulin gene mutations as a cause of permanent neonatal diabetes. *Proc. Natl. Acad. Sci. USA* **2007**, *104*, 15040–15044. [CrossRef]
39. Wabitsch, M.; Pridzun, L.; Ranke, M.; von Schnurbein, J.; Moss, A.; Brandt, S.; Kohlsdorf, K.; Moepps, B.; Schaab, M.; Funcke, J.B.; et al. Measurement of immunofunctional leptin to detect and monitor patients with functional leptin deficiency. *Eur. J. Endocrinol.* **2017**, *176*, 315–322. [CrossRef]
40. Curat, C.A.; Wegner, V.; Sengenes, C.; Miranville, A.; Tonus, C.; Busse, R.; Bouloumie, A. Macrophages in human visceral adipose tissue: Increased accumulation in obesity and a source of resistin and visfatin. *Diabetologia* **2006**, *49*, 744–747. [CrossRef]
41. Stromsdorfer, K.L.; Yamaguchi, S.; Yoon, M.J.; Moseley, A.C.; Franczyk, M.P.; Kelly, S.C.; Qi, N.; Imai, S.I.; Yoshino, J. NAMPT-Mediated NAD+ Biosynthesis in Adipocytes Regulates Adipose Tissue Function and Multi-Organ Insulin Sensitivity in Mice. *Cell Rep.* **2016**, *16*, 1851–1860. [CrossRef] [PubMed]

42. Campbell, C.D.; Lyon, H.N.; Nemesh, J.; Drake, J.A.; Tuomi, T.; Gaudet, D.; Zhu, X.; Cooper, R.S.; Ardlie, K.G.; Groop, L.C.; et al. Association studies of BMI and type 2 diabetes in the neuropeptide Y pathway: A possible role for NPY2R as a candidate gene for type 2 diabetes in men. *Diabetes* **2007**, *56*, 1460–14607. [CrossRef] [PubMed]
43. Blaner, W.S. Vitamin A signaling and homeostasis in obesity, diabetes, and metabolic disorders. *Pharmacol. Ther.* **2019**, *197*, 153–178. [CrossRef] [PubMed]
44. Qi, Q.; Menzaghi, C.; Smith, S.; Liang, L.; de Rekeneire, N.; Garcia, M.E.; Lohman, K.K.; Miljkovic, I.; Strotmeyer, E.S.; Cummings, S.R.; et al. Genome-wide association analysis identifies TYW3/CRYZ and NDST4 loci associated with circulating resistin levels. *Hum. Mol. Genet.* **2012**, *21*, 4774–4780. [CrossRef] [PubMed]
45. Rathwa, N.; Patel, R.; Palit, S.P.; Ramachandran, A.V.; Begum, R. Genetic variants of resistin and its plasma levels: Association with obesity and dyslipidemia related to type 2 diabetes susceptibility. *Genomics* **2019**, *111*, 980–985. [CrossRef]
46. Schnabl, K.; Li, Y.; Klingenspor, M. The gut hormone secretin triggers a gut-brown fat-brain axis in the control of food intake. *Exp. Physiol.* **2020**, *105*, 1206–1213. [CrossRef]
47. Oliveira, M.S.; Rheinheimer, J.; Moehlecke, M.; Rodrigues, M.; Assmann, T.S.; Leitão, C.B.; Trindade, M.R.M.; Crispim, D.; de Souza, B.M. UCP2, IL18, and miR-133a-3p are dysregulated in subcutaneous adipose tissue of patients with obesity. *Mol. Cell. Endocrinol.* **2020**, *509*, 110805. [CrossRef]
48. Available online: https://pubmed.ncbi.nlm.nih.gov (accessed on 14 November 2022).
49. Khoramipour, K.; Chamari, K.; Hekmatikar, A.A.; Ziyaiyan, A.; Taherkhani, S.; Elguindy, N.M.; Bragazzi, N.L. Adiponectin: Structure, Physiological Functions, Role in Diseases, and Effects of Nutrition. *Nutrients* **2021**, *13*, 1180. [CrossRef]
50. Pruitt, K.D.; Tatusova, T.; Brown, G.R.; Maglott, D.R. NCBI Reference Sequences (RefSeq): Current Status, New Features and Genome Annotation Policy. *Nucleic. Acids Res.* **2012**, *40*, D130–D135. [CrossRef]
51. Achari, A.E.; Jain, S.K. Adiponectin, a Therapeutic Target for Obesity, Diabetes, and Endothelial Dysfunction. *Int. J. Mol. Sci.* **2017**, *18*, 1321. [CrossRef]
52. Bueno, A.C.; Sun, K.; Martins, C.S.; Elias, J.; Miranda, W.; Tao, C.; Foss-Freitas, M.C.; Barbieri, M.A.; Bettiol, H.; de Castro, M.; et al. A Novel ADIPOQ Mutation (p.M40K) Impairs Assembly of High-Molecular-Weight Adiponectin and Is Associated with Early-Onset Obesity and Metabolic Syndrome. *J. Clin. Endocrinol. Metab.* **2014**, *99*, E683–E693. [CrossRef] [PubMed]
53. Apalasamy, Y.D.; Rampal, S.; Salim, A.; Moy, F.M.; Bulgiba, A.; Mohamed, Z. Association of ADIPOQ Gene with Obesity and Adiponectin Levels in Malaysian Malays. *Mol. Biol. Rep.* **2014**, *41*, 2917–2921. [CrossRef] [PubMed]
54. Olusegun, E.; Ogundele, O.E.; Adekoya, K.O.; Osinubi, A.A.A.; Awofala, A.A.; Oboh, B.O. Association of Adiponectin Gene (ADIPOQ) Polymorphisms with Measures of Obesity in Nigerian Young Adults. *Egypt. J. Med. Hum. Genet.* **2018**, *19*, 123–127. [CrossRef]
55. Siitonen, N.; Pulkkinen, L.; Lindström, J.; Kolehmainen, M.; Eriksson, J.G.; Venojärvi, M.; Ilanne-Parikka, P.; Keinänen-Kiukaanniemi, S.; Tuomilehto, J.; Uusitupa, M. Association of ADIPOQ Gene Variants with Body Weight, Type 2 Diabetes and Serum Adiponectin Concentrations: The Finnish Diabetes Prevention Study. *BMC Med. Genet.* **2011**, *12*, 5. [CrossRef] [PubMed]
56. Palit, S.P.; Patel, R.; Jadeja, S.D.; Rathwa, N.; Mahajan, A.; Ramachandran, A.V.; Dhar, M.K.; Sharma, S.; Begum, R. A Genetic Analysis Identifies a Haplotype at Adiponectin Locus: Association with Obesity and Type 2 Diabetes. *Sci. Rep.* **2020**, *10*, 2904. [CrossRef]
57. Vasseur, F.; Helbecque, N.; Dina, C.; Lobbens, S.; Delannoy, V.; Gaget, S.; Boutin, P.; Vaxillaire, M.; Leprêtre, F.; Dupont, S.; et al. Single-Nucleotide Polymorphism Haplotypes in the Both Proximal Promoter and Exon 3 of the APM1 Gene Modulate Adipocyte-Secreted Adiponectin Hormone Levels and Contribute to the Genetic Risk for Type 2 Diabetes in French Caucasians. *Hum. Mol. Genet.* **2002**, *11*, 2607–2614. [CrossRef] [PubMed]
58. Kondo, H.; Shimomura, I.; Matsukawa, Y.; Kumada, M.; Takahashi, M.; Matsuda, M.; Ouchi, N.; Kihara, S.; Kawamoto, T.; Sumitsuji, S.; et al. Association of Adiponectin Mutation With Type 2 Diabetes A Candidate Gene for the Insulin Resistance Syndrome. *Diabetes* **2002**, *51*, 2325–2328. [CrossRef]
59. Hammad, S.S.; Eck, P.; Sihag, J.; Chen, X.; Connelly, P.W.; Lamarche, B.; Couture, P.; Guay, V.; Maltais-Giguère, J.; West, S.G.; et al. Common Variants in Lipid Metabolism-Related1 Genes Associate with Fat Mass Changes in Response to Dietary Monounsaturated Fatty Acids in Adults with Abdominal Obesity. *J. Nutr.* **2019**, *149*, 1749–1756. [CrossRef]
60. ADRB3 Adrenoceptor Beta 3 [*Homo sapiens* (Human)]. Available online: https://www.ncbi.nlm.nih.gov/gene/155 (accessed on 14 November 2022).
61. Takenaka, A.; Nakamura, S.; Mitsunaga, F.; Inoue-Murayama, M.; Udono, T.; Suryobroto, B. Human-specific SNP in obesity genes, adrenergic receptor beta2 (ADRB2), Beta3 (ADRB3), and PPAR γ2 (PPARG), during primate evolution. *PLoS ONE* **2012**, *7*, e43461. [CrossRef]
62. Kadowaki, H.; Yasuda, K.; Iwamoto, K.; Otabe, S.; Shimokawa, K.; Silver, K.; Walston, J.; Yoshinaga, H.; Kosaka, K.; Yamada, N.; et al. A Mutation in the B3-Adrenergic Receptor Gene Is Associated with Obesity and Hyperinsulinemia in Japanese Subjects. *Biochem. Biophys. Res. Commun* **1995**, *215*, 555–560. [CrossRef]
63. Xie, C.; Hua, W.; Zhao, Y.; Rui, J.; Feng, J.; Chen, Y.; Liu, Y.; Liu, J.; Yang, X.; Xu, X. The ADRB3 Rs4994 Polymorphism Increases Risk of Childhood and Adolescent Overweight/Obesity for East Asia's Population: An Evidence-Based Meta-Analysis. *Adipocyte* **2020**, *9*, 77–86. [CrossRef] [PubMed]

64. Ryukm, J.A.; Zhang, X.; Ko, B.S.; Daily, J.W.; Park, S. Association of β3-adrenergic receptor rs4994 polymorphisms with the risk of type 2 diabetes: A systematic review and meta-analysis. *Diabetes Res. Clin. Pract.* 2017, *129*, 86–96. [CrossRef] [PubMed]
65. Huang, Q.; Yang, T.L.; Tang, B.S.; Chen, X.; Huang, X.; Luo, X.H.; Zhu, Y.S.; Chen, X.P.; Hu, P.C.; Chen, J.; et al. Two Novel Functional Single Nucleotide Polymorphisms of ADRB3 Are Associated with Type 2 Diabetes in the Chinese Population. *J. Clin. Endocrinol. Metab.* 2013, *98*, E1272–E1277. [CrossRef] [PubMed]
66. Zhong, J.C.; Zhang, Z.Z.; Wang, W.; McKinnie, S.M.K.; Vederas, J.C.; Oudit, G.Y. Targeting the Apelin Pathway as a Novel Therapeutic Approach for Cardiovascular Diseases. *Biochim. Biophys. Acta Mol. Basis. Dis.* 2017, *1863*, 1942–1950. [CrossRef]
67. Zheng, H.; Fan, X.; Li, X.; Zhang, Y.; Fan, Y.; Zhang, N.; Song, Y.; Ren, F.; Shen, C.; Shen, J.; et al. The Association between Single Nucleotide Polymorphisms of the Apelin Gene and Diabetes Mellitus in a Chinese Population. *J. Pediatr. Endocrinol. Metab.* 2016, *29*, 1397–1402. [CrossRef]
68. Liao, Y.C.; Chou, W.W.; Li, Y.N.; Chuang, S.C.; Lin, W.Y.; Lakkakula, B.V.K.S.; Yu, M.L.; Juo, S.H.H. Apelin gene polymorphism influences apelin expression and obesity phenotypes in Chinese women. *Am. J. Clin. Nutr.* 2011, *94*, 921–928. [CrossRef]
69. Zhang, M.; Peng, F.; Lin, L.; Yu, M.; Huang, C.; Hu, D.; Guo, Q.; Xu, C.; Lin, J.; Zhang, M.; et al. Association Study of Apelin-APJ System Genetic Polymorphisms with Incident Metabolic Syndrome in a Chinese Population: A Case-Control Study. *Oncotarget* 2019, *10*, 3807–3817. [CrossRef]
70. Galon-Tilleman, H.; Yang, H.; Bednarek, M.A.; Spurlock, S.M.; Paavola, K.J.; Ko, B.; To, C.; Luo, J.; Tian, H.; Jermutus, L.; et al. Apelin-36 Modulates Blood Glucose and Body Weight Independently of Canonical APJ Receptor Signaling. *J. Biol. Chem.* 2017, *292*, 1925–1933. [CrossRef]
71. Yoshikawa, M.; Asaba, K.; Nakayama, T. The APLNR gene polymorphism rs7119375 is associated with an increased risk of development of essential hypertension in the Chinese population: A meta-analysis. *Medicine* 2020, *99*, e22418. [CrossRef]
72. Available online: https://www.ncbi.nlm.nih.gov/gene/ (accessed on 14 November 2022).
73. Mikhailova, S.V.; Ivanoshchuk, D.E. Innate-Immunity Genes in Obesity. *J. Pers. Med.* 2021, *11*, 1201. [CrossRef]
74. Guzmán-Ornelas, M.O.; Petri, M.H.; Vázquez-Del Mercado, M.; Chavarría-Ávila, E.; Corona-Meraz, F.I.; Ruíz-Quezada, S.L.; Madrigal-Ruíz, P.M.; Castro-Albarrán, J.; Sandoval-García, F.; Navarro-Hernández, R.E. CCL2 Serum Levels and Adiposity Are Associated with the Polymorphic Phenotypes -2518A on CCL2 and 64ILE on CCR2 in a Mexican Population with Insulin Resistance. *J. Diabetes Res.* 2016, *2016*, 5675739. [CrossRef] [PubMed]
75. Teler, J.; Tarnowski, M.; Safranow, K.; Maciejewska, A.; Sawczuk, M.; Dziedziejko, V.; Sluczanowska-Glabowska, S.; Pawlik, A. CCL2, CCL5, IL4 and IL15 Gene Polymorphisms in Women with Gestational Diabetes Mellitus. *Horm. Metab. Res.* 2017, *49*, 10–15. [CrossRef] [PubMed]
76. Huber, J.; Kiefer, F.W.; Zeyda, M.; Ludvik, B.; Silberhumer, G.R.; Prager, G.; Zlabinger, G.J.; Stulnig, T.M. CC Chemokine and CC Chemokine Receptor Profiles in Visceral and Subcutaneous Adipose Tissue Are Altered in Human Obesity. *J. Clin. Endocrinol. Metab.* 2008, *93*, 3215–3221. [CrossRef] [PubMed]
77. Sindhu, S.; Thomas, R.; Kochumon, S.; Wilson, A.; Abu-Farha, M.; Bennakhi, A.; Al-Mulla, F.; Ahmad, R. Increased Adipose Tissue Expression of Interferon Regulatory Factor (IRF)-5 in Obesity: Association with Metabolic Inflammation. *Cells* 2019, *8*, 1418. [CrossRef]
78. Wei, J.; Liu, F.; Lu, Z.; Fei, Q.; Ai, Y.; He, P.C.; Shi, H.; Cui, X.; Su, R.; Klungland, A.; et al. Differential m 6 A, m 6 A m, and m 1 A Demethylation Mediated by FTO in the Cell Nucleus and Cytoplasm. *Mol. Cell* 2018, *71*, 973–985.e5. [CrossRef]
79. Povel, C.M.; Boer, J.M.; Onland-Moret, N.C.; Dollé, M.E.; Feskens, E.J.; van der Schouw, Y.T. Single nucleotide polymorphisms (SNPs) involved in insulin resistance, weight regulation, lipid metabolism and inflammation in relation to metabolic syndrome: An epidemiological study. *Cardiovasc. Diabetol.* 2012, *11*, 133. [CrossRef]
80. Hinney, A.; Nguyen, T.T.; Scherag, A.; Friedel, S.; Brönner, G.; Müller, T.D.; Grallert, H.; Illig, T.; Wichmann, H.E.; Rief, W.; et al. Genome Wide Association (GWA) Study for Early Onset Extreme Obesity Supports the Role of Fat Mass and Obesity Associated Gene (FTO) Variants. *PLoS ONE* 2007, *2*, e1361. [CrossRef]
81. Scott, L.J.; Mohlke, K.L.; Bonnycastle, L.L.; Willer, C.J.; Li, Y.; Duren, W.L.; Erdos, M.R.; Stringham, H.M.; Chines, P.S.; Jackson, A.U.; et al. A Genome-Wide Association Study of Type 2 Diabetes in Finns Detects Multiple Susceptibility Variants. *Science* 2007, *316*, 1341–1345. [CrossRef]
82. Larsson, S.C.; Burgess, S.; Michaëlsson, K. Genetic association between adiposity and gout: A Mendelian randomization study. *Rheumatology* 2018, *57*, 2145–2148. [CrossRef]
83. Fox, C.S.; Liu, Y.; White, C.C.; Feitosa, M.; Smith, A.V.; Heard-Costa, N.; Lohman, K.; GIANT Consortium; MAGIC Consortium; GLGC Consortium; et al. Genome-wide association for abdominal subcutaneous and visceral adipose reveals a novel locus for visceral fat in women. *PLoS Genet.* 2012, *8*, e1002695. [CrossRef]
84. Chauhan, G.; Tabassum, R.; Mahajan, A.; Dwivedi, O.P.; Mahendran, Y.; Kaur, I.; Nigam, S.; Dubey, H.; Varma, B.; Madhu, S.V.; et al. Common Variants of FTO and the Risk of Obesity and Type 2 Diabetes in Indians. *J. Hum. Genet.* 2011, *56*, 720–726. [CrossRef]
85. Baturin, A.K.; Sorokina, E.Y.; Pogozheva, A.V.; Keshabyants, E.E.; Kobelkova, I.v.; Kambarov, A.O.; Elizarova, E.v.; Tutelyan, V.A. The Association of Rs993609 Polymorphisms of Gene FTO and Rs659366 Polymorphisms of Gene UCP2 with Obesity among Arctic Russian Population. *Vopr. Pitan.* 2017, *86*, 32–39. [CrossRef]
86. Matsuo, T.; Nakata, Y.; Hotta, K.; Tanaka, K. The FTO genotype as a useful predictor of body weight maintenance: Initial data from a 5-year follow-up study. *Metabolism* 2014, *63*, 912–917. [CrossRef]

87. Kamura, Y.; Iwata, M.; Maeda, S.; Shinmura, S.; Koshimizu, Y.; Honoki, H.; Fukuda, K.; Ishiki, M.; Usui, I.; Fukushima, Y.; et al. FTO Gene Polymorphism Is Associated with Type 2 Diabetes through Its Effect on Increasing the Maximum BMI in Japanese Men. *PLoS ONE* **2016**, *11*, e0165523. [CrossRef] [PubMed]
88. Cyrus, C.; Ismail, M.H.; Chathoth, S.; Vatte, C.; Hasen, M.; al Ali, A. Analysis of the Impact of Common Polymorphisms of the FTO and MC4R Genes with the Risk of Severe Obesity in Saudi Arabian Population. *Genet. Test Mol. Biomark.* **2018**, *22*, 170–177. [CrossRef] [PubMed]
89. Xi, B.; Cheng, H.; Shen, Y.; Chandak, G.R.; Zhao, X.; Hou, D.; Wu, L.; Wang, X.; Mi, J. Study of 11 BMI-associated loci identified in GWAS for associations with central obesity in the Chinese children. *PLoS ONE* **2013**, *8*, e56472. [CrossRef] [PubMed]
90. Salim, S.; Kartawidjajaputra, F.; Suwanto, A. Association of FTO rs9939609 and CD36 rs1761667 with Visceral Obesity. *J. Nutr. Sci. Vitam.* **2020**, *66*, S329–S335. [CrossRef] [PubMed]
91. Kring, S.I.; Holst, C.; Zimmermann, E.; Jess, T.; Berentzen, T.; Toubro, S.; Hansen, T.; Astrup, A.; Pedersen, O.; Sørensen, T.I. FTO gene associated fatness in relation to body fat distribution and metabolic traits throughout a broad range of fatness. *PLoS ONE* **2008**, *3*, e2958. [CrossRef] [PubMed]
92. Ağagündüz, D.; Gezmen-Karadağ, M. Association of FTO common variant (rs9939609) with body fat in Turkish individuals. *Lipids Health Dis.* **2019**, *18*, 212. [CrossRef]
93. Kong, X.; Xing, X.; Zhang, X.; Hong, J.; Yang, W. Sexual Dimorphism of a Genetic Risk Score for Obesity and Related Traits among Chinese Patients with Type 2 Diabetes. *Obes. Facts* **2019**, *12*, 328–343. [CrossRef]
94. Moore, S.C.; Gunter, M.J.; Daniel, C.R.; Reddy, K.S.; George, P.S.; Yurgalevitch, S.; Devasenapathy, N.; Ramakrishnan, L.; Chatterjee, N.; Chanock, S.J.; et al. Common genetic variants and central adiposity among Asian-Indians. *Obesity* **2012**, *20*, 1902–1908. [CrossRef] [PubMed]
95. Monnereau, C.; Santos, S.; van der Lugt, A.; Jaddoe, V.W.V.; Felix, J.F. Associations of adult genetic risk scores for adiposity with childhood abdominal, liver and pericardial fat assessed by magnetic resonance imaging. *Int. J. Obes.* **2018**, *42*, 897–904. [CrossRef] [PubMed]
96. Monnereau, C.; Vogelezang, S.; Kruithof, C.J.; Jaddoe, V.W.; Felix, J.F. Associations of genetic risk scores based on adult adiposity pathways with childhood growth and adiposity measures. *BMC Genet.* **2016**, *17*, 120. [CrossRef] [PubMed]
97. Winkler, T.W.; Justice, A.E.; Graff, M.; Barata, L.; Feitosa, M.F.; Chu, S.; Czajkowski, J.; Esko, T.; Fall, T.; Kilpeläinen, T.O.; et al. The Influence of Age and Sex on Genetic Associations with Adult Body Size and Shape: A Large-Scale Genome-Wide Interaction Study. *PLoS Genet.* **2015**, *11*, e1005378. [CrossRef] [PubMed]
98. GCG Glucagon [*Homo sapiens* (Human)]. Available online: https://www.ncbi.nlm.nih.gov/gene/2641 (accessed on 14 November 2022).
99. Torekov, S.S.; Ma, L.; Grarup, N.; Hartmann, B.; Hainerová, I.A.; Kielgast, U.; Kissow, H.; Rosenkilde, M.; Lebl, J.; Witte, D.R.; et al. Homozygous Carriers of the G Allele of Rs4664447 of the Glucagon Gene (GCG) Are Characterised by Decreased Fasting and Stimulated Levels of Insulin, Glucagon and Glucagon-like Peptide (GLP)-1. *Diabetologia* **2011**, *54*, 2820–2831. [CrossRef] [PubMed]
100. GLP1R Glucagon Like Peptide 1 Receptor [*Homo sapiens* (Human)]. Available online: https://www.ncbi.nlm.nih.gov/gene/2740 (accessed on 14 November 2022).
101. Tokuyama, Y.; Matsui, K.; Egashira, T.; Nozaki, O.; Ishizuka, T.; Kanatsuka, A. Five Missense Mutations in Glucagon-like Peptide 1 Receptor Gene in Japanese Population. *Diabetes Res. Clin. Pract.* **2004**, *66*, 63–69. [CrossRef]
102. Li, P.; Tiwari, H.K.; Lin, W.Y.; Allison, D.B.; Chung, W.K.; Leibel, R.L.; Yi, N.; Liu, N. Genetic Association Analysis of 30 Genes Related to Obesity in a European American Population. *Int. J. Obes.* **2014**, *38*, 724–729. [CrossRef]
103. de Luis, D.A.; Aller, R.; de la Fuente, B.; Primo, D.; Conde, R.; Izaola, O.; Sagrado, M.G. Relation of the Rs6923761 Gene Variant in Glucagon-like Peptide 1 Receptor with Weight, Cardiovascular Risk Factor, and Serum Adipokine Levels in Obese Female Subjects. *J. Clin. Lab. Anal.* **2015**, *29*, 100–105. [CrossRef]
104. Michałowska, J.; Miller-Kasprzak, E.; Seraszek-Jaros, A.; Mostowska, A.; Bogdański, P. Association of GLP1R Variants Rs2268641 and Rs6923761 with Obesity and Other Metabolic Parameters in a Polish Cohort. *Front. Endocrinol.* **2022**, *13*, 1000185. [CrossRef]
105. Wessel, J.; Chu, A.Y.; Willems, S.M.; Wang, S.; Yaghootkar, H.; Brody, J.A.; Dauriz, M.; Hivert, M.F.; Raghavan, S.; Lipovich, L.; et al. Low-Frequency and Rare Exome Chip Variants Associate with Fasting Glucose and Type 2 Diabetes Susceptibility. *Nat. Commun.* **2015**, *6*, 5897. [CrossRef]
106. Li, W.; Li, P.; Li, R.; Yu, Z.; Sun, X.; Ji, G.; Yang, X.; Zhu, L.; Zhu, S. GLP1R Single-Nucleotide Polymorphisms Rs3765467 and Rs10305492 Affect β Cell Insulin Secretory Capacity and Apoptosis through GLP-1. *DNA Cell Biol.* **2020**, *39*, 1700–1710. [CrossRef] [PubMed]
107. El Eid, L.; Reynolds, C.A.; Tomas, A.; Jones, B. Biased Agonism and Polymorphic Variation at the GLP-1 Receptor: Implications for the Development of Personalised Therapeutics. *Pharmacol. Res.* **2022**, *184*, 106411. [CrossRef] [PubMed]
108. GHRL Ghrelin and Obestatin Prepropeptide [*Homo sapiens* (Human)]. Available online: https://www.ncbi.nlm.nih.gov/gene/51738 (accessed on 14 November 2022).
109. Jiao, Z.T.; Luo, Q. Molecular Mechanisms and Health Benefits of Ghrelin: A Narrative Review. *Nutrients* **2022**, *14*, 4191. [CrossRef] [PubMed]
110. Ukkola, O.; Ravussin, E.; Jacobson, P.; Snyder, E.E.; Chagnon, M.; SjÖstrÖm, L.; Bouchard, C. RAPID COMMUNICATIONS: Mutations in the Preproghrelin/Ghrelin Gene Associated with Obesity in Humans. *J. Clin. Endocrinol. Metab.* **2001**, *86*, 3996–3999. [CrossRef]

111. Steinle, N.I.; Pollin, T.I.; O'Connell, J.R.; Mitchell, B.D.; Shuldiner, A.R. Variants in the Ghrelin Gene Are Associated with Metabolic Syndrome in the Old Order Amish. *J. Clin. Endocrinol. Metab.* **2005**, *90*, 6672–6677. [CrossRef] [PubMed]
112. Gueorguiev, M.; Lecoeur, C.; Meyre, D.; Benzinou, M.; Mein, C.A.; Hinney, A.; Vatin, V.; Weill, J.; Heude, B.; Hebebrand, J.; et al. Association Studies on Ghrelin and Ghrelin Receptor Gene Polymorphisms with Obesity. *Obesity* **2009**, *17*, 745–754. [CrossRef]
113. Chung, W.K.; Patki, A.; Matsuoka, N.; Boyer, B.B.; Liu, N.; Musani, S.K.; Goropashnaya, A.V.; Tan, P.L.; Katsanis, N.; Johnson, S.B.; et al. Analysis of 30 Genes (355 SNPS) Related to Energy Homeostasis for Association with Adiposity in European-American and Yup'ik Eskimo Populations. *Hum. Hered.* **2009**, *67*, 193–205. [CrossRef]
114. Imaizumi, T.; Ando, M.; Nakatochi, M.; Yasuda, Y.; Honda, H.; Kuwatsuka, Y.; Kato, S.; Kondo, T.; Iwata, M.; Nakashima, T.; et al. Effect of Dietary Energy and Polymorphisms in BRAP and GHRL on Obesity and Metabolic Traits. *Obes. Res. Clin. Pract.* **2018**, *12*, 39–48. [CrossRef]
115. Wang, X.; Qu, F.; Wang, C.; Wang, Y.; Wang, D.; Zhao, M.; Yun, X.; Zheng, Q.; Xu, L. Variation Analysis of Ghrelin Gene in Chinese Patients with Obesity, Having Polycystic Ovarian Syndrome. *Gynecol. Endocrinol.* **2020**, *36*, 594–598. [CrossRef]
116. Ando, T.; Komaki, G.; Naruo, T.; Okabe, K.; Takii, M.; Kawai, K.; Konjiki, F.; Takei, M.; Oka, T.; Takeuchi, K.; et al. Possible Role of Preproghrelin Gene Polymorphisms in Susceptibility to Bulimia Nervosa. *Am. J. Med. Genet. Part B Neuropsychiatr. Genet.* **2006**, *141*, 929–934. [CrossRef]
117. GIP Gastric Inhibitory Polypeptide [*Homo sapiens* (Human)]. Available online: https://www.ncbi.nlm.nih.gov/gene/2695 (accessed on 14 November 2022).
118. Chang, C.L.; Cai, J.J.; Cheng, P.J.; Chueh, H.Y.; Hsu, S.Y.T. Identification of Metabolic Modifiers That Underlie Phenotypic Variations in Energy-Balance Regulation. *Diabetes* **2011**, *60*, 726–734. [CrossRef] [PubMed]
119. Nakayama, K.; Watanabe, K.; Boonvisut, S.; Makishima, S.; Miyashita, H.; Iwamoto, S. Common variants of GIP are associated with visceral fat accumulation in Japanese adults. *Am. J. Physiol. Gastrointest. Liver. Physiol.* **2014**, *307*, G1108–G1114. [CrossRef] [PubMed]
120. INS Insulin [*Homo sapiens* (Human)]. Available online: https://www.ncbi.nlm.nih.gov/gene/3630 (accessed on 14 November 2022).
121. Liu, M.; Weiss, M.A.; Arunagiri, A.; Yong, J.; Rege, N.; Sun, J.; Haataja, L.; Kaufman, R.J.; Arvan, P. Biosynthesis, Structure, and Folding of the Insulin Precursor Protein. *Diabetes Obes. Metab.* **2018**, *20*, 28–50. [CrossRef]
122. Vakilian, M.; Tahamtani, Y.; Ghaedi, K. A Review on Insulin Trafficking and Exocytosis. *Gene* **2019**, *706*, 52–61. [CrossRef]
123. Ghosh, S.; Mahalanobish, S.; Sil, P.C. Diabetes: Discovery of Insulin, Genetic, Epigenetic and Viral Infection Mediated Regulation. *Nucleus* **2021**, *65*, 283–297. [CrossRef] [PubMed]
124. Liu, M.; Sun, J.; Cui, J.; Chen, W.; Guo, H.; Barbetti, F.; Arvan, P. INS-Gene Mutations: From Genetics and Beta Cell Biology to Clinical Disease. *Mol. Aspects Med.* **2015**, *42*, 3–18. [CrossRef]
125. Arneth, B. Insulin Gene Mutations and Posttranslational and Translocation Defects: Associations with Diabetes. *Endocrine* **2020**, *70*, 488–497. [CrossRef]
126. Edghill, E.L.; Flanagan, S.E.; Patch, A.M.; Boustred, C.; Parrish, A.; Shields, B.; Shepherd, M.H.; Hussain, K.; Kapoor, R.R.; Malecki, M.; et al. Insulin Mutation Screening in 1044 Patients with Diabetes Mutations in the INS Gene Are a Common Cause of Neonatal Diabetes but a Rare Cause of Diabetes Diagnosed in Childhood or Adulthood. *Diabetes* **2008**, *57*, 1034–1042. [CrossRef]
127. Boesgaard, T.W.; Pruhova, S.; Andersson, E.A.; Cinek, O.; Obermannova, B.; Lauenborg, J.; Damm, P.; Bergholdt, R.; Pociot, F.; Pisinger, C.; et al. Further Evidence That Mutations in INS Can Be a Rare Cause of Maturity-Onset Diabetes of the Young (MODY). *BMC Med. Genet.* **2010**, *11*, 42. [CrossRef]
128. LEP Leptin [*Homo sapiens* (Human)]. Available online: https://www.ncbi.nlm.nih.gov/gene/3952 (accessed on 23 December 2022).
129. Caldeira, R.S.; Panissa, V.L.G.; Inoue, D.S.; Campos, E.Z.; Monteiro, P.A.; Giglio, B.D.M.; Pimentel, G.D.; Hofmann, P.; Lira, F.S. Impact to short-term high intensity intermittent training on different storages of body fat, leptin and soluble leptin receptor levels in physically active non-obese men: A pilot investigation. *Clin. Nutr. ESPEN* **2018**, *28*, 186–192. [CrossRef]
130. Hamilton, K.; Harvey, J. The neuronal actions of leptin and the implications for treating alzheimer's disease. *Pharmaceuticals* **2021**, *14*, 52. [CrossRef] [PubMed]
131. Guzmán, A.; Hernández-Coronado, C.G.; Rosales-Torres, A.M.; Hernández-Medrano, J.H. Leptin regulates neuropeptides associated with food intake and GnRH secretion. *Ann. Endocrinol.* **2019**, *80*, 38–46. [CrossRef] [PubMed]
132. Marcos, P.; Coveñas, R. Neuropeptidergic control of feeding: Focus on the galanin family of peptides. *Int. J. Mol. Sci.* **2021**, *22*, 2544. [CrossRef] [PubMed]
133. P41159 LEP_HUMAN. Available online: https://www.uniprot.org/uniprotkb/P41159/entry (accessed on 23 December 2022).
134. Eikelis, N.; Lambert, G.; Wiesner, G.; Kaye, D.; Schlaich, M.; Morris, M.; Hastings, J.; Socratous, F.; Esler, M. Extra-adipocyte leptin release in human obesity and its relation to sympathoadrenal function. *Am. J. Physiol. Endocrinol. Metab* **2004**, *286*, E744–E752. [CrossRef]
135. Funcke, J.B.; von Schnurbein, J.; Lennerz, B.; Lahr, G.; Debatin, K.M.; Fischer-Posovszky, P.; Wabitsch, M. Monogenic forms of childhood obesity due to mutations in the leptin gene. *Mol. Cell. Pediatr.* **2014**, *1*, 3. [CrossRef]
136. Dasgupta, S.; Salman, M.; Siddalingaiah, L.B.; Lakshmi, G.L.; Xaviour, D.; Sreenath, J. Genetic variants in leptin: Determinants of obesity and leptin levels in South Indian population. *Adipocyte* **2014**, *4*, 135–140. [CrossRef]
137. Aljanabi, M.A.; Alfaqih, M.A.; Khanfar, M.; Amarin, Z.O.; Elsalem, L.; Saadeh, R.; Al-Mughales, F. Leptin and the GA genotype of rs2167270 of the LEP gene increase the risk of prediabetes. *Biomed. Rep.* **2021**, *14*, 44. [CrossRef]

138. Lombard, Z.; Crowther, N.J.; van der Merwe, L.; Pitamber, P.; Norris, S.A.; Ramsay, M. Appetite regulation genes are associated with body mass index in black South African adolescents: A genetic association study. *BMJ Open.* **2012**, *2*, e000873. [CrossRef]
139. Manju, S.K.; Anilkumar, T.R.; Vysakh, G.; Leena, B.K.; Lekshminarayan, V.; Kumar, P.G.; Shenoy, T.K. A Case-Control Study of the Association of Leptin Gene Polymorphisms with Plasma Leptin Levels and Obesity in the Kerala Population. *J. Obes.* **2022**, *2022*, 1040650. [CrossRef]
140. Ashraf, R.; Khan, M.; Lone, S.; Bhat, M.; Rashid, S.; Majid, S.; Bashir, H. Implication of Leptin and Leptin Receptor Gene Variations in Type 2 Diabetes Mellitus: A Case-Control Study. *J. Endocrinol. Metab.* **2022**, *12*, 19–31. [CrossRef]
141. Enns, J.E.; Taylor, C.G.; Zahradka, P. Variations in Adipokine Genes AdipoQ, Lep, and LepR are Associated with Risk for Obesity-Related Metabolic Disease: The Modulatory Role of Gene-Nutrient Interactions. *J. Obes.* **2011**, *2011*, 168659. [CrossRef] [PubMed]
142. Yaghootkar, H.; Zhang, Y.; Spracklen, C.N.; Karaderi, T.; Huang, L.O.; Bradfield, J.; Schurmann, C.; Fine, R.S.; Preuss, M.H.; Kutalik, Z.; et al. Genetic Studies of Leptin Concentrations Implicate Leptin in the Regulation of Early Adiposity. *Diabetes* **2020**, *69*, 2806–2818. [CrossRef] [PubMed]
143. Haglund, E.; Nguyen, L.; Schafer, N.P.; Lammert, H.; Jennings, P.A.; Onuchic, J.N. Uncovering the molecular mechanisms behind disease-associated leptin variants. *J. Biol. Chem.* **2018**, *293*, 12919–12933. [CrossRef] [PubMed]
144. NAMPT Nicotinamide Phosphoribosyltransferase [*Homo sapiens* (Human)]. Available online: https://www.ncbi.nlm.nih.gov/gene/10135 (accessed on 14 November 2022).
145. Fagerberg, L.; Hallstrom, B.M.; Oksvold, P.; Kampf, C.; Djureinovic, D.; Odeberg, J.; Habuka, M.; Tahmasebpoor, S.; Danielsson, A.; Edlund, K.; et al. Analysis of the Human Tissue-Specific Expression by Genome-Wide Integration of Transcriptomics and Antibody-Based Proteomics. *Mol. Cell. Proteom.* **2014**, *13*, 397–406. [CrossRef]
146. Böttcher, Y.; Teupser, D.; Enigk, B.; Berndt, J.; Klöting, N.; Schön, M.R.; Thiery, J.; Blüher, M.; Stumvoll, M.; Kovacs, P. Genetic Variation in the Visfatin Gene (PBEF1) and Its Relation to Glucose Metabolism and Fat-Depot-Specific Messenger Ribonucleic Acid Expression in Humans. *J. Clin. Endocrinol. Metab.* **2006**, *91*, 2725–2731. [CrossRef]
147. Johansson, L.M.; Johansson, L.E.; Ridderstråle, M. The Visfatin (PBEF1) G-948T Gene Polymorphism Is Associated with Increased High-Density Lipoprotein Cholesterol in Obese Subjects. *Metabolism* **2008**, *57*, 1558–1562. [CrossRef]
148. Blakemore, A.I.F.; Meyre, D.; Delplanque, J.; Vatin, V.; Lecoeur, C.; Marre, M.; Tichet, J.; Balkau, B.; Froguel, P.; Walley, A.J. A Rare Variant in the Visfatin Gene (Nampt/Pbef1) Is Associated with Protection from Obesity. *Obesity* **2009**, *17*, 1549–1553. [CrossRef]
149. Tabassum, R.; Mahendran, Y.; Dwivedi, O.P.; Chauhan, G.; Ghosh, S.; Marwaha, R.K.; Tandon, N.; Bharadwaj, D. Common Variants of IL6, LEPR, and PBEF1 Are Associated with Obesity in Indian Children. *Diabetes* **2012**, *61*, 626–631. [CrossRef]
150. Rong, J.; Chu, M.; Xing, B.; Zhu, L.; Wang, S.; Tao, T.; Zhao, Y.; Jiang, L. Variations in the PBEF1 Gene Are Associated with Body Mass Index: A Population-Based Study in Northern China. *Meta Gene* **2015**, *6*, 65–68. [CrossRef]
151. Zhou, Q.; Chen, B.; Ji, T.; Luo, M.; Luo, J. Association of Genetic Variants in RETN, NAMPT and ADIPOQ Gene with Glycemic, Metabolic Traits and Diabetes Risk in a Chinese Population. *Gene* **2018**, *642*, 439–446. [CrossRef]
152. Kim, J.-E.; Kim, J.-S.; Jo, M.-J.; Cho, E.; Ahn, S.-Y.; Kwon, Y.-J.; Ko, G.-J.T.; Roles, A.; Kim, J.-E.; Kim, J.-S.; et al. The Roles and Associated Mechanisms of Adipokines in Development of Metabolic Syndrome. *Molecules* **2022**, *27*, 334. [CrossRef]
153. PPY Pancreatic Polypeptide [*Homo sapiens* (Human)]. Available online: https://www.ncbi.nlm.nih.gov/gene/5539 (accessed on 14 November 2022).
154. PYY Peptide YY [*Homo sapiens* (Human)]. Available online: https://www.ncbi.nlm.nih.gov/gene/5697 (accessed on 14 November 2022).
155. Simpson, K.; Parker, J.; Plumer, J.; Bloom, S. CCK, PYY and PP: The Control of Energy Balance. *Handb. Exp. Pharmacol.* **2012**, *209*, 209–230. [CrossRef]
156. Friedlander, Y.; Li, G.; Fornage, M.; Williams, O.D.; Lewis, C.E.; Schreiner, P.; Pletcher, M.J.; Enquobahrie, D.; Williams, M.; Siscovick, D.S. Candidate Molecular Pathway Genes Related to Appetite Regulatory Neural Network, Adipocyte Homeostasis and Obesity: Results from the CARDIA Study. *Ann. Hum. Genet.* **2010**, *74*, 387–398. [CrossRef] [PubMed]
157. Siddiq, A.; Gueorguiev, M.; Samson, C.; Hercberg, S.; Heude, B.; Levy-Marchal, C.; Jouret, B.; Weill, J.; Meyre, D.; Walley, A.; et al. Single Nucleotide Polymorphisms in the Neuropeptide Y2 Receptor (NPY2R) Gene and Association with Severe Obesity in French White Subjects. *Diabetologia* **2007**, *50*, 574–584. [CrossRef]
158. Ahituv, N.; Kavaslar, N.; Schackwitz, W.; Ustaszewska, A.; Martin, J.; Hébert, S.; Doelle, H.; Ersoy, B.; Kryukov, G.; Schmidt, S.; et al. Medical Sequencing at the Extremes of Human Body Mass. *Am. J. Hum. Genet.* **2007**, *80*, 779–791. [CrossRef]
159. Perez-Frances, M.; van Gurp, L.; Abate, M.V.; Cigliola, V.; Furuyama, K.; Bru-Tari, E.; Oropeza, D.; Carreaux, T.; Fujitani, Y.; Thorel, F.; et al. Pancreatic Ppy-Expressing γ-Cells Display Mixed Phenotypic Traits and the Adaptive Plasticity to Engage Insulin Production. *Nat. Commun.* **2021**, *12*, 4458. [CrossRef] [PubMed]
160. Kim, H.J.; Lee, S.Y.; Kim, C.M. Association between Gene Polymorphisms and Obesity and Physical Fitness in Korean Children. *Biol. Sport* **2018**, *35*, 21–27. [CrossRef]
161. RBP4 Retinol Binding Protein 4 [*Homo sapiens* (Human)]. Available online: https://www.ncbi.nlm.nih.gov/gene/5950 (accessed on 14 November 2022).
162. Yang, Q.; Graham, T.E.; Mody, N.; Preitner, F.; Peroni, O.D.; Zabolotny, J.M.; Kotani, K.; Quadro, L.; Kahn, B.B. Serum Retinol Binding Protein 4 Contributes to Insulin Resistance in Obesity and Type 2 Diabetes. *Nature* **2005**, *436*, 356–362. [CrossRef]

163. Craig, R.L.; Chu, W.S.; Elbein, S.C. Retinol Binding Protein 4 as a Candidate Gene for Type 2 Diabetes and Prediabetic Intermediate Traits. *Mol. Genet. Metab.* **2007**, *90*, 338–344. [CrossRef]
164. Wu, Y.; Li, H.; Loos, R.J.F.; Qi, Q.; Hu, F.B.; Liu, Y.; Lin, X. RBP4 Variants Are Significantly Associated with Plasma RBP4 Levels and Hypertriglyceridemia Risk in Chinese Hans. *J. Lipid. Res.* **2009**, *50*, 1479–1486. [CrossRef]
165. Codoñer-Franch, P.; Carrasco-Luna, J.; Allepuz, P.; Codoñer-Alejos, A.; Guillem, V. Association of RBP4 Genetic Variants with Childhood Obesity and Cardiovascular Risk Factors. *Pediatr. Diabetes* **2016**, *17*, 576–583. [CrossRef]
166. Hu, S.; Ma, S.; Li, X.; Tian, Z.; Liang, H.; Yan, J.; Chen, M.; Tan, H. Relationships of SLC2A4, RBP4, PCK1, and PI3K Gene Polymorphisms with Gestational Diabetes Mellitus in a Chinese Population. *Biomed. Res. Int.* **2019**, *2019*, 7398063. [CrossRef]
167. RETN Resistin [*Homo sapiens* (Human)]. Available online: https://www.ncbi.nlm.nih.gov/gene/56729 (accessed on 14 November 2022).
168. Tripathi, D.; Kant, S.; Pandey, S.; Ehtesham, N.Z. Resistin in Metabolism, Inflammation, and Disease. *FEBS J.* **2020**, *287*, 3141–3149. [CrossRef] [PubMed]
169. Hishida, A.; Wakai, K.; Okada, R.; Morita, E.; Hamajima, N.; Hosono, S.; Higaki, Y.; Turin, T.C.; Suzuki, S.; Motahareh, K.; et al. Significant Interaction between RETN -420 G/G Genotype and Lower BMI on Decreased Risk of Type 2 Diabetes Mellitus (T2DM) in Japanese–the J-MICC Study. *Endocr. J.* **2013**, *60*, 237–243. [CrossRef] [PubMed]
170. Zayani, N.; Omezzine, A.; Boumaiza, I.; Achour, O.; Rebhi, L.; Rejeb, J.; ben Rejeb, N.; ben Abdelaziz, A.; Bouslama, A. Association of ADIPOQ, Leptin, LEPR, and Resistin Polymorphisms with Obesity Parameters in Hammam Sousse Sahloul Heart Study. *J. Clin. Lab. Anal.* **2017**, *31*, e22148. [CrossRef] [PubMed]
171. Beckers, S.; Zegers, D.; van Camp, J.K.; Boudin, E.; Nielsen, T.L.; Brixen, K.; Andersen, M.; van Hul, W. Resistin Polymorphisms Show Associations with Obesity, but Not with Bone Parameters in Men: Results from the Odense Androgen Study. *Mol. Biol. Rep.* **2013**, *40*, 2467–2472. [CrossRef]
172. Chung, C.M.; Lin, T.H.; Chen, J.W.; Leu, H.B.; Yin, W.H.; Ho, H.Y.; Sheu, S.H.; Tsai, W.C.; Chen, J.H.; Lin, S.J.; et al. Common Quantitative Trait Locus Downstream of RETN Gene Identified by Genome-Wide Association Study Is Associated with Risk of Type 2 Diabetes Mellitus in Han Chinese: A Mendelian Randomization Effect. *Diabetes Metab. Res. Rev.* **2014**, *30*, 232–240. [CrossRef]
173. Ortega, L.; Navarro, P.; Riestra, P.; Gavela-Pérez, T.; Soriano-Guillén, L.; Garcés, C. Association of Resistin Polymorphisms with Resistin Levels and Lipid Profile in Children. *Mol. Biol. Rep.* **2014**, *41*, 7659–7664. [CrossRef]
174. Nakatochi, M.; Ichihara, S.; Yamamoto, K.; Ohnaka, K.; Kato, Y.; Yokota, S.; Hirashiki, A.; Naruse, K.; Asano, H.; Izawa, H.; et al. Epigenome-Wide Association Study Suggests That SNPs in the Promoter Region of RETN Influence Plasma Resistin Level via Effects on DNA Methylation at Neighbouring Sites. *Diabetologia* **2015**, *58*, 2781–2790. [CrossRef]
175. Elkhattabi, L.; Morjane, I.; Charoute, H.; Amghar, S.; Bouafi, H.; Elkarhat, Z.; Saile, R.; Rouba, H.; Barakat, A. In Silico Analysis of Coding/Noncoding SNPs of Human RETN Gene and Characterization of Their Impact on Resistin Stability and Structure. *J. Diabetes Res.* **2019**, *2019*, 4951627. [CrossRef]
176. SCT Secretin [*Homo sapiens* (Human)]. Available online: https://www.ncbi.nlm.nih.gov/gene/6343 (accessed on 14 November 2022).
177. Laurila, S.; Rebelos, E.; Honka, M.J.; Nuutila, P. Pleiotropic Effects of Secretin: A Potential Drug Candidate in the Treatment of Obesity? *Front Endocrinol.* **2021**, *12*, 1259. [CrossRef]
178. Laurila, S.; Sun, L.; Lahesmaa, M.; Schnabl, K.; Laitinen, K.; Klén, R.; Li, Y.; Balaz, M.; Wolfrum, C.; Steiger, K.; et al. Secretin Activates Brown Fat and Induces Satiation. *Nat. Metab.* **2021**, *3*, 798–809. [CrossRef] [PubMed]
179. UCP2 Uncoupling Protein 2 [*Homo sapiens* (Human)]. Available online: https://www.ncbi.nlm.nih.gov/gene/7351 (accessed on 14 November 2022).
180. Demine, S.; Renard, P.; Arnould, T. Mitochondrial Uncoupling: A Key Controller of Biological Processes in Physiology and Diseases. *Cells* **2019**, *8*, 795. [CrossRef] [PubMed]
181. Esterbauer, H.; Schneitler, C.; Oberkofler, H.; Ebenbichler, C.; Paulweber, B.; Sandhofer, F.; Ladurner, G.; Hell, E.; Strosberg, A.D.; Patsch, J.R.; et al. A Common Polymorphism in the Promoter of UCP2 Is Associated with Decreased Risk of Obesity in Middle-Aged Humans. *Nat. Genet.* **2001**, *28*, 178–183. [CrossRef] [PubMed]
182. Bulotta, A.; Ludovico, O.; Coco, A.; di Paola, R.; Quattrone, A.; Carella, M.; Pellegrini, F.; Prudente, S.; Trischitta, V. The Common -866G/A Polymorphism in the Promoter Region of the UCP-2 Gene Is Associated with Reduced Risk of Type 2 Diabetes in Caucasians from Italy. *J. Clin. Endocrinol. Metab.* **2005**, *90*, 1176–1180. [CrossRef]
183. Andersen, G.; Dalgaard, L.T.; Justesen, J.M.; Anthonsen, S.; Nielsen, T.; Thørner, L.W.; Witte, D.; Jørgensen, T.; Clausen, J.O.; Lauritzen, T.; et al. The Frequent UCP2-866G>A Polymorphism Protects against Insulin Resistance and Is Associated with Obesity: A Study of Obesity and Related Metabolic Traits among 17 636 Danes. *Int. J. Obes.* **2013**, *37*, 175–181. [CrossRef]
184. Salopuro, T.; Pulkkinen, L.; Lindström, J.; Kolehmainen, M.; Tolppanen, A.M.; Eriksson, J.G.; Valle, T.T.; Aunola, S.; Ilanne-Parikka, P.; Keinänen-Kiukaanniemi, S. Variation in the UCP2 and UCP3 genes associates with abdominal obesity and serum lipids: The Finnish Diabetes Prevention Study. *BMC Med. Genet.* **2009**, *10*, 94. [CrossRef]
185. Oktavianthi, S.; Trimarsanto, H.; Febinia, C.A.; Suastika, K.; Saraswati, M.R.; Dwipayana, P.; Arindrarto, W.; Sudoyo, H.; Malik, S.G. Uncoupling Protein 2 Gene Polymorphisms Are Associated with Obesity. *Cardiovasc. Diabetol.* **2012**, *11*, 41. [CrossRef]

186. Martinez-Hervas, S.; Mansego, M.L.; de Marco, G.; Martinez, F.; Alonso, M.P.; Morcillo, S.; Rojo-Martinez, G.; Real, J.T.; Ascaso, J.F.; Redon, J.; et al. Polymorphisms of the UCP2 Gene Are Associated with Body Fat Distribution and Risk of Abdominal Obesity in Spanish Population. *Eur. J. Clin. Invest.* **2012**, *42*, 171–178. [CrossRef]
187. Xu, L.; Chen, S.; Zhan, L. Association of Uncoupling Protein-2 -866G/A and Ala55Val Polymorphisms with Susceptibility to Type 2 Diabetes Mellitus: A Meta-Analysis of Case-Control Studies. *Medicine* **2021**, *100*, e24464. [CrossRef]
188. Fall, T.; Mendelson, M.; Speliotes, E.K. Recent Advances in Human Genetics and Epigenetics of Adiposity: Pathway to Precision Medicine? *Gastroenterology* **2017**, *152*, 1695–1706. [CrossRef] [PubMed]
189. Christakoudi, S.; Tsilidis, K.K.; Evangelou, E.; Riboli, E. A Body Shape Index (ABSI), hip index, and risk of cancer in the UK Biobank cohort. *Cancer Med.* **2021**, *10*, 5614–5628. [CrossRef] [PubMed]
190. Wu, S.; Hsu, L.-A.; Teng, M.-S.; Chou, H.-H.; Ko, Y.-L. Differential Genetic and Epigenetic Effects of the KLF14 Gene on Body Shape Indices and Metabolic Traits. *Int. J. Mol. Sci.* **2022**, *23*, 4165. [CrossRef] [PubMed]
191. Nagayama, D.; Sugiura, T.; Choi, S.Y.; Shirai, K. Various Obesity Indices and Arterial Function Evaluated with CAVI—Is Waist Circumference Adequate to Define Metabolic Syndrome? *Vasc. Health Risk. Manag.* **2022**, *18*, 721–733. [CrossRef] [PubMed]
192. Nagayama, D.; Fujishiro, K.; Watanabe, Y.; Yamaguchi, T.; Suzuki, K.; Saiki, A.; Shirai, K. A Body Shape Index (ABSI) as a Variant of Conicity Index Not Affected by the Obesity Paradox: A Cross-Sectional Study Using Arterial Stiffness Parameter. *J. Pers. Med.* **2022**, *12*, 2014. [CrossRef]
193. Young, K.L.; Graff, M.; Fernandez-Rhodes, L.; North, K.E. Genetics of Obesity in Diverse Populations. *Curr. Diab. Rep.* **2018**, *18*, 145. [CrossRef] [PubMed]
194. Locke, A.E.; Kahali, B.; Berndt, S.I.; Justice, A.E.; Pers, T.H.; Day, F.R.; Powell, C.; Vedantam, S.; Buchkovich, M.L.; Yang, J.; et al. Genetic studies of body mass index yield new insights for obesity biology. *Nature* **2015**, *518*, 197–206. [CrossRef]
195. Pan, D.Z.; Miao, Z.; Comenho, C.; Rajkumar, S.; Koka, A.; Lee, S.H.T.; Alvarez, M.; Kaminska, D.; Ko, A.; Sinsheimer, J.S.; et al. Identification of TBX15 as an adipose master trans regulator of abdominal obesity genes. *Genome Med.* **2021**, *13*, 123. [CrossRef]
196. Larsson, S.C.; Bäck, M.; Rees, J.M.B.; Mason, A.M.; Burgess, S. Body mass index and body composition in relation to 14 cardiovascular conditions in UK Biobank: A Mendelian randomization study. *Eur. Heart J.* **2020**, *41*, 221–226. [CrossRef]
197. Beaney, K.E.; Cooper, J.A.; Shahid, S.U.; Ahmed, W.; Qamar, R.; Drenos, F.; Crockard, M.A.; Humphries, S.E. Clinical Utility of a Coronary Heart Disease Risk Prediction Gene Score in UK Healthy Middle-Aged Men and in the Pakistani Population. *PLoS ONE* **2015**, *10*, e0130754. [CrossRef]
198. Iribarren, C.; Lu, M.; Jorgenson, E.; Martínez, M.; Lluis-Ganella, C.; Subirana, I.; Salas, E.; Elosua, R. Weighted Multi-marker Genetic Risk Scores for Incident Coronary Heart Disease among Individuals of African, Latino and East-Asian Ancestry. *Sci. Rep.* **2018**, *8*, 6853. [CrossRef]
199. Semaev, S.; Shakhtshneider, E. Genetic Risk Score for Coronary Heart Disease: Review. *J. Pers. Med.* **2020**, *10*, 239. [CrossRef] [PubMed]
200. Benbaibeche, H.; Bounihi, A.; Koceir, E.A. Leptin level as a biomarker of uncontrolled eating in obesity and overweight. *Ir. J. Med. Sci.* **2020**, *190*, 155–161. [CrossRef] [PubMed]
201. Poetsch, M.S.; Strano, A.; Guan, K. Role of Leptin in Cardiovascular Diseases. *Front. Endocrinol.* **2020**, *11*, 354. [CrossRef]
202. Reyes-Barrera, J.; Sainz-Escárrega, V.H.; Medina-Urritia, A.X.; Jorge-Galarza, E.; Osorio-Alonso, H.; Torres-Tamayo, M.; Leal-Escobar, G.; Posadas-Romero, C.; Torre-Villalvazo, I.; Juárez-Rojas, J.G. Dysfunctional adiposity index as a marker of adipose tissue morpho-functional abnormalities and metabolic disorders in apparently healthy subjects. *Adipocyte* **2021**, *10*, 142–152. [CrossRef] [PubMed]
203. Trinh, T.; Broxmeyer, H.E. Role for Leptin and Leptin Receptors in Stem Cells During Health and Diseases. *Stem. Cell Rev. Rep.* **2021**, *17*, 511–522. [CrossRef]

Disclaimer/Publisher's Note: The statements, opinions and data contained in all publications are solely those of the individual author(s) and contributor(s) and not of MDPI and/or the editor(s). MDPI and/or the editor(s) disclaim responsibility for any injury to people or property resulting from any ideas, methods, instructions or products referred to in the content.

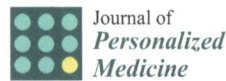
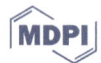

Article

The Mutation Spectrum of Rare Variants in the Gene of Adenosine Triphosphate (ATP)-Binding Cassette Subfamily C Member 8 in Patients with a MODY Phenotype in Western Siberia

Dinara Ivanoshchuk [1,2,*], Elena Shakhtshneider [1,2], Svetlana Mikhailova [1], Alla Ovsyannikova [2], Oksana Rymar [2], Emil Valeeva [1], Pavel Orlov [1,2] and Mikhail Voevoda [1]

1. Federal Research Center Institute of Cytology and Genetics, Siberian Branch of Russian Academy of Sciences, Prospekt Lavrentyeva 10, 630090 Novosibirsk, Russia
2. Institute of Internal and Preventive Medicine—Branch of Institute of Cytology and Genetics, Siberian Branch of Russian Academy of Sciences, Bogatkova Str. 175/1, 630004 Novosibirsk, Russia
* Correspondence: dinara@bionet.nsc.ru; Tel.: +7-(383)-363-4963; Fax: +7-(383)-333-1278

Abstract: During differential diagnosis of diabetes mellitus, the greatest difficulties are encountered with young patients because various types of diabetes can manifest themselves in this age group (type 1, type 2, and monogenic types of diabetes mellitus, including maturity-onset diabetes of the young (MODY)). The MODY phenotype is associated with gene mutations leading to pancreatic-β-cell dysfunction. Using next-generation sequencing technology, targeted sequencing of coding regions and adjacent splicing sites of MODY-associated genes (*HNF4A*, *GCK*, *HNF1A*, *PDX1*, *HNF1B*, *NEUROD1*, *KLF11*, *CEL*, *PAX4*, *INS*, *BLK*, *KCNJ11*, *ABCC8*, and *APPL1*) was carried out in 285 probands. Previously reported missense variants c.970G>A (p.Val324Met) and c.1562G>A (p.Arg521Gln) in the *ABCC8* gene were found once each in different probands. Variant c.1562G>A (p.Arg521Gln) in *ABCC8* was detected in a compound heterozygous state with a pathogenic variant of the *HNF1A* gene in a diabetes patient and his mother. Novel frameshift mutation c.4609_4610insC (p.His1537ProfsTer22) in this gene was found in one patient. All these variants were detected in available family members of the patients and cosegregated with diabetes mellitus. Thus, next-generation sequencing of MODY-associated genes is an important step in the diagnosis of rare MODY subtypes.

Keywords: 15]maturity-onset diabetes of the young; MODY; diabetes mellitus; next-generation sequencing; *ABCC8*; SUR1; single-nucleotide variant

Citation: Ivanoshchuk, D.; Shakhtshneider, E.; Mikhailova, S.; Ovsyannikova, A.; Rymar, O.; Valeeva, E.; Orlov, P.; Voevoda, M. The Mutation Spectrum of Rare Variants in the Gene of Adenosine Triphosphate (ATP)-Binding Cassette Subfamily C Member 8 in Patients with a MODY Phenotype in Western Siberia. *J. Pers. Med.* **2023**, *13*, 172. https://doi.org/10.3390/jpm13020172

Academic Editor: Oscar Campuzano

Received: 9 December 2022
Revised: 10 January 2023
Accepted: 17 January 2023
Published: 19 January 2023

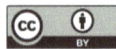

Copyright: © 2023 by the authors. Licensee MDPI, Basel, Switzerland. This article is an open access article distributed under the terms and conditions of the Creative Commons Attribution (CC BY) license (https://creativecommons.org/licenses/by/4.0/).

1. Introduction

Maturity-onset diabetes of the young (MODY) is a rare monogenic type of diabetes mellitus with autosomal dominant inheritance and includes 14 subtypes, which are classified by causative genes: *HNF4A*, *GCK*, *HNF1A*, *NEUROD1*, *PDX1*, *HNF1B*, *KLF11*, *CEL*, *PAX4*, *INS*, *BLK*, *KCNJ11*, *ABCC8*, or *APPL1* [1]. The complexity of diagnosing MODY is due to the similarity of its clinical signs with type 1 diabetes mellitus (T1DM) and type 2 diabetes mellitus (T2DM) [2]. Patients with monogenic types of diabetes mellitus require a personalized approach to the selection of a proper treatment [3]. Verification of these types of diabetes is possible only through molecular genetic testing. Without this analysis, up to 80% of cases of monogenic diabetes can be misdiagnosed or may go undiagnosed [4]. Most MODY cases (70%) are due to mutations in the *GCK* or *HNF1A* gene, whereas pathogenic variants in other genes are rarer [5]. The gene of adenosine triphosphate (ATP)-binding cassette subfamily C member 8 (*ABCC8*) is reported to be associated with the MODY12 subtype, permanent or transient neonatal diabetes mellitus, and an opposite phenotype: hyperinsulinemic hypoglycemia [6–8]. This gene is located on the short arm of chromosome 11, consists of 39 exons, and encodes a protein of 1581 amino acid residues. The product of

ABCC8 is a sulfonylurea receptor (SUR1), a regulatory subunit of the ATP-sensitive K$^+$ channel in membranes of pancreatic β-cells. This channel is composed of four inward-rectifier potassium ion pore-forming subunits (Kir6.2) and four SUR1 subunits combined into a hetero-octameric complex [9]. One of the main functions of this channel is the regulation of insulin secretion through changes in the membrane potential of the cell [10]. When the glucose level rises, the ATP/adenosine diphosphate (ADP) ratio increases in β-cells, thus leading to the closure of the K$^+$ channel with the subsequent opening of a voltage-gated calcium channel. Insulin secretion goes up as a consequence [10]. An increase in ADP concentration influences SUR1 by forcing the channel to open and preventing an insulin release [11]. SUR1 is known to be a multidomain protein that includes transmembrane-domain 0 (TMD0, exons 1–4), loop 0 (L0, exons 5 and 6), transmembrane domain 1 (TMD1, exons 6–12), a part of nucleotide-binding domain 1 (NBD1, exons 13–15), and a sulfonylurea receptor motif (exons 2, 3, 5, and 7). Exons 17 to 39 code for P-loop-containing nucleoside triphosphate hydrolase, transmembrane domain 2 (TMD2), and nucleotide-binding domain 2 (NBD2) [12]. More than 400 mutations in the *ABCC8* gene have been described, most of which are located in coding parts of the gene (www.hgmd.org, accessed on 2 November 2022). Hyperinsulinism of various severity levels is usually induced by inactivating mutations in *ABCC8* [13]. Activating mutations in the *ABCC8* gene reduces the sensitivity of the channel to the inhibitory effect of ATP and enhances its sensitivity to ADP, thereby leading to the channel opening regardless of glucose levels. Such mutations can cause permanent or transient neonatal diabetes, MODY, or T2DM [14–16]. Most patients with *ABCC8* mutations have diabetes only; however, a greater decrease in the channel's sensitivity to ATP gives rise to a more severe clinical phenotype, which may include neurological features, such as a developmental delay, seizures, epilepsy, mild dystonia, tonic posture, and muscle weakness [14,15].

The *ABCC8*-associated phenotype may depend on the type of mutation: variants activating the channel cause diabetes mellitus, whereas inactivating ones usually induce hyperinsulinism [13,14]. Few cases are described where the carriage of the same substitution in the same residue causes hyperglycemia or congenital hyperinsulinism in different patients [17,18]. There are also cases when congenital hyperinsulinism transforms into diabetes mellitus later in life [19–21]. An association of common variant rs757110 G of the *ABCC8* gene with the risk of T2DM has also been shown in the global population [22]. Clinical variability of symptoms and genetic heterogeneity of patients carrying mutations in the *ABCC8* gene complicates MODY12 diagnosis. Most cases of *ABCC8*-dependent diabetes are misdiagnosed as other types of diabetes mellitus, and insulin is mistakenly prescribed, which can result in poor control of carbohydrate metabolism [23]. Therefore, genetic testing is required for the identification of a causative gene in patients with a family history of diabetes.

In this study, the screening of rare genetic variants in *ABCC8* was performed using next-generation sequencing (NGS) technology in patients with hyperglycemia accompanied by the absence of antibodies against pancreas islet cells and glutamic acid decarboxylase and without ketoacidosis. The pathogenicity of the genetic variants was evaluated according to the standards of the American College of Medical Genetics (ACMG) and Genomics and the Association for Molecular Pathology [24], available databases, and literature data.

2. Materials and Methods

2.1. Study Subjects

The study protocol was approved by the local Ethics Committee of the Institute of Internal and Preventive Medicine (a branch of the Institute of Cytology and Genetics, the Siberian Branch of the Russian Academy of Sciences, Novosibirsk, Russia), protocol number 7 of 22 June 2008.

The total group of unrelated patients consisted of 285 persons (23.1 ± 11.7 years old [mean ± SD]; 37.9% males) examined at the Clinical Department of the Institute of Internal and Preventive Medicine from the year 2014 to 2022. Diabetes mellitus was diagnosed according to the criteria of the American Diabetes Association (Arlington County, VI, USA): HbA1C ≥ 6.5%, or fasting plasma glucose ≥ 126 mg/dL (7.0 mmol/L), or 2-h plasma glucose ≥ 200 mg/dL (11.1 mmol/L) during an oral glucose tolerance test (in the absence of unequivocal hyperglycemia; the result had to be confirmed by repeat testing), or a patient with classic symptoms of hyperglycemia or a hyperglycemic crisis with a random plasma glucose level ≥ 200 mg/dL (11.1 mmol/L) [25]; a debut of the disease in probands at the age of 35 years or earlier; a family history of diabetes mellitus; the absence of obesity; the absence of antibodies against pancreas islet cells and glutamic acid decarboxylase; intact secretory function of β-cells; normal or mildly reduced C-peptide levels; no need of insulin therapy; and the absence of ketoacidosis at the onset of the disease. The study population could include patients with MODY as well as T1DM patients with a negative antibody test result and an early onset of T2DM. Patients with clinical features of atypical diabetes mellitus (differing from those of T1DM and T2DM) and, in some cases, lacking a family history were included in this study [26]. Patients with tuberculosis or human immunodeficiency virus infection, as well as those who underwent antiviral therapy for hepatitis B or C, who abused psychoactive substances or alcohol within 2 years prior to the study, were excluded.

2.2. Sequencing of MODY-Associated Genes and Bioinformatic Analysis

After informed consent was obtained, venous blood (5 mL) was collected from all the studied patients. DNA was extracted from the venous blood using phenol–chloroform extraction [27]. The quantity and quality of the DNA were assessed on an Epoch microplate spectrophotometer (BioTek, Winooski, VT, USA). The first step of the preparation of a DNA library included DNA fragmentation using the KAPA HyperPlus Kit (Roche, Switzerland). SeqCap EZ Prime Choice Probes (Roche, Basel, Switzerland) were employed for NGS target enrichment. Targeted regions included coding regions and adjacent splicing sites of the following MODY-associated genes: *HNF4A, GCK, HNF1A, PDX1, HNF1B, NEUROD1, KLF11, CEL, PAX4, INS, BLK, KCNJ11, ABCC8*, and *APPL1*. The HyperCap Target Enrichment Kit (Roche, Switzerland) was used for the recovery of captured DNA regions. The quality of the analyzed DNA and of the prepared libraries was evaluated by means of a capillary electrophoresis system, Agilent 2100 Bioanalyzer (Agilent Technologies Inc., Santa Clara, CA, USA). The prepared DNA samples were sequenced on the Illumina MiSeq platform (Illumina, San Diego, CA, USA) at the multi-access center Proteome Analysis (Federal Research Center of Fundamental and Translational Medicine, Novosibirsk, Russia). Automated processing and annotation of the obtained NGS data were carried out on the NGS Wizard platform (genomenal.com, accessed on 19 May 2021).

Data on the clinical significance and pathogenicity prediction of the annotated single-nucleotide variants (SNVs), ClinVar and VarSome, and literature data were employed for the analysis. Allele frequencies were annotated using databases GnomAD v3.1.2 [28] and RUSeq, 2 November 2022 (http://ruseq.ru/). Variants described in ClinVar or VarSome or predicted in silico to be benign/likely benign, as well as variants with minor allele frequency higher than 0.01% according to gnomAD and RUSeq, were excluded from the analysis. The pathogenicity of new variants was assessed in accordance with the recommendations of the ACMG and Genomics and the Association for Molecular Pathology [24].

The present study is focused on the spectrum of rare variants in the *ABCC8* gene.

2.3. ABCC8 Confirmation Analysis

The detected substitutions c.970G>A (p.Val324Met), c.1562G>A (p.Arg521Gln), and c.4609_4610insC (p.His1537Profs*22) in the *ABCC8* gene (NM_000352.6) were verified by Sanger sequencing of the corresponding DNA fragments of the *ABCC8* gene in probands and their relatives available for the analysis. The oligonucleotide primers used are shown in Table 1. The design of the oligonucleotides was performed in the Primer-Blast software 19 May 2021 (https://www.ncbi.nlm.nih.gov/tools/primer-blast/). The sequencing reaction was performed on an ABI 3500 instrument (Thermo Fisher Scientific, Waltham, MA, USA) using the BigDye Terminator v3.1 Cycle Sequencing Kit (Thermo Fisher Scientific, USA) in accordance with the manufacturer's protocol. The sequences were analyzed in Chromas, 2 June 2021 (http://technelysium.com.au/wp/) and Vector NTI® Advance 11 (Thermo Fisher Scientific, USA) software; a fragment of the *ABCC8* gene (NG_008867.1) served as a reference sequence for alignment.

Table 1. Sequencing primers used with the identified variants.

SNV	Forward Primer 5′-3′	Revers Primer 5′-3′	Product Length
c.970G>A (p.Val324Met)	GCCCAGCCGTGAATTAGCC	CCTCTGGCATTTCTGTTGACCA	429
c.1562G>A (p.Arg521Gln)	CTTTGAGTAGGCCACTTCACCT	CAGAGCCAGTTTGAGGCTCC	501
c.4609_4610insC (p.His1537Profs*22)	CCTGTCCCAAGGCCTTATATGT	GTATGGGCAGGGTCCGAATG	502

3. Results

The search for pathogenic variants was carried out in 14 MODY-associated genes. No such variants were identified in *PDX1, NEUROD1, KLF11, CEL, PAX4, INS, BLK, KCNJ11,* and *APPL1*. In total, 55 out of the 285 probands proved to be carriers of pathogenic or probably pathogenic (previously described in ref. [29,30] or new) variants in *GCK, HNF1A, HNF4A, HNF1B,* and *ABCC8* (Supplementary Materials; Table S1.). Among these 55, only 3 probands are carriers of rare variants in the *ABCC8* gene.

3.1. Variants in Genes GCK, HNF1A, HNF4A, and HNF1B

A total of 36 probands out of the 55 were found to be carriers of pathogenic and probably pathogenic variants (nonsense mutations, small deletions, missense mutations, or splice site mutations) in the *GCK* gene, and 13 probands are carriers of variants in the *HNF1A* gene.

Among the additionally examined patients, previously described *GCK* variants were identified: two patients (P398 and P412) turned out to be carriers of c.238G>A (p.Gly80Ser) in exon 2; c.556C>T (p.Arg186*) and c.562G>A (p.Ala188Thr) in exon 5 were found in probands P186 and P188, respectively; c.659G>A (p.Cys220Tyr) in exon 6 and c.683C>T (p.Thr228Met) in exon 7 was detected in probands P384 and P433, respectively (Supplementary Materials; Table S1). Novel dinucleotide deletion AC c.11_12del (p.Asp4Glufs*47) was revealed in one proband (P437) in exon 1 of the *GCK* gene (Supplementary Materials; Table S1).

In the *HNF1A* gene, novel variant c.335delA (p.Pro112Argfs*43) and previously described c.872dupC (p.Gly292Argfs*25) and c.872delC (p.Pro291Glnfs*51) were identified (Supplementary Materials; Table S1). Proband P73 is a carrier of the c.160C>T (p.Arg54*) variant in the *HNF1A* gene and c.1562G>A (p.Arg521Gln) in the *ABCC8* gene (Supplementary Materials; Table S1). Novel single-nucleotide deletion c.85delC (p.Asn30Thrfs*74) in the *HNF4A* gene was detected in a heterozygous state in one proband: P381. We described the patient's medical history and clinical features in ref. [31].

Two unrelated participants with diabetes and negative for autoimmunity (P27 and P400) carry previously described variant c.1006C>A (p.His336Asp) in the *HNF1B* gene. Some variants of this gene are associated with the MODY5 subtype and congenital anomalies of the kidneys and urinary tract and, less often, of the pancreas or genitalia [32]. In P27's family, variant p.His336Asp did not cosegregate with a pathological phenotype. Family members of P400, other than the healthy mother, were not available for genetic analysis, and we had no information about any kidney or other anomalies among them. There are no published data with clear evidence of p.His336Asp pathogenicity [33,34], and it has been classified as a variant of uncertain significance in the LOVD database or a variant with conflicting interpretations of pathogenicity in ClinVar.

3.2. Variants in ABCC8

Because the MODY12 subtype is extremely rare in most populations [35], it is of interest to analyze variants in the *ABCC8* gene in patients with diabetes mellitus.

Earlier, we published a detailed clinical case of proband P12 [36].

The *ABCC8* gene variants identified in this study in the 285 probands (including three rare variants detected in this study) are presented in Table 2. Some common variants of this gene are reported in the literature to be associated with T2DM, but these results are ethnospecific [37]. No potentially pathogenic variants were identified here in adjacent regions of splice sites of this gene. Variants c.354C>T (p.Val118=), c.1678G>A (p.Val560Met), and c.2274G>A (p.Ala758=) were not included in the analysis because they were identified as benign in ClinVar (Variation ID: 255930, 188919, and 1097104, respectively) and in VarSome. Three heterozygous variants c.970G>A (p.Val324Met), c.1562G>A (p.Arg521Gln), and c.4609_4610insC (p.His1537ProfsTer22) were selected for further analysis.

Table 2. The genetic variants in *ABCC8* exons identified in our patients, their minor allele frequencies in our group of patients and according to the gnomAD and RUSeq databases, and associated phenotypes according to the literature data.

dbSNP ID	Substitution (NM_000352.6)	Nucleotide Changes (NM_000352.6)	Minor Allele Frequency (Our Study)	Minor Allele Frequency (gnomADv3.1.2)	Minor Allele Frequency (RUSeq)	Associated Phenotype [Reference *]
rs1048099	p.Pro69=	c.207T > C	0.468	0.459	0.478	-
rs8192695	p.Ala110=	c.330C>T	0.046	0.065	0.043	-
rs137873871	p.Val118=	c.354C>T	0.008	0.004	0.009	-
rs2301703	-	c.579 + 14C>T	0.390	0.470	0.384	-
rs1328072266	p. Val324Met	c.970G>A	0.002	-	-	ND/TND [38–40]
rs368114790	p.Arg521Gln	c.1562G>A	0.002	0.000	0.000	DM [41,42]
rs2074308	-	c.1672-74G>A	0.159	0.121	0.153	T2DM [43]
rs4148619	p.Val560Met	c.1678G>A	0.002	0.000	0.000	-
rs1799857	p.His562=	c.1686C>T	0.390	0.441	0.408	-
rs1799858	p.Lys649=	c.1947G>A	0.131	0.166	0.142	T2DM [43]
rs1799854	-	c.2117-3C>T	0.523	0.372	0.480	T2DM [44]
rs761258571	p.Ala758=	c.2274G>A	0.002	0.000	-	-
rs1801261	p.Thr759=	c.2277C>T	0.002	0.028	-	T2DM [45]
rs1805036	p.Leu829=	c.2485C>T	0.079	0.140	0.099	-
rs1799859	p.Arg1273=	c.3819G>A	0.295	0.387	0.273	T2DM [46]
rs757110	p.Ala1369Ser	c.4105G>T	0.605	0.712	0.622	T2DM [22]
rs72559717	p.Ala1457Thr	c.4369G>A	0.002	0.000	-	MODY [36]
New	p.His1537Profs*22	c.4609_4610insC	0.002	-	-	-
rs8192690	p.Val1572Ile	c.4714G>A	0.055	0.051	0.069	-

DM: diabetes mellitus, ND: neonatal diabetes, T2DM: type 2 diabetes mellitus, TND: transient neonatal diabetes mellitus; * an association is reported in the literature.

3.3. The Phenotype of Patients with MODY12

Diabetes mellitus was diagnosed at ages of up to 27 in probands and up to 50 among their family members. At the onset of the disease, fasting hyperglycemia was determined during a routine examination or during pregnancy. There were no islet cell cytoplasmic antibodies (ICA), insulin antibodies (IAA), antibodies to glutamate decarboxylase (GAD), tyrosine phosphatase (IA2), antibodies to the zinc transporter (ZnT8A), and there were no symptoms of ketoacidosis at the onset of the disease. The weight of all patients was within the age norm (body–mass index (BMI): 18.2–22.6). In all the families examined, there was a family history of pathology of carbohydrate metabolism.

When observed for 3 years (2019–2022), hyperglycemia ranged from asymptomatic to significant decompensation of carbohydrate metabolism in the probands. Macro- and microvascular complications were not detectable at the time of examination and observation. All three probands (P293, P73, and P330) were on insulin therapy. Available family members of the three probands were examined for the presence of corresponding variants in the *ABCC8* gene (Figure 1).

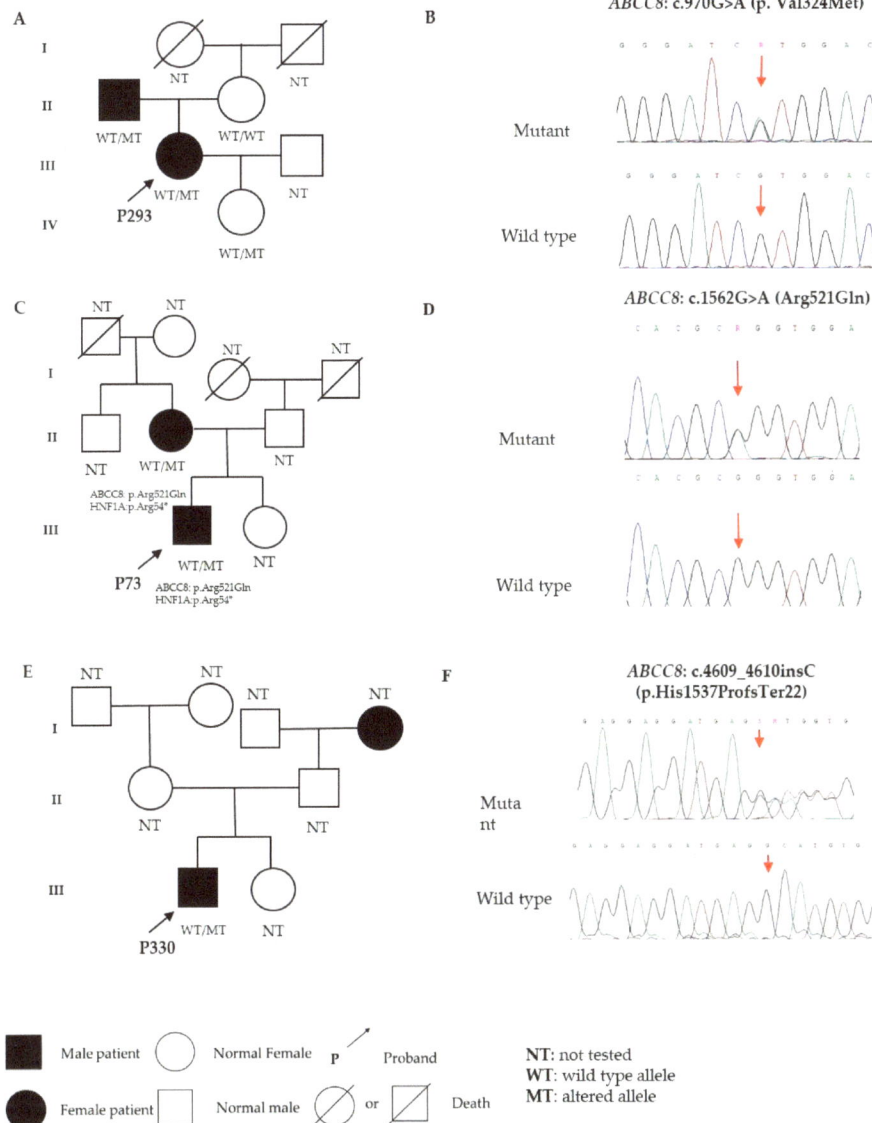

Figure 1. The screened families with identified variants. (**A,B**) c.970G>A (p.Val324Met), (**C,D**) c.1562G>A (p.Arg521Gln), and (**E,F**) c.4609_4610insC (p.His1537Profs*22) in the *ABCC8* gene.

Heterozygous missense mutation c.970G>A (p.Val324Met) in *ABCC8* was identified in proband P293, her affected father, and little daughter (Figure 1A,B) and was absent in the proband's healthy mother. Close monitoring of carbohydrate metabolism parameters in proband P293's daughter was recommended because of the high risk of diabetes mellitus. We did not find other pathogenic variants in other MODY-associated genes in the proband. This variant is classified as pathogenic in ClinVar (Variation ID: 1338342) and VarSome (ACMG: PS3, PP3, PP5, PM1, and PM2). The variant was absent in databases gnomAD and RUSeq (Table 2).

Heterozygous missense mutation c.1562G>A (p.Arg521Gln) in the *ABCC8* gene was identified in proband P73 and his affected mother (Figure 1C,D). Other family members were unavailable for the examination. The proband and his mother also proved to be carriers of pathogenic variant c.160C>T (p.Arg54*) in the *HNF1A* gene [29]. Arg521Gln in the *ABCC8* gene is classified as "conflicting interpretations of pathogenicity" in ClinVar (Variation ID: 157683) and as "Uncertain Significance" in VarSome (ACMG: PM1, PM2, PP5, and BP4). This variant is described in gnomAD v3.1.2 with minor allele frequency (MAF) = 0.0001117 and RUSeq (MAF) = 0.0004160, eastern Russia) (Table 2). In both databases, this variant is described only in a heterozygous state. In the proband and his mother, the variant cosegregated with the disease (criterion PP1).

In proband P330, the c.4609_4610insC (p.His1537Profs*22) variant of the *ABCC8* gene was identified (Figure 1E,F). It is not described in databases gnomAD v3.1.2 and RUSeq (criterion PM2) or in the literature. The patient's relatives were not available for the analysis. The c.4609_4610insC variant (p.His1537Profs*22) is a single-nucleotide deletion of cytosine that results in a frameshift and probably a premature stop codon. Loss-of-function mutations in the *ABCC8* gene have been repeatedly described and are pathologically significant (criterion PVS1). In silico analysis showed that the variant is damaging (criterion PP3). Thus, according to the set of criteria (PVS1, PM2, and PP3), p.His1537Profs*22 was assumed to be pathogenic.

4. Discussion

MODY was suspected in the probands owing to the age of onset of diabetes mellitus before 45 years, the presence of relevant family history, the absence of ketoacidosis at the onset of the disease, the absence of relevant antibodies, and the absence of symptoms of insulin resistance. We did not find any MODY12-specific symptoms common among the three probands and their relatives other than the usual clinical signs of MODY.

The c.970G>A (p.Val324Met) substitution is located in the transmembrane domain TMD1 of SUR1. There is a report of heterozygous carriage of this mutation in a female patient (age at diagnosis: 2 days) with transient neonatal diabetes mellitus without relapse at the time of examination (22 weeks) [47]. The substitution was inherited on the maternal side, but the proband's mother had no signs of diabetes. A male patient with neonatal diabetes and a severe developmental delay at 74 days of life has been described who carries substitutions c.970G>A (p.Val324Met) and Arg1394Leu in the *ABCC8* gene; at the age of 6, he still had diabetes (C-peptide level 0.07, HbA1c 61 mmol/mol, and the absence of relevant antibodies), and his treatment was changed to sulfonylureas [38]. Carriage of a c.970G>A (p.Val324Met) and the Trp688Arg compound heterozygous variant in the *ABCC8* gene was associated with permanent neonatal diabetes mellitus in a 17-year-old Italian female (age of manifestation: 15 days) [39]. A successful treatment change from insulin to sulfonylureas was reported. It is likely that the patient's deceased mother was a carrier of the c.970G>A (p.Val324Met) variant because the 74-year-old grandfather of the proband is a carrier of this variant and has diabetes mellitus (2 h plasma glucose: 14 mmol/L). The paternal grandmother of the proband is a carrier of the Trp688Arg variant and features impaired glucose tolerance (2 h plasma glucose: 8.4 mmol/L) [39]. A heterozygous male carrier of c.970G>A (p.Val324Met) with transient neonatal diabetes mellitus (absence of relevant antibodies, glucose at 24 mmol/L, and presence of ketoacidosis) and a developmental speech delay has been described [40]. The diabetes relapsed at age 9, and treatment with insulin was prescribed. After identification of the mutation, the treatment was switched successfully to glibenclamide [40]. Functional studies on a cell line have shown that the c.970G>A (p.Val324Met) variant causes a severe activating gating defect and reduces SUR1 expression on the cell surface, followed by attenuation of its functional effect on β-cells [48].

Variants responsible for the development of late-onset autosomal dominant diabetes in genes of ATP-sensitive K$^+$ channels have rarely been described [42]. Heterozygous variant c.1562G>A (p.Arg521Gln) in the *ABCC8* gene has been found in a man with nonimmune diabetes mellitus and a family history of diabetes; the age of manifestation is 34 [41]. The same variant has been identified by laboratory tests in another person with diabetes mellitus [42]. The same as p.Val324Met, p.Arg521Gln is located in transmembrane domain 1 of the SUR1 protein; this domain is involved in ATP binding. In proband P73 and his mother (Figure 1C), this variant was found to be combined with a substitution in the *HNF1A* gene. In terms of the clinical phenotype, carriers of pathogenic *ABCC8* gene variants are similar to patients with *HNF1A* and *HNF4A* MODY [7]; therefore, it was not possible to identify a contribution of a specific mutation to the clinical signs.

Heterozygous variant c.4609_4610insC (p.His1537Profs*22) was found in proband P330. During the survey, a family history of disorders of carbohydrate metabolism was revealed (Figure 1E), but his relatives were not available for the analysis. The detected variant is located in NBD2, which is responsible for the binding of Mg-nucleotides and, as a result, channel opening and membrane hyperpolarization, which leads to the prevention of insulin secretion. Known mutations in *ABCC8* that cause diabetes mellitus either increase the activation of the Mg-nucleotide-mediated channel or alter the intrinsic gating [49]. Functional studies on this variant have not yet been conducted, and there are no data on this variant in the literature and databases.

Thus, in patients with a MODY phenotype in the Russian population, 18 previously described and one novel [c.4609_4610insC (p.His1537ProfsTer22)] variant as revealed in the *ABCC8* gene. Among them, we identified four potentially causative variants [c.970G>A (p.Val324Met), c.1562G>A (p.Arg521Gln), c.4369G>C (p.Ala1457Thr), and c.4609_4610insC (p.His1537Profs*r22)], which cosegregated with diabetes mellitus in the available family members of the patients.

Limitations

This study has some limitations due to the unavailability of information about some family members.

5. Conclusions

Our results suggest that variants c.970G>A (p.Val324Met), c.1562G>A (p.Arg521Gln), and c.4609_4610insC (p.His1537ProfsTer22) in *ABCC8* could be the cause of MODY-*ABCC8* in the Russian population. We did not detect any specific clinical features of MODY among patients carrying pathogenic variants of *ABCC8*, thereby confirming the need for genetic testing of patients with a MODY phenotype using NGS for correct diagnosis and treatment as well as for counseling the patients' relatives.

Supplementary Materials: The following supporting information can be downloaded at: https://www.mdpi.com/article/10.3390/jpm13020172/s1, Table S1: The genetic variants identified in Western Siberian patients with a phenotype of maturity-onset diabetes of the young (MODY) and new genetic variants.

Author Contributions: Conceptualization, M.V.; data curation, E.S., O.R. and A.O.; investigation, D.I.; methodology, D.I. and E.V.; project administration, M.V.; validation, S.M. and P.O.; writing—original draft, D.I. and A.O.; writing—review and editing, D.I., S.M. and E.S. All authors have read and agreed to the published version of the manuscript.

Funding: The molecular genetic study was conducted within the framework of the main topic in state assignment No. FWNR-2022-0003.

Institutional Review Board Statement: The study was conducted in accordance with the Declaration of Helsinki, and approved by the local Ethics Committee of the Institute of Internal and Preventive Medicine (a branch of the Institute of Cytology and Genetics, the Siberian Branch of the Russian Academy of Sciences, Novosibirsk, Russia), protocol number 7 of 22 June 2008.

Informed Consent Statement: Written informed consent to be examined and to participate in the study was obtained from each patient or his/her parent or legal guardian.

Data Availability Statement: The data presented in this study are available on request from the corresponding author.

Acknowledgments: The authors thank the patients for the participation in this study.

Conflicts of Interest: The authors declare no conflict of interest.

References

1. Firdous, P.; Nissar, K.; Ali, S.; Ganai, B.A.; Shabir, U.; Hassan, T.; Masoodi, S.R. Genetic Testing of Maturity-Onset Diabetes of the Young Current Status and Future Perspectives. *Front. Endocrinol.* **2018**, *9*, 253. [CrossRef] [PubMed]
2. Lachance, C.H. Practical Aspects of Monogenic Diabetes: A Clinical Point of View. *Can. J. Diabetes* **2016**, *40*, 368–375. [CrossRef] [PubMed]
3. Mohan, V.; Radha, V. Precision Diabetes Is Slowly Becoming a Reality. *Med. Princ. Pract.* **2019**, *28*, 1–9. [CrossRef] [PubMed]
4. Shields, B.M.; Hicks, S.; Shepherd, M.H.; Colclough, K.; Hattersley, A.T.; Ellard, S. Maturity-onset diabetes of the young (MODY): How many cases are we missing? *Diabetologia* **2010**, *53*, 2504–2508. [CrossRef] [PubMed]
5. Ellard, S.; Bellanné-Chantelot, C.; Hattersley, A.T. European Molecular Genetics Quality Network (EMQN) MODY group. Best practice guidelines for the molecular genetic diagnosis of maturity-onset diabetes of the young. *Diabetologia* **2008**, *51*, 546–553. [CrossRef]
6. Ellard, S.; Flanagan, S.E.; Girard, C.A.; Patch, A.M.; Harries, L.W.; Parrish, A.; Edghill, E.L.; Mackay, D.J.; Proks, P.; Shimomura, K.; et al. Permanent neonatal diabetes caused by dominant, recessive, or compound heterozygous SUR1 mutations with opposite functional effects. *Am. J. Hum. Genet.* **2007**, *81*, 375–382. [CrossRef]
7. Bowman, P.; Flanagan, S.E.; Edghill, E.L.; Damhuis, A.; Shepherd, M.H.; Paisey, R.; Hattersley, A.T.; Ellard, S. Heterozygous ABCC8 mutations are a cause of MODY. *Diabetologia* **2012**, *55*, 123–127. [CrossRef]
8. Nessa, A.; Rahman, S.A.; Hussain, K. Hyperinsulinemic Hypoglycemia—The Molecular Mechanisms. *Front. Endocrinol.* **2016**, *7*, 29. [CrossRef]
9. Shyng, S.; Nichols, C.G. Octameric stoichiometry of the KATP channel complex. *J. Gen. Physiol.* **1997**, *110*, 655–664. [CrossRef]
10. Ashcroft, F.M.; Rorsman, P. Electrophysiology of the pancreatic beta-cell. *Prog. Biophys. Mol. Biol.* **1989**, *54*, 87–143. [CrossRef] [PubMed]
11. Tucker, S.J.; Gribble, F.M.; Zhao, C.; Trapp, S.; Ashcroft, F.M. Truncation of Kir6.2 produces ATP-sensitive K+ channels in the absence of the sulphonylurea receptor. *Nature* **1997**, *387*, 179–183. [CrossRef] [PubMed]
12. Jha, R.M.; Koleck, T.A.; Puccio, A.M.; Okonkwo, D.O.; Park, S.Y.; Zusman, B.E.; Clark, R.S.B.; Shutter, L.A.; Wallisch, J.S.; Empey, P.E.; et al. Regionally clustered ABCC8 polymorphisms in a prospective cohort predict cerebral oedema and outcome in severe traumatic brain injury. *J. Neurol. Neurosurg. Psychiatry* **2018**, *89*, 1152–1162. [CrossRef] [PubMed]
13. Galcheva, S.; Demirbilek, H.; Al-Khawaga, S.; Hussain, K. The Genetic and Molecular Mechanisms of Congenital Hyperinsulinism. *Front. Endocrinol.* **2019**, *10*, 111. [CrossRef] [PubMed]
14. Ashcroft, F.M.; Puljung, M.C.; Vedovato, N. Neonatal Diabetes and the KATP Channel: From Mutation to Therapy. *Trends Endocrinol. Metab.* **2017**, *28*, 377–387. [CrossRef] [PubMed]
15. Patch, A.M.; Flanagan, S.E.; Boustred, C.; Hattersley, A.T.; Ellard, S. Mutations in the ABCC8 gene encoding the SUR1 subunit of the KATP channel cause transient neonatal diabetes, permanent neonatal diabetes or permanent diabetes diagnosed outside the neonatal period. *Diabetes Obes. Metab.* **2007**, *9*, 28–39. [CrossRef]
16. Bonnefond, A.; Boissel, M.; Bolze, A.; Durand, E.; Toussaint, B.; Vaillant, E.; Gaget, S.; Graeve, F.; Dechaume, A.; Allegaert, F.; et al. Pathogenic variants in actionable MODY genes are associated with type 2 diabetes. *Nat. Metab.* **2020**, *2*, 1126–1134. [CrossRef]
17. Koufakis, T.; Sertedaki, A.; Tatsi, E.-B.; Trakatelli, C.-M.; Karras, S.N.; Manthou, E.; Kanaka-Gantenbein, C.; Kotsa, K. First Report of Diabetes Phenotype due to a Loss-of-Function ABCC8 Mutation Previously Known to Cause Congenital Hyperinsulinism. *Case Rep. Genet.* **2019**, *2019*, 3654618. [CrossRef]
18. Männikkö, R.; Flanagan, S.E.; Sim, X.; Segal, D.; Hussain, K.; Ellard, S.; Hattersley, A.T.; Ashcroft, F.M. Mutations of the same conserved glutamate residue in NBD2 of the sulfonylurea receptor 1 subunit of the KATP channel can result in either hyperinsulinism or neonatal diabetes. *Diabetes* **2011**, *60*, 1813–1822. [CrossRef]
19. Işık, E.; Demirbilek, H.; Houghton, J.A.; Ellard, S.; Flanagan, S.E.; Hussain, K. Congenital Hyperinsulinism and Evolution to Sulfonylurearesponsive Diabetes Later in Life due to a Novel Homozygous p.L171F ABCC8 Mutation. *J. Clin. Res. Pediatr. Endocrinol.* **2019**, *11*, 82–87. [CrossRef]

20. Abdulhadi-Atwan, M.; Bushman, J.; Tornovsky-Babaey, S.; Perry, A.; Abu-Libdeh, A.; Glaser, B.; Shyng, S.L.; Zangen, D.H. Novel de novo mutation in sulfonylurea receptor 1 presenting as hyperinsulinism in infancy followed by overt diabetes in early adolescence. *Diabetes* **2008**, *57*, 1935–4190. [CrossRef]
21. Kapoor, R.R.; Flanagan, S.E.; James, C.T.; McKiernan, J.; Thomas, A.M.; Harmer, S.C.; Shield, J.P.; Tinker, A.; Ellard, S.; Hussain, K. Hyperinsulinaemic hypoglycaemia and diabetes mellitus due to dominant ABCC8/KCNJ11 mutations. *Diabetologia* **2011**, *10*, 2575–2583. [CrossRef]
22. Qin, L.J.; Lv, Y.; Huang, Q.Y. Meta-analysis of association of common variants in the KCNJ11-ABCC8 region with type 2 diabetes. *Genet. Mol. Res.* **2013**, *12*, 2990–3002. [CrossRef] [PubMed]
23. Delvecchio, M.; Pastore, C.; Giordano, P. Treatment Options for MODY Patients: A Systematic Review of Literature. *Diabetes Ther.* **2020**, *11*, 1667–1685. [CrossRef]
24. Richards, S.; Aziz, N.; Bale, S.; Bick, D.; Das, S.; Gastier-Foster, J.; Grody, W.W.; Hegde, M.; Lyon, E.; Spector, E.; et al. Standards and guidelines for the interpretation of sequence variants: A joint consensus recommendation of the American College of Medical Genetics and Genomics and the Association for Molecular Pathology. *Genet. Med.* **2015**, *17*, 405–423. [CrossRef]
25. American Diabetes Association. Diagnosis and classification of diabetes mellitus. *Diabetes Care* **2005**, *28*, 37–42. [CrossRef] [PubMed]
26. Stanik, J.; Dusatkova, P.; Cinek, O.; Valentinova, L.; Huckova, M.; Skopkova, M.; Dusatkova, L.; Stanikova, D.; Pura, M.; Klimes, I.; et al. De novo mutations of GCK, HNF1A and HNF4A may be more frequent in MODY than previously assumed. *Diabetologia* **2014**, *57*, 480–484. [CrossRef]
27. Sambrook, J.; Russell, D.W. Purification of nucleic acids by extraction with phenol: Chloroform. *Cold Spring Harb. Protoc.* **2006**, *2006*, 4455. [CrossRef] [PubMed]
28. Karczewski, K.J.; Francioli, L.C.; Tiao, G.; Cummings, B.B.; Alföldi, J.; Wang, Q.; Collins, R.L.; Laricchia, K.M.; Ganna, A.; Birnbaum, D.P.; et al. The mutational constraint spectrum quantified from variation in 141,456 humans. *Nature* **2020**, *581*, 434–443. [CrossRef]
29. Ivanoshchuk, D.E.; Shakhtshneider, E.V.; Rymar, O.D.; Ovsyannikova, A.K.; Mikhailova, S.V.; Fishman, V.S.; Valeev, E.S.; Orlov, P.S.; Voevoda, M.I. The Mutation Spectrum of Maturity Onset Diabetes of the Young (MODY)-Associated Genes among Western Siberia Patients. *J. Pers. Med.* **2021**, *11*, 57. [CrossRef]
30. In Supplimentary Wang, Z.; Diao, C.; Liu, Y.; Li, M.; Zheng, J.; Zhang, Q.; Yu, M.; Zhang, H.; Ping, F.; Li, M.; et al. Identification and functional analysis of GCK gene mutations in 12 Chinese families with hyperglycemia. *J. Diabetes Investig.* **2019**, *10*, 963–971. [CrossRef] [PubMed]
31. Ivanoshchuk, D.E.; Ovsyannikova, A.K.; Mikhailova, S.V.; Shakhtshneider, E.V.; Valeev, E.S.; Rymar, O.D.; Orlov, P.S.; Voevoda, M.I. Variants of the HNF4A and HNF1A genes in patients with impaired glucose metabolism and dyslipidemia. *Aterscleroz* **2022**, *17*, 11–19. [CrossRef]
32. Madariaga, L.; García-Castaño, A.; Ariceta, G.; Martínez-Salazar, R.; Aguayo, A.; Castaño, L.; Spanish Group for the Study of HNF1B Mutations. Variable phenotype in HNF1B mutations: Extrarenal manifestations distinguish affected individuals from the population with congenital anomalies of the kidney and urinary tract. *Clin. Kidney J.* **2018**, *12*, 373–379. [CrossRef] [PubMed]
33. Urrutia, I.; Martínez, R.; Rica, I.; Martínez de LaPiscina, I.; García-Castaño, A.; Aguayo, A.; Calvo, B.; Castaño, L. Spanish Pediatric Diabetes Collaborative Group. Negative autoimmunity in a Spanish pediatric cohort suspected of type 1 diabetes, could it be monogenic diabetes? *PLoS ONE* **2019**, *14*, e02206342019. [CrossRef]
34. Hohendorff, J.; Kwiatkowska, M.; Pisarczyk-Wiza, D.; Ludwig-Słomczyńska, A.; Milcarek, M.; Kapusta, P.; Zapała, B.; Kieć-Wilk, B.; Trznadel-Morawska, I.; Szopa, M.; et al. Mutation search within monogenic diabetes genes in Polish patients with long-term type 1 diabetes and preserved kidney function. *Pol. Arch. Intern. Med.* **2022**, *132*, 16143. [CrossRef]
35. Reilly, F.; Sanchez-Lechuga, B.; Clinton, S.; Crowe, G.; Burke, M.; Ng, N.; Colclough, K.; Byrne, M.M. Phenotype, genotype and glycaemic variability in people with activating mutations in the ABCC8 gene: Response to appropriate therapy. *Diabet. Med.* **2020**, *37*, 876–884. [CrossRef] [PubMed]
36. Ovsyannikova, A.K.; Rymar, O.D.; Shakhtshneider, E.V.; Klimontov, V.V.; Koroleva, E.A.; Myakina, N.E.; Voevoda, M.I. ABCC8-Related Maturity-Onset Diabetes of the Young (MODY12): Clinical Features and Treatment Perspective. *Diabetes Ther.* **2016**, *7*, 591–600. [CrossRef] [PubMed]
37. Liu, C.; Lai, Y.; Guan, T.; Zhan, J.; Pei, J.; Wu, D.; Ying, S.; Shen, Y. Associations of ATP-Sensitive Potassium Channel's Gene Polymorphisms With Type 2 Diabetes and Related Cardiovascular Phenotypes. *Front. Cardiovasc. Med.* **2022**, *23*, 816847. [CrossRef]
38. Globa, E.; Zelinska, N.; Mackay, D.J.; Temple, K.I.; Houghton, J.A.; Hattersley, A.T.; Flanagan, S.E.; Ellard, S. Neonatal diabetes in Ukraine: Incidence, genetics, clinical phenotype and treatment. *J. Pediatr. Endocrinol. Metab.* **2015**, *28*, 1279–1286. [CrossRef]
39. Russo, L.; Iafusco, D.; Brescianini, S.; Nocerino, V.; Bizzarri, C.; Toni, S.; Cerutti, F.; Monciotti, C.; Pesavento, R.; Iughetti, L.; et al. Permanent diabetes during the first year of life: Multiple gene screening in 54 patients. *Diabetologia* **2011**, *54*, 1693–1701. [CrossRef]
40. Vaxillaire, M.; Dechaume, A.; Busiah, K.; Cavé, H.; Pereira, S.; Scharfmann, R.; de Nanclares, G.P.; Castano, L.; Froguel, P.; Polak, M.; et al. New ABCC8 mutations in relapsing neonatal diabetes and clinical features. *Diabetes* **2007**, *56*, 1737–1741. [CrossRef]

41. Rego, S.; Dagan-Rosenfeld, O.; Zhou, W.; Sailani, M.R.; Limcaoco, P.; Colbert, E.; Avina, M.; Wheeler, J.; Craig, C.; Salins, D.; et al. High-frequency actionable pathogenic exome variants in an average-risk cohort. *Cold Spring Harb. Mol. Case Stud.* **2018**, *4*, a003178. [CrossRef] [PubMed]
42. De Franco, E.; Saint-Martin, C.; Brusgaard, K.; Knight Johnson, A.E.; Aguilar-Bryan, L.; Bowman, P.; Arnoux, J.B.; Larsen, A.R.; Sanyoura, M.; Greeley, S.A.W.; et al. Update of variants identified in the pancreatic β-cell KATP channel genes KCNJ11 and ABCC8 in individuals with congenital hyperinsulinism and diabetes. *Hum. Mutat.* **2020**, *41*, 884–905. [CrossRef] [PubMed]
43. Odgerel, Z.; Lee, H.S.; Erdenebileg, N.; Gandbold, S.; Luvsanjamba, M.; Sambuughin, N.; Sonomtseren, S.; Sharavdorj, P.; Jodov, E.; Altaisaikhan, K.; et al. Genetic variants in potassium channels are associated with type 2 diabetes in a Mongolian population. *J. Diabetes* **2012**, *4*, 238–242. [CrossRef] [PubMed]
44. Engwa, G.A.; Nwalo, F.N.; Chikezie, C.C.; Onyia, C.O.; Ojo, O.O.; Mbacham, W.F.; Ubi, B.E. Possible association between ABCC8 C49620T polymorphism and type 2 diabetes in a Nigerian population. *BMC Med. Genet.* **2018**, *19*, 78. [CrossRef]
45. Matharoo, K.; Arora, P.; Bhanwer, A.J. Association of adiponectin (AdipoQ) and sulphonylurea receptor (ABCC8) gene polymorphisms with Type 2 Diabetes in North Indian population of Punjab. *Gene* **2013**, *527*, 228–234. [CrossRef]
46. Reis, A.F.; Ye, W.Z.; Dubois-Laforgue, D.; Bellanné-Chantelot, C.; Timsit, J.; Velho, G. Association of a variant in exon 31 of the sulfonylurea receptor 1 (SUR1) gene with type 2 diabetes mellitus in French Caucasians. *Hum. Genet.* **2000**, *107*, 138–144. [CrossRef]
47. Flanagan, S.E.; Patch, A.M.; Mackay, D.; Edghill, E.L.; Gloyn, A.L.; Robinson, D.; Shield, J.P.; Temple, K.; Ellard, S.; Hattersley, A.T. Mutations in ATP-sensitive K+ channel genes cause transient neonatal diabetes and permanent diabetes in childhood or adulthood. *Diabetes* **2007**, *56*, 1930–1937. [CrossRef]
48. Zhou, Q.; Garin, I.; Castaño, L.; Argente, J.; Muñoz-Calvo, M.; Perez de Nanclares, G.; Shyng, S.L. Neonatal diabetes caused by mutations in sulfonylurea receptor 1: Interplay between expression and Mg-nucleotide gating defects of ATP-sensitive potassium channels. *J. Clin. Endocrinol. Metab.* **2010**, *95*, 473–478. [CrossRef]
49. Edghill, E.L.; Flanagan, S.E.; Ellard, S. Permanent neonatal diabetes due to activating mutations in ABCC8 and KCNJ11. *Rev. Endocr. Metab. Disord.* **2010**, *11*, 193–198. [CrossRef]

Disclaimer/Publisher's Note: The statements, opinions and data contained in all publications are solely those of the individual author(s) and contributor(s) and not of MDPI and/or the editor(s). MDPI and/or the editor(s) disclaim responsibility for any injury to people or property resulting from any ideas, methods, instructions or products referred to in the content.

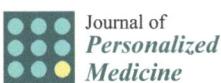

Brief Report

Diagnostic Accuracy of Methods for Detection of Antibodies against Type I Interferons in Patients with Endocrine Disorders

Nurana Nuralieva [1], Marina Yukina [1], Leila Sozaeva [1], Maxim Donnikov [2], Liudmila Kovalenko [2], Ekaterina Troshina [1], Elizaveta Orlova [1], Dmitry Gryadunov [3], Elena Savvateeva [3,*] and Ivan Dedov [1]

1. Endocrinology Research Centre, Ministry of Health of Russia, 117036 Moscow, Russia
2. Medical Institute, Surgut State University, 628416 Surgut, Russia
3. Center for Precision Genome Editing and Genetic Technologies for Biomedicine, Engelhardt Institute of Molecular Biology, Russian Academy of Sciences, 119991 Moscow, Russia
* Correspondence: len.savv@gmail.com

Abstract: Autoantibodies against type 1 interferons (IFN-I) are a highly specific marker for type 1 autoimmune polyglandular syndrome (APS-1). Moreover, determination of antibodies to omega-interferon (IFN-ω) and alpha2-interferon (IFN-α2) allows a short-term diagnosis in patients with isolated and atypical forms of APS-1. In this study, a comparison of three different methods, namely multiplex microarray-based, cell-based and enzyme-linked immunosorbent assays for detection of antibodies against omega-interferon and alpha2-interferon, was carried out. A total of 206 serum samples from adult patients with APS-1, APS-2, isolated autoimmune endocrine pathologies or non-autoimmune endocrine disorders, and healthy individuals were analyzed. In the APS-1 patient cohort ($n = 18$), there was good agreement between the results of anti-IFN-I antibody tests performed by three methods, with 100% specificity and sensitivity for microarray-based assay. Although only the cell-based assay can determine the neutralizing activity of autoantibodies, the microarray-based assay can serve as a highly specific and sensitive screening test to identify anti-IFN-I antibody positive patients.

Keywords: autoantibodies; type I interferon; interferon-ω; interferon-α2; multiplex assay; protein microarray; cell-based autoantibody assay; ELISA

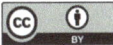

1. Introduction

Autoantibodies against type 1 interferons (IFN-I) are highly specific for type 1 autoimmune polyglandular syndrome (APS-1), a monogenic disease caused by a mutation in the *AIRE* gene [1]. The formation of these autoantibodies (auto-Abs) is presumably caused by a disorder in the negative selection for IFN-I-specific T-lymphocytes in the thymus [2]. For APS-1 patients, it has been shown that Abs against omega-interferon (IFN-ω) are 100% specific and antibodies against alpha2-interferon (IFN-α2) are 99.9% specific [3]. However, such auto-Abs are also typical for patients with myasthenia gravis and/or thymoma [4], and can be detected in patients with systemic lupus erythematosus, rheumatoid arthritis [5], Sjogren's syndrome [6], and incontinentia pigmenti [7].

Nevertheless, recent data indicate that anti-interferon auto-Abs are more common in the population than previously thought. Over the past two years, the role of auto-Abs against IFN-I in SARS-CoV-2 infection has been demonstrated [7]; moreover, they have been shown to underlie severe side effects after vaccination with a live attenuated yellow fever virus vaccine [8]. Multiple studies have shown that more than 10% of patients with neutralizing auto-Abs against IFN-I had life-threatening COVID-19 pneumonia [9–11]. The presence of auto-Abs against IFN-I appears to remain clinically asymptomatic in people prior to their infection with SARS-CoV-2. To date, a case of APS-1 was diagnosed in two brothers, 7-year-old and 13-year-old, with life-threatening pneumonia caused by COVID-19. Due to the severity of COVID-19 and their medical history, APS-1 was suspected and the patients underwent appropriate molecular testing. In addition to a mutation in the *AIRE* gene, the patients were found to carry auto-Abs against IFN-I [12]. Thus, the long-standing opinion that there is no increased susceptibility to viral infections in patients with APS-1, despite the presence of auto-Abs against IFN-I [13], is refuted. Currently, there are also suggestions about the possible role of autoantibodies against IFN-I in other severe viral and malignant diseases, especially in the elderly [14].

At the same time, the work on the development and implementation of screening tests for anti-cytokine antibodies, including antibodies against IFN-1 for patients with endocrine diseases, is in progress. For instance, recently, Sjøgren et al., using screening tests for auto-Abs against IFN-ω and interleukin-22 (IL-22) on a large cohort of patients with endocrine diseases, followed by subsequent genetic testing of positive samples, identified patients with undiagnosed APS-1 as well as several patients with previously unknown monogenic or oligogenic causes of organ-specific autoimmunity and immunodeficiency [15]. Identification of patients with endocrine autoimmune conditions is important to ensure targeted treatment and personalized follow-up aimed at preventing complications. Thus, the development of new effective methods for the detection of auto-Abs against IFN-I is extremely important. The simplicity of the assay and its availability is a priority for conducting exploratory research and screening tests.

There are various methods for detecting auto-Abs against IFN-I, for example, antiviral interferon neutralizing assay [1], time-resolved immunofluorometric assay [2], radioimmunoassay [16], magnetic-beads-based assay [17] and microarray-based assay [18], as well as some commercially available enzyme-linked immunosorbent assays (ELISA). Until now, in Russia, the study of auto-Abs against IFN-I was carried out for the purpose of APS-1 diagnostics using a cell-based autoantibody assay (CBAA) [19]. Orlova et al., who introduced the method for the qualitative determination of auto-Abs against IFN-ω and IFN-α using the human embryonic kidney (HEK)-blue cell culture in Russia, confirmed its high sensitivity and specificity for APS-1 [20,21]. However, due to the need for cell cultivation, this method is rather laborious.

Earlier, our research group developed and tested a microarray to detect auto-Abs associated with endocrine autoimmune diseases, both organ-specific (auto-Abs against thyroperoxidase (TPO), thyroglobulin (Tg), glutamic acid decarboxylase (GAD-65), islet cell cytoplasmic antigen (ICA), tyrosine phosphatase-like protein (IA2) and steroid 21-hydroxylase (21-OH)) and anti-cytokine autoantibodies (anti-IFN-ω, anti-IFN-α-2a and anti-interleukin 22(IL-22)-auto-Abs) [22]. Using this microarray, we detected a characteristic triplet of anti-cytokine auto-Abs in 89% of patients with APS-1 in the studied cohort; 100% of them were found to carry auto-Abs against IFN-I. However, a method to compare auto-Abs against IFN-I was not available in this study. The aim of this work was to compare the specificity and sensitivity of anti-IFN-I auto-Abs detection using various methods: multiplex microarray analysis, CBAA and a commercially available ELISA.

2. Materials and Methods

2.1. Patients, Healthy Donors and Serum Samples

The study included 206 participants: the main group—18 patients with APS-1 (group 1), and three control groups—89 patients with autoimmune endocrine pathology (group 2), 71 patients with non-autoimmune endocrine pathology (group 3) and 28 healthy individuals (group 4).

Group 2 included patients with the following pathologies:
- Autoimmune polyendocrine syndrome type 2, $n = 38$;
- Autoimmune thyropathies (autoimmune thyroiditis (AIT) and Graves' disease), $n = 23$;
- Type 1 diabetes mellitus (T1D)/latent autoimmune diabetes in adults (LADA), $n = 21$;
- Hypergonadotropic hypogonadism (HH) of autoimmune origin, $n = 4$;
- Autoimmune adrenal insufficiency (AAI), $n = 3$.

Group 3 included patients with the following pathologies:
- Non-autoimmune thyroid diseases, $n = 5$;

- Non-autoimmune diabetes, n = 5;
- Non-autoimmune HH, n = 6;
- Non-autoimmune adrenal insufficiency (AI), n = 17;
- Non-autoimmune pathology of the parathyroid glands, n = 6;
- Multiple endocrine pathology of non-autoimmune origin, n = 32.

Group 4 included healthy individuals, in particular, carriers of antibodies that are markers of autoimmune damage of the pancreatic islet apparatus without carbohydrate metabolism disorders. In addition, group 4 included the parents of a patient with APS-1 (#194 in Table S1) who were heterozygous carriers of a mutation in the *AIRE* gene without any diagnosed autoimmune diseases.

Criteria for inclusion and exclusion from this study are summarized in Table S2. The characteristics of the participants are provided in Tables S1 and S3. Before inclusion into the study, a comprehensive examination of all patients and healthy individuals was carried out. To clarify the genesis of the disease, all participants underwent an examination of the level of organ-specific autoantibodies using the following assays: ELISA (anti-21-OH (BioVendor, Czech Republic), anti-GAD (Euroimmun, Germany), anti-IA2 (Medipan Gmbh, Berlin, Germany), anti-ICA (Medipan Gmbh, Berlin, Germany)) and chemiluminescent cicroparticle immunoassay (CMIA) (anti-TPO (Abbott Laboratories, Chicago, IL, USA), anti-TG (Roche Diagnostics, Switzerland)) (Table S1).

Patient serum samples were frozen and stored at $-80\ °C$ until analysis.

2.2. Microarray-Based Assay

Hydrogel microarrays with immobilized antigens, including IFN-ω (Cat # 300-02J, Pepro-Tech, Cranbury, NJ, USA) and IFN-α-2a (Cat # 11100-1, PBL Assay Science, Piscataway, NJ, USA), were manufactured as described previously [22]. Each antigen was immobilized in 4 repetitions to increase the reproducibility of the assay results. Patient serum samples were diluted 1:100 (100 mM Tris-HCl buffer with 0.1% Triton X-100, Sigma-Aldrich, St. Louis, MO, USA) and applied to the microarray (100 µL). After overnight incubation at 37 °C, intermediate washing for 20 min (PBS with 0.1% Tween 20, Sigma-Aldrich, St. Louis, MO, USA), rinsing and drying, the microarrays were developed with fluorescently labeled anti-species antibodies. As detecting antibodies, we used F(ab')2-Goat anti-Human IgG Fc gamma Secondary Antibody (Cat # 31163, Invitrogen, Waltham, MA, USA) labeled with Cy5 cyanine dye. After incubation for 30 min at 37 °C, the microarrays were washed (PBS with 0.1% Tween 20, 30 min), rinsed and dried by centrifugation. Registration of fluorescent images of microarrays and calculation of fluorescent signals were performed using a microarray analyzer and software developed at the Engelhardt Institute of Molecular Biology, Moscow. Interpretation of the results of analysis on a microarray with the determination of the presence/absence of auto-Abs against IFN-ω and IFN-α-2a in blood serum were performed as described previously [22]. The determination of anti-IFN-ω and anti-IFN-α-2a by the microarray-based multiplex analysis was carried out in serum samples from all participants in the study (Table S1).

2.3. Anti-IFN-ω Cell-Based Autoantibody Assay

The study of auto-Abs against IFN-ω was carried out by the method of qualitative determination using the HEK-blue cell culture according to a previously developed method [19]. The method is based on the ability of cells to synthesize alkaline phosphatase in the presence of IFN. With a high titer of neutralizing IFN antibodies in the patient's serum, the ability of the cell to synthesize alkaline phosphatase is suppressed, which in turn is registered by measuring the optical density. The presence of secreted alkaline phosphatase is determined using a spectrometer with the determination of the optical density of the test liquid at a wavelength of 650 nm (Abs650). IFN inhibition is given as a percentage of neutralization (Abs index) and is calculated by the formula:

$$\text{Abs index} = \frac{\text{Abs650 negative control} - \text{Abs650 sample}}{\text{Abs650 negative control} - \text{Abs650 positive control}}$$

Determination of auto-Abs against IFN-ω using the HEK-blue cell culture was carried out in 200 study participants: group 1—17 patients with APS-1, and control groups (groups 2–4)—87 patients with autoimmune endocrine pathology, 68 patients with non-autoimmune endocrine pathology and 28 healthy individuals, respectively (Table S1).

2.4. Anti-IFN-α Autoantibodies ELISA

To detect autoantibodies against IFN alpha, serum samples were tested by ELISA according to the manufacturer's instructions (Cat # BMS217, Invitrogen, Waltham, MA, USA). The determination of auto-Abs against IFN-α by ELISA was carried out for positive samples identified using a microarray-based assay, and selectively for 10 negative samples. In total, the determination of auto-Abs against IFN-α by ELISA was carried out for 29 study participants: 17 patients with APS-1 (group 1), 2 patients with non-autoimmune endocrine pathology (group 3) and 10 healthy individuals (group 4) (Table S1).

3. Results and Discussion

3.1. Autoantibodies against IFN-I among APS-1 Patients

In this work, a comparison of three different methods, namely multiplex microarray-based, cell-based and enzyme-linked immunosorbent assays for anti-IFN-I antibody detection, was carried out on a sample of APS-1 patients, patients with autoimmune endocrine pathologies and non-autoimmune endocrine pathologies, and healthy individuals. The results of detection of autoantibodies against IFN-I using microarray-based assay, CBBA and ELISA for APS-1 patients are summarized in Table 1.

Table 1. Characteristics of the type I autoimmune polyglandular syndrome (APS-1) patients and results of testing serum samples for the presence of anti-omega-interferon (IFN-ω) and anti-alpha-interferon (IFN-α) autoantibodies using microarray-based, cell-based and enzyme-linked immunosorbent immunoassays.

| Sample # | Age | Gender | AIRE Mutations | APS-1 Components – Endocrine ||||||| APS-1 Components – Non-Endocrine | Anti-IFN-ω Auto-Abs || Anti-IFN-α Auto-Abs ||
				AAI *	Hypoparathyroidism	TDI/LADA	AIT	HH	CMC	Other pathology	Microarray	CBAA	Microarray	ELISA
3	49	m	R257X/R257X	+	+	−	−	−	+	−	+	+	+	n/a
49	20	f	R257X/R257X	+	+	−	+	+	+	Malabsorption syndrome, tooth enamel hypoplasia, total alopecia, vitiligo	+	+	+	+
51	18	f	R257X/−	+	+	−	−	+	+	−	+	+	+	+
64	29	f	p.R257*/p.W78R	+	+	−	−	+	+	Atrophic gastritis, cataract	+	+	+	+
103	18	f	R257X/R257X	+	+	−	−	+	+	Atrophic gastritis, cataract	+	+	+	+
115	30	f	R257X/R257X	+	+	+	+	−	+	Total alopecia, atrophic gastritis	+	+	+	+

Table 1. Cont.

| Sample # | Age | Gender | AIRE Mutations | APS-1 Components ||||||| Anti-IFN-ω Auto-Abs || Anti-IFN-α Auto-Abs ||
| | | | | Endocrine ||||| Non-Endocrine || | | | |
				AAI*	Hypoparathyroidism	T1D/LADA	AIT	HH	CMC	Other pathology	Microarray	CBAA	Microarray	ELISA
124	18	m	R257X/A58V	+	−	−	−	−	+	B12 deficiency anemia, malabsorption syndrome, tooth enamel hypoplasia, spleen hypoplasia	+	+	+	+
125	45	f	not studied	+	+	−	+	−	+	Atrophic gastroduodenitis, vitiligo, cataract, corneal dystrophy	+	+	+	+
129	45	m	not studied	+	+	−	−	−	+	Alopecia areata	+	+	+	+
133	27	m	−	+	+	−	+	−	+	Autoimmune fibrosing alveolitis, total alopecia	+	n/a	+	+
135	30	f	R257X/R257X	+	+	−	−	+	+	Vitiligo, malabsorption syndrome, corneal dystrophy, partial eyelid ptosis, asplenia, atrophic gastroduodenitis, autoimmune hepatitis	+	−	+	+
136	28	f	R257X/c.931delT	+	+	−	−	+	+	Corneal dystrophy, atrophic gastritis	+	+	+	+
152	27	f	R257X/-	+	+	−	−	+	+	Subtotal alopecia, tooth enamel dysplasia, chronic tubulointerstitial nephritis	+	+	+	+
156	36	m	not studied	+	+	−	−	−	+	−	+	+	+	+
168	32	f	R257X/R257X	+	+	−	−	+	+	Diffuse alopecia, vitiligo	+	+	+	+
189	31	f	R257X/R257X	+	+	−	−	+	+	Atrophic gastroduodenitis, malabsorption syndrome, tooth enamel hypoplasia, retinitis pigmentosa, cataract, strabismus	+	+	+	+
191	44	f	R257X/R257X	+	+	−	−	+	+	Cataract	+	+	+	+
194	25	f	R257X/c.821delG	+	+	−	+	+	+	Atrophic gastritis	+	+	+	+

* Abbreviations: m—male; f—female; AAI—autoimmune adrenal insufficiency; T1D/LADA—type 1 diabetes mellitus/latent autoimmune diabetes in adults; AIT—autoimmune thyroiditis; HH—hypergonadotropic hypogonadism; CMC—chronic mucocutaneous candidiasis; CBAA—cell-based autoantibody assay; ELISA—enzyme-linked immunosorbent assay.

Samples from 206 patients were analyzed using a previously developed microarray for multiplex detection of auto-Abs [22]. All APS-1 patients (n = 18) were positive for auto-Abs against IFN-ω and IFN-α-2a. As an example, Figure 1a shows a fluorescent image of a microarray after assay with an APS-1 patient sample. According to the previously described algorithm for interpreting the results [22], positive signals indicating the presence of auto-Abs in blood serum were detected for groups of elements containing IFN-ω and IFN-α-2a, as well as for groups of elements containing IL-22, 21-OH, GAD-65, TG and TPO (not considered in this work). Figure 1b shows the results of microarray-based assay with serum from a patient with multiple endocrine neoplasia type 1. Positive signals indicating the presence of autoantibodies in serum were detected only for a group of elements containing IFN-α-2a.

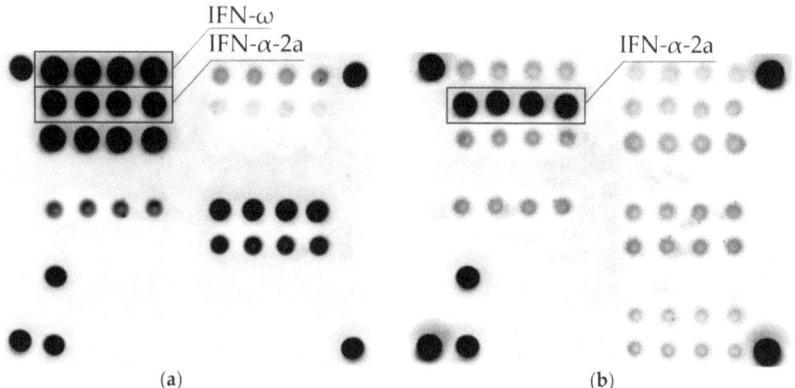

Figure 1. Fluorescence images of microarrays after assay with serum samples from: an APS-1 patient (**a**), a patient with multiple endocrine neoplasia type 1 (**b**). Groups of elements with immobilized omega-interferon (IFN-ω) and alpha2a-interferon (IFN-α-2a) are indicated by solid lines.

Using the CBAA method [19], samples from 200 patients were analyzed for auto-Abs against IFN-ω. All analyzed APS-1 samples (n = 17), except for one, were anti–IFN–ω auto-Abs positive. A negative anti-IFN-ω auto-Abs result was detected using CBAA in APS-1 patient #135 with a common *AIRE* mutation and the classic triad (Table 1). For technical reasons, it was not possible to re-examine this sample by CBAA. On the one hand, the results are consistent with data of other researchers: for example, the absence of auto-Abs against IFN-ω in patients with mutations in *AIRE* and only one component of APS-1 (hypoparathyroidism) was observed in the work of Cervato et al. [23]. On the other hand, patient #135 was shown by microarray-based multiplex assay to carry both auto-Abs against IFN-ω and auto-Abs against IFN-α; the presence of the latter was also confirmed by ELISA.

Using a commercially available ELISA, samples from 29 patients (among them, 17 APS-1 patients) were analyzed for auto-Abs against IFN-α. For anti-IFN-α auto-Abs, an agreement between the results of the two methods (microarray-based assay and ELISA) was observed; all analyzed APS-1 patient samples were anti-IFN-α auto-Abs positive for both methods (Table 1). Since the ELISA kit was quantitative, it is worth noting that all positive samples were oversaturated (>1 µg/mL) on initial analysis. For individual samples, the concentration was estimated at a 5000-fold dilution or more, resulting in a concentration of anti-IFN-α antibodies in the samples, on average, of about 1 mg/mL, taking into account the dilution.

3.2. Anti-IFN-I Autoantibodies among Control Groups

The microarray-based assay identified two patients who were anti-IFN-ω and/or anti-IFN-α-2a auto-Abs positive among patients from groups without diagnosed APS-1. Sample #56 (male, 70 years old) was positive for both anti-IFN-ω and anti-IFN-α-2a auto-Abs, and sample #147 (female, 45 years old) was positive for auto-Abs against IFN-α-2a. These two serum samples were also shown to be anti-IFN-α auto-Abs positive by ELISA. However, serum sample #56 was found to be anti-IFN-ω auto-Abs negative using CBAA. The frequency of detection of anti-IFN-I auto-Abs in the groups by different methods is summarized in Table 2.

Table 2. Anti-IFN-I positive patients by group (n/n total), sensitivity and specificity of assays.

Group	Anti-IFN-ω Auto-Abs Microarray	Anti-IFN-ω Auto-Abs CBAA	Anti-IFN-α Auto-Abs Microarray	Anti-IFN-α Auto-Abs ELISA
1	18/18	16/17	18/18	17/17
2	0/89	0/87	0/89	n/a
3	1/71	0/68	2/71	2/2
4	0/28	0/28	0/28	0/10
Total number of samples tested	206	200	206	29
Sensitivity, 95% CI	100.0% [78.9%; 100.0%]	94.1% [70.7%; 100.0%]	100.0% [78.9%; 100.0%]	Not determined. The assay was used as a comparative test
Specificity, 95% CI	99.5% [96.7%; 100.0%]	100.0% [97.5%; 100.0%]	98.9% [95.9%; 99.9%]	Not determined. The assay was used as a comparative test

Anti-IFN-I auto-Abs positive patients from control group 3 had severe and complex medical conditions. For instance, patient #56, who was tested positive for anti-IFN-ω auto-Abs using the microarray-based assay, was diagnosed with adrenal insufficiency of non-autoimmune origin as a result of adrenal metastasis (presumably, the primary tumor was lymphoma). Using multiplex analysis, auto-Abs against IFN-α2 were also detected in the patient, later confirmed by ELISA. The patient denied that he underwent therapy with IFN drugs, as well as the presence of a thymoma in anamnesis, which may be the cause of the formation of anti-IFN-I auto-Abs [4,24]. During an ophthalmological examination, the presence of myasthenia gravis was not detected.

Anti-IFN-α auto-Abs positive patient #147 (by microarray-based assay and by ELISA) had a genetically proven syndrome of multiple endocrine neoplasia type 1 (multiple insulinomas, non-functioning tumors of the pancreas, duodenal gastrinomas, primary hyperparathyroidism, lung carcinoids, multifocal hormonally inactive formations in both adrenal glands, hyperprolactinemia). The formation of anti-IFN-α auto-Abs in this patient can also be related to antiviral therapy for hepatitis C 17 years prior to participation in this study; similar cases have been described previously [25]. In light of an emerging assumption about a possible role for anti-IFN-I auto-Abs in severe viral or malignant diseases [14], these anti-IFN-I auto-Abs positive patients identified by microarray-based assay are of great interest.

APS-1 is an orphan disease. The prevalence of APS-1 in different European countries averages from 1:90,000 to 1:200,000 [26]. Unfortunately, there are currently no data on the frequency of occurrence of APS-1 in the population in Russia. The largest Russian APS-1 cohort described to date included 112 patients [27]. Since the symptoms may debut at intervals of several years and non-specific clinical manifestations can occur, diagnosis is often delayed. Autoantibodies against IFN-ω and IFN-α2 are specific and sensitive markers of APS-1, which makes it possible to use them for screening diagnostics of patients with autoimmune diseases to exclude atypical forms of the disease. Although there are a number of research tests for the detection of antibodies against IFN-I, including those that allow the determination of the neutralizing activity of autoantibodies, studies aimed at comparing the specificity and sensitivity of these methods in the diagnostics of APS-1 are extremely limited. The main problem of such studies is the small sample of APS-1 patients, which makes it difficult to validate the results. In the present study on a small cohort of APS-1 patients, there was a good agreement between results of the tests for anti-IFN-1 antibodies performed by microarray-based assay and previously validated cell-based autoantibody and enzyme-linked immunosorbent assays. The results indicated that microarray-based assay can serve as a highly specific and sensitive screening test to identify anti-IFN-1 antibody positive patients. The introduction of such tests into clinical practice would make it possible to increase the availability of testing for antibodies against IFN-I in diagnostically difficult cases, as well as to study larger cohorts of patients with various severe viral and malignant diseases.

4. Conclusions

Microarray-based assay showed almost 100% sensitivity and specificity in detection of anti-IFN-I antibodies in patients with endocrine disorders. Determination of antibodies to IFN-ω and IFN-α2 can be used as an inexpensive and rapid way to diagnose APS-1. Thanks to these antibodies, the number of people who need to undergo genetic analysis can be reduced, i.e., in patients who do not have antibodies to IFN-ω and IFN-α2, the diagnosis of APS-1 can be ruled out without testing for the *AIRE* gene. In addition, this analysis may be recommended for individuals who do not fully meet the diagnostic criteria: patients who failed to detect a second mutation in the *AIRE* gene, or patients with dominant-negative mutations.

Supplementary Materials: The following supporting information can be downloaded at: https://www.mdpi.com/article/10.3390/jpm12121948/s1, Table S1: Patient characteristics and results of testing serum samples for the presence of autoantibodies using microarray-based assay, CBAA, ELISA and CMIA. Table S2: Criteria for inclusion and exclusion from this study; Table S3: Age and gender in groups of participants.

Author Contributions: N.N., M.Y. and L.S. conducted the patient interviews and sample collection, and contributed to the design and implementation of the research; L.S. and E.O. obtained CBAA data; M.D. and L.K. provided resources for ELISA data; E.T. and E.O. designed and directed the project; D.G. and E.S. realized microarray manufacturing, obtained microarray-based data, wrote the manuscript in consultation with N.N. and M.Y.; I.D. supervised the project. All authors have read and agreed to the published version of the manuscript.

Funding: This study was supported by the Foundation for Scientific and Technological Development of Yugra, agreement No 2022-05-01/2022 (development of microarray-based assay) and by the Ministry of Science and Higher Education of the Russian Federation to the EIMB Center for Precision Genome Editing and Genetic Technologies for Biomedicine, agreement number 075-15-2019-1660 (determination of auto-Abs against IFN-α by ELISA).

Institutional Review Board Statement: This study was conducted according to the guidelines of the Declaration of Helsinki and approved by the local ethics committee of the Endocrinology Research Centre, Ministry of Health of Russia, Moscow, Russia (protocol No 17 and date of approval 27 September 2017).

Informed Consent Statement: Informed consent was obtained from all subjects involved in the study. Written informed consent was obtained from the patients for the publication of this article.

Data Availability Statement: The authors confirm that the data supporting the findings of this study are available within the article and/or its Supplementary Materials.

Conflicts of Interest: The authors declare no conflict of interest.

References

1. Meager, A.; Visvalingam, K.; Peterson, P.; Möll, K.; Murumägi, A.; Krohn, K.; Eskelin, P.; Perheentupa, J.; Husebye, E.; Kadota, Y.; et al. Anti-interferon autoantibodies in autoimmune polyendocrinopathy syndrome type 1. *PLoS Med.* **2006**, *3*, 1152–1164. [CrossRef]
2. Zhang, L.; Barker, J.M.; Babu, S.; Su, M.; Stenerson, M.; Cheng, M.; Shum, A.; Zamir, E.; Badolato, R.; Law, A.; et al. A robust immunoassay for anti-interferon autoantibodies that is highly specific for patients with autoimmune polyglandular syndrome type 1. *Clin. Immunol.* **2007**, *125*, 131–137. [CrossRef] [PubMed]
3. Meloni, A.; Furcas, M.; Cetani, F.; Marcocci, C.; Falorni, A.; Perniola, R.; Pura, M.; Bøe Wolff, A.S.; Husebye, E.S.; Lilic, D.; et al. Autoantibodies against type I interferons as an additional diagnostic criterion for autoimmune polyendocrine syndrome type I. *J. Clin. Endocrinol. Metab.* **2008**, *93*, 4389–4397. [CrossRef] [PubMed]

4. Meager, A.; Wadhwa, M.; Dilger, P.; Bird, C.; Thorpe, R.; Newsom-Davis, J.; Willcox, N. Anti-cytokine autoantibodies in autoimmunity: Preponderance of neutralizing autoantibodies against interferon-alpha, interferon-omega and interleukin-12 in patients with thymoma and/or myasthenia gravis. *Clin. Exp. Immunol.* **2003**, *132*, 128–136. [CrossRef]
5. Gupta, S.; Tatouli, I.P.; Rosen, L.B.; Hasni, S.; Alevizos, I.; Manna, Z.G.; Rivera, J.; Jiang, C.; Siegel, R.M.; Holland, S.M.; et al. Distinct functions of autoantibodies against interferon in systemic lupus erythematosus: A comprehensive analysis of anticytokine autoantibodies in common rheumatic diseases. *Arthritis Rheumatol.* **2016**, *68*, 1677–1687. [CrossRef]
6. Burbelo, P.D.; Browne, S.; Holland, S.M.; Iadarola, M.J.; Alevizos, I. Clinical features of Sjögren's syndrome patients with autoantibodies against interferons. *Clin. Transl. Med.* **2019**, *8*, e1. [CrossRef]
7. Bastard, P.; Rosen, L.B.; Zhang, Q.; Michailidis, E.; Hoffmann, H.H.; Zhang, Y.; Dorgham, K.; Philippot, Q.; Rosain, J.; Béziat, V.; et al. Autoantibodies against type I IFNs in patients with life-threatening COVID-19. *Science* **2020**, *370*. [CrossRef] [PubMed]
8. Bastard, P.; Michailidis, E.; Hoffmann, H.H.; Chbihi, M.; Le Voyer, T.; Rosain, J.; Philippot, Q.; Seeleuthner, Y.; Gervais, A.; Materna, M.; et al. Auto-antibodies to type I IFNs can underlie adverse reactions to yellow fever live attenuated vaccine. *J. Exp. Med.* **2021**, *218*, e20202486. [CrossRef]
9. Bastard, P.; Gervais, A.; Le Voyer, T.; Rosain, J.; Philippot, Q.; Manry, J.; Michailidis, E.; Hoffmann, H.-H.; Eto, S.; Garcia-Prat, M.; et al. Autoantibodies neutralizing type I IFNs are present in ~4% of uninfected individuals over 70 years old and account for ~20% of COVID-19 deaths. *Sci. Immunol.* **2021**, *6*, eabl4340. [CrossRef] [PubMed]
10. Troya, J.; Bastard, P.; Casanova, J.L.; Abel, L.; Pujol, A. Low lymphocytes and IFN-neutralizing autoantibodies as biomarkers of COVID-19 mortality. *J. Clin. Immunol.* **2022**, *42*, 738–741. [CrossRef] [PubMed]
11. Savvateeva, E.; Filippova, M.; Valuev-Elliston, V.; Nuralieva, N.; Yukina, M.; Troshina, E.; Baklaushev, V.; Ivanov, A.; Gryadunov, D. Microarray-based detection of antibodies against SARS-CoV-2 proteins, common respiratory viruses and type I interferons. *Viruses* **2021**, *13*, 2553. [CrossRef]
12. Schidlowski, L.; Iwamura, A.P.D.; Condino-Neto, A.; Prando, C. Diagnosis of APS-1 in two siblings following life-threatening COVID-19 pneumonia. *J. Clin. Immunol.* **2022**, *42*, 749–752. [CrossRef] [PubMed]
13. Kisand, K.; Link, M.; Wolff, A.S.B.; Meager, A.; Tserel, L.; Org, T.; Murumägi, A.; Uibo, R.; Willcox, N.; Podkrajšek, K.T.; et al. Interferon autoantibodies associated with *AIRE* deficiency decrease the expression of IFN-stimulated genes. *Blood* **2008**, *112*, 2657–2666. [CrossRef] [PubMed]
14. Puel, A.; Bastard, P.; Bustamante, J.; Casanova, J.L. Human autoantibodies underlying infectious diseases. *J. Exp. Med.* **2022**, *219*, e20211387. [CrossRef] [PubMed]
15. Sjøgren, T.; Bratland, E.; Røyrvik, E.C.; Grytaas, M.A.; Benneche, A.; Knappskog, P.M.; Kämpe, O.; Oftedal, B.E.; Husebye, E.S.; Wolff, A.S.B. Screening patients with autoimmune endocrine disorders for cytokine autoantibodies reveals monogenic immune deficiencies. *J. Autoimmun.* **2022**, *133*, 102917. [CrossRef]
16. Oftedal, B.E.; Bøe Wolff, A.S.; Bratland, E.; Kämpe, O.; Perheentupa, J.; Myhre, A.G.; Meager, A.; Purushothaman, R.; Ten, S.; Husebye, E.S. Radioimmunoassay for autoantibodies against interferon omega; its use in the diagnosis of autoimmune polyendocrine syndrome type I. *Clin. Immunol.* **2008**, *129*, 163–169. [CrossRef]
17. Ding, L.; Mo, A.; Jutivorakool, K.; Pancholi, M.; Holland, S.M.; Browne, S.K. Determination of human anticytokine autoantibody profiles using a particle-based approach. *J. Clin. Immunol.* **2012**, *32*, 238–245. [CrossRef]
18. Rosenberg, J.M.; Price, J.V.; Barcenas-Morales, G.; Ceron-Gutierrez, L.; Davies, S.; Kumararatne, D.S.; Döffinger, R.; Utz, P.J. Protein microarrays identify disease-specific anti-cytokine autoantibody profiles in the landscape of immunodeficiency. *J. Allergy Clin. Immunol.* **2016**, *137*, 204–213.e3. [CrossRef]
19. Breivik, L.; Oftedal, B.E.V.; Bøe Wolff, A.S.; Bratland, E.; Orlova, E.M.; Husebye, E.S. A novel cell-based assay for measuring neutralizing autoantibodies against type I interferons in patients with autoimmune polyendocrine syndrome type 1. *Clin. Immunol.* **2014**, *153*, 220–227. [CrossRef] [PubMed]
20. Orlova, E.M.; Sozaeva, L.S.; Karmanov, M.E.; Breivik, L.E.; Husebye, E.S.; Kareva, M.A. The new immunological methods for diagnostics of type 1 autoimmune polyendocrine syndrome (the first experience in Russia). *Probl. Endocrinol.* **2015**, *61*, 9–13. [CrossRef]
21. Sozaeva, L.S. The new immunological methods for diagnostics of type 1 autoimmune polyendocrine syndrome. *Probl. Endocrinol.* **2015**, *61*, 43–46. [CrossRef]
22. Savvateeva, E.N.; Yukina, M.Y.; Nuralieva, N.F.; Filippova, M.A.; Gryadunov, D.A.; Troshina, E.A. Multiplex autoantibody detection in patients with autoimmune polyglandular syndromes. *Int. J. Mol. Sci.* **2021**, *22*, 5502. [CrossRef]
23. Cervato, S.; Morlin, L.; Albergoni, M.P.; Masiero, S.; Greggio, N.; Meossi, C.; Chen, S.; Del Pilar Larosa, M.; Furmaniak, J.; Rees Smith, B.; et al. AIRE gene mutations and autoantibodies to interferon omega in patients with chronic hypoparathyroidism without APECED. *Clin. Endocrinol.* **2010**, *73*, 630–636. [CrossRef]
24. Antonelli, G.; Currenti, M.; Turriziani, O.; Dianzani, F. Neutralizing antibodies to interferon-α: Relative frequency in patients treated with different interferon preparations. *J. Infect. Dis.* **1991**, *163*, 882–885. [CrossRef]
25. Antonelli, G.; Simeoni, E.; Currenti, M.; De Pisa, F.; Colizzi, V.; Pistello, M.; Dianzani, F. Interferon antibodies in patients with infectious diseases. *Biotherapy* **1997**, *10*, 7–14. [CrossRef] [PubMed]

26. Guo, C.J.; Leung, P.S.C.; Zhang, W.; Ma, X.; Gershwin, M.E. The immunobiology and clinical features of type 1 autoimmune polyglandular syndrome (APS-1). *Autoimmun. Rev.* **2018**, *17*, 78–85. [CrossRef] [PubMed]
27. Orlova, E.M.; Sozaeva, L.S.; Kareva, M.A.; Oftedal, B.E.; Wolff, A.S.B.; Breivik, L.; Zakharova, E.Y.; Ivanova, O.N.; Kämpe, O.; Dedov, I.I.; et al. Expanding the phenotypic and genotypic landscape of autoimmune polyendocrine syndrome type 1. *J. Clin. Endocrinol. Metab.* **2017**, *102*, 3546–3556. [CrossRef] [PubMed]

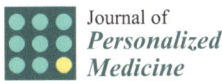

Article

Markers for the Prediction of Probably Sarcopenia in Middle-Aged Individuals

Yulia G. Samoilova [1], Mariia V. Matveeva [1,*], Ekaterina A. Khoroshunova [1], Dmitry A. Kudlay [2,3], Oxana A. Oleynik [1] and Liudmila V. Spirina [1]

1. Federal State Budgetary Educational Institution of Higher Education «Siberian State Medical University» of the Ministry of Health of Russia, Moskovsky Trakt 2, 634050 Tomsk, Russia
2. Federal State Autonomous Educational Institution of Higher Education "First Moscow State Medical University Named after I.I. THEM. Sechenov" of the Ministry of Health of Russia (Sechenov University), St. Trubetskaya 8, Building 2, 119048 Moscow, Russia
3. Federal State Budgetary Institution "State Research Center "Institute of Immunology"" FMBA of Russia, Kashirskoe sh., 24, 115478 Moscow, Russia
* Correspondence: matveeva.mariia@yandex.ru; Tel.: +7-913-815-2552

Citation: Samoilova, Y.G.; Matveeva, M.V.; Khoroshunova, E.A.; Kudlay, D.A.; Oleynik, O.A.; Spirina, L.V. Markers for the Prediction of Probably Sarcopenia in Middle-Aged Individuals. *J. Pers. Med.* 2022, *12*, 1830. https://doi.org/10.3390/jpm12111830

Academic Editors: Yuliya I. Ragino and Oksana D. Rymar

Received: 12 October 2022
Accepted: 31 October 2022
Published: 3 November 2022

Publisher's Note: MDPI stays neutral with regard to jurisdictional claims in published maps and institutional affiliations.

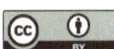

Copyright: © 2022 by the authors. Licensee MDPI, Basel, Switzerland. This article is an open access article distributed under the terms and conditions of the Creative Commons Attribution (CC BY) license (https://creativecommons.org/licenses/by/4.0/).

Abstract: Sarcopenia is a condition that is characterized by a progressive loss of muscle mass, strength, and function, resulting in reduced quality of life. The aim of the study was to analyze the significance of pro-inflammatory markers in the prognostic diagnosis of sarcopenia. The participants were divided into two groups: the main group of 146 people and the control—75 people. The complex of examinations included neuropsychological testing (Hospital Anxiety and Depression Scale (HADS), quality-of-life questionnaire for patients with sarcopenia (SarQoL), and short health assessment form (MOS SF-36)), a 6 m walking speed test, manual dynamometry, bioimpedancemetry, and metabolic markers (nitrates, fibroblast growth factor 21, and malondialdehyde). When analyzing metabolic markers in the main group, a twofold increase in nitrates in the main group was recorded in a subsequent analysis adjusted for multiple variables, there was a negative association between the nitrate levels for weak grip strength and appendicular muscle mass. An additional analysis revealed that the complaint of pain in the lower extremities was more frequent in patients of the main group, as well as constipation and the pathology of thyroid gland, and they were more frequently diagnosed with arterial hypertension. At the same time, patients from the main group more frequently took vitamin D. When conducting body composition, the main group recorded a higher weight visceral fat content, as well as a decrease in appendicular and skeletal muscle mass; these changes were accompanied by a decrease in protein and minerals. Among the markers that differed significantly were nitrates, and it was this that was associated with decreased muscle strength and appendicular mass, which may indicate both a possible mechanism and a possible predictive marker. The results of this study can be used to develop a screening method for diagnosing sarcopenia at the outpatient stage.

Keywords: pro-inflammatory markers; probably sarcopenia; middle-aged individuals

1. Introduction

Every year, the number of people in the world increases by 250 thousand people, mainly due to the elderly [1]. According to experts of the United Nations Organization, the number of the elderly will increase to 21% by 2050 and will amount to 2.1 billion people [2]. One condition that worsens prognosis and quality is sarcopenia. Sarcopenia is a progressive and generalized skeletal muscle disorder involving the accelerated loss of muscle mass and function that is associated with increased adverse outcomes, including falls, functional decline, frailty, and mortality. It occurs commonly as an age-related process in older people, influenced not only by contemporaneous risk factors, but also by genetic and lifestyle factors operating across the life course. It can also occur in mid-life in association with a range of conditions. The prevalence of sarcopenia in persons 60–70 years old is 5–13%, and in the group over 80 years old, it increases to 50% [3]. Currently, the number of patients with sarcopenia in the world is 50 million people, and this figure is predicted to quadruple in 40 years [4]. According to studies, presarcopenia is more susceptible to men over the age of 60 years and women over 80 years old [5]. The prevalence of sarcopenia is 10–15% lower than in Russia [6].

The pathogenesis of sarcopenia is quite complex; at present, many factors have been identified that affect the decrease in muscle mass, among which endocrine ones play a significant role. At the same time, the prognosis remains unfavorable since there are no registered pathogenetic drugs for the treatment of sarcopenia [7].

Severe sarcopenia is known to be associated with decreased quality of life and symptoms of depression, which requires mandatory diagnosis in the examination, but there is no information on such changes in probable sarcopenia, which is also interesting to study [8].

As one of the biomarkers, we consider fibroblast growth factor 21 (FGF21), which, in a healthy population, is responsible for many processes, including muscle function [9]. In one study, FGF21 was identified as another independent biomarker of successful aging, increased by a counterregulatory mechanism when compensating for metabolic stress, including in muscle tissue [10]. Circulating levels of FGF21 are elevated in patients with mitochondrial disorders affecting skeletal muscle [11]. Thus, FGF21 may be involved in the regulation of body muscle and in the modulation of metabolism, and thus be associated with presarcopenia.

Other promising metabolites are nitrates. In the human body, nitric oxide (NO) is one of the key endogenous regulators of the cardiovascular and other systems. The endothelium can be considered a giant endocrine organ in which the cells are not collected together, as in the endocrine glands, but dispersed, in the vessels. Its activation is mainly associated with hemodynamic changes occurring in the body [12]. Many articles have been published information about the effect of nitrates on the cardiovascular system. However, there are no large-scale studies in patients with sarcopenia. Nitric oxide synthase inhibitors (iNOS) have been studied as a therapeutic point [13]. This scientific work revealed a mutual correlation of high iNOS expression with activation of cytokine-induced storm. Inhibitors of iNOS activity had a positive effect on the prevention of muscle mass reduction [14]. The main consequence of the decrease in NO in the muscle is a decrease in the flow of vasodilation, which directly correlates with muscle strength and physical functioning, respectively, can influence the development of sarcopenia [15].

Malonic dialdehyde is a produced form of peroxidation of polyunsaturated fatty acids. This marker easily reacts with proteins, forming a wide range of intra- and intermolecular covalent adducts. These metabolic products gradually accumulate in the vascular system, leading to cellular dysfunction and tissue damage [16]. Loss of muscle mass in healthy older adults is associated with the development of lipid peroxidation, and taking antioxidants or exercising improves muscle-system parameters, indicating a possible evaluation of antioxidant system parameters in the preclinical stage of sarcopenia [17,18].

Currently, there is evidence that the loss of muscle mass occurs much earlier, starting as early as age 55 in men and 45 in women, respectively [19]. The diagnosis of sarcopenia rests on muscle-mass measurements and on functional tests that evaluate either muscle strength or physical performance (walking and balance). No specific biomarkers have been identified to date. The identification of a single metabolic marker or a panel of markers can verify a decrease in muscle mass in the preclinical stage, when preventive and rehabilitative measures are effective. The aim of the study was to analyze the significance of pro-inflammatory markers in the prognostic probably sarcopenia in middle-aged adults.

2. Materials and Methods

The study was performed in accordance with Good Clinical Practice and the principles of the Declaration of Helsinki. The study protocol was approved by the ethical committee of Siberian State Medical University No. 8888 dated 29 November 2021. Prior to inclusion in the study, written informed consent was obtained from all participants.

The study was conducted in the medical prevention office of the Center for Public Health and Medical Prevention for one-quarter of 2022. All patients who were 45–85 years old, who have signed informed consents, with no exclusion criteria were included in the study (Figure 1). Of the many criteria, those that could affect the results of the study have been chosen, meaning that it is they, not sarcopenia, that will determine the results obtained even as early as the first stage of randomization, which would violate the purity of the experiment. Vital functions, including blindness, can affect physical activity and muscle mass. In this regard, the status of these functions was necessarily taken into account during randomization. Exclusion criteria: pregnant women, alcohol abusers, patients with liver diseases, respiratory and cardiovascular systems, gastrointestinal tract in decompensation stage, musculoskeletal pathology, moderate-or-severe cognitive impairment, and immobilization in the last 6 months. A total of 460 patients were included in the study. Of all included patients, 158 were excluded due to musculoskeletal pathology, 56 had cognitive impairment of moderate severity or dementia, 15 had blindness, and 16 had stroke. A total of 221 people aged 45 to 85 years participated, including 145 women and 56 men (the predominance of women in the study is associated with more frequent use of medical care for disease prevention).

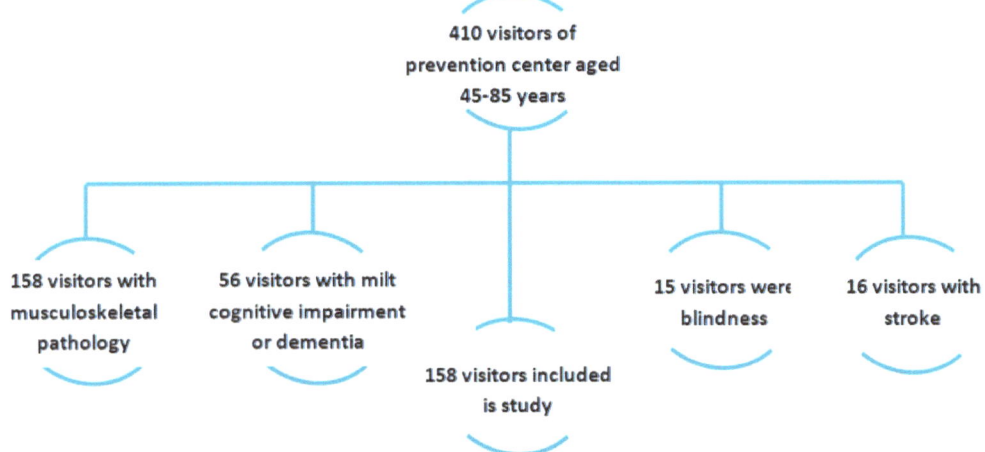

Figure 1. Recruitment protocol for the patients.

The patients were divided into 2 groups according AWGS 2019: the main group with reduced muscle mass of 146 people (118 women and 28 men) and the control group of 75 people (47 women and 28 men) based on testing [20]. A dynamometer and walking-speed test were used as primary testing to differentiate into groups. Patients were divided into groups according to the results of physical strength and function assessment, thus belonging to the group according to the classification features "probable sarcopenia". The protocol included measuring handgrip strength while taking maximum readings in two trials, using both arms in isometric contraction with maximum force; the standard was sitting position with 90° elbow extension for the dynamometer. The diagnostic criteria for low handgrip muscle strength was <28.0 kg for men and <18.0 kg for women [20]. To assess the functions, we measured the time taken to walk 6 m at a normal pace from the start without slowing down and took the average result of at least two trials, using a handheld stopwatch, as the recorded speed. A level ≤ 0.8 m/s to <1.0 m/s, independent of floor, was used for the criteria.

A screening test SarQol for probable sarcopenia was performed on everyone, but because the patients included in the pain study were younger than the generally accepted age for sarcopenia, it was not used as a cutoff point. To exclude the influence of neuropsychological parameters on the development of sarcopenia, all patients underwent an assessment. For this purpose, we used the hospital anxiety assessment scale (HADS), as well as the general quality of life questionnaire (SF36 SF36).

All participants underwent bioimpedance measurement with the help of an Inbody 770 device (Korea), with an evaluation of the following parameters: analysis of proteins, minerals, total body water, total weight, fat mass, skeletal muscle mass, muscle mass, analysis of extracellular and intracellular fluid, analysis of fat tissue by segments (right arm, left arm, trunk, right leg, and left leg), and appendicular skeletal mass index. The appendicular skeletal mass index (SMI) was calculated by the ratio of lean muscle mass of all to the height parameter in square meters. Measurements were taken according to the manufacturer's manual, in a vertical position, with the legs and arms in contact with the base electrodes and the capture electrodes, respectively. AWGS 2019 low muscle mass values of <7.0 kg/m^2 and <5.7 kg/m^2 for men and women, respectively, were used as cutoff points [19].

For the study of metabolic markers, blood was taken, with further laboratory analysis: fibroblast growth factor 21, nitrates, malondialdehyde (MDA), and lactate dehydrogenase by enzyme immunoassay.

A statistical analysis and data processing were performed by using SPSS Statistica software. For sample-size calculations, we took limb extremities' muscle mass as the outcome index and used the mean and standard deviation values in Shahar et al. with a fixed power of 80% and an α level of 5% for the main variable [21]. This gave a sample size of 70 subjects for each group. However, by taking into account the exclusion criteria and possible dropout from the study, the main and control groups were increased in size. The methods of descriptive statistics were quartiles—for non-normally distributed data. Testing of statistical hypotheses of normally distributed quantitative parameters was performed by using the following parametric criteria: Student's t-test for paired comparison. The correlation analysis was assessed by using Pearson's criterion. To assess reliability of differences in qualitative characteristics, we used conjugation tables with the calculation of χ^2 (chi-square). The null hypothesis was rejected at the level of statistical significance $p < 0.05$.

3. Results

This section presents the results of the examination of patients with probable sarcopenia, who were divided according to gender (because there are gender differences and norms) in the tables.

The characteristics of the patients are presented in Table 1.

Table 1. Characteristics of included patients stratified by gender.

Parameters	Women			Men		
	Main Group (n = 118)	Control Group (n = 28)	p	Main Group (n = 47)	Control Group (n = 28)	p
Age, years	54 [48–65]	55 [48–66]	0.453	53 [49–59]	52 [47–56.5]	0.534
Body mass index kg/m^2	28.5 [25.1–31.8]	28.5 [25.1–31.8]	0.285	28.5 [25.1–31.8]	28.5 [25.1–31.8]	0.285
Waist-to-hip ratio	0.97 [0.93–1.01]	0.96 [0.9–1.02]	0.435	0.94 [0.8–1.02]	0.95 [0.8–1.05]	0.435
Right hand, kg	24 [19–31]	40 [38–53]	0.001	17 [15–24]	35 [27–39]	0.001
Left hand, kg	23 [19–29]	38 [33–51]	0.001	15 [13–22]	33 [25–36]	0.001
Gait speed, m/s	0.95 [0.8–1.25]	1.15 [0.8–1.4]	<0.001	1.0 [0.9–1.3]	1.2 [0.9–1.5]	<0.001
Glycemia, mmol/L	4.9 [4.6–5.3]	4.95 [4.6–5.3]	0.834	4.7 [4.3–5.2]	4.5 [4.2–5.0]	0.745

We analyzed neuropsychological characteristics, namely depression and quality of life, and the groups did not differ (Table 2).

Table 2. Parameters of neuropsychological testing in the main and control groups.

Options	Main Group	Control Group	p
SarQol	80.54 [67.89–86.895]	78.03 [63.81–89.19]	0.833
HADS (anaxiety)	4 [2–7]	4 [2–6]	0.108
HADS (depression)	4 [2–6]	3 [1–5]	0.142
SF36, physical component	55 [49–59]	56 [50–60]	0.228
SF36, psychological component	45 [42–48]	46 [43–49]	0.499

Table 3 presents data on the composition of the body.

Table 3. Bioimpedancemetry parameters in the main and control groups.

Parameters	Women			Men		
	Main Group (n = 118)	Control Group (n = 28)	p	Main Group (n = 47)	Control Group (n = 28)	p
Body fat mass (kg)	28 [25.1–36]	26.5 [20.65–35]	0.011	30 [26.1–38]	26.5 [20.65–35]	0.002
Body fat percentage (%)	35.9 [35.4–41.3]	33.7 [29.85–40.1]	0.0001	39.7 [35.6–44.8]	35.1 [29.7–40.5]	0.0001
Visceral fat area (cm^2)	144.2 [128.3–176.1]	129.1 [92.2–169.25]	0.002	154.7 [128.3–198.4]	132.3 [95.3–183.5]	0.002
Skeletal muscle mass (kg^2)	25.5 [23.4–27.9]	28.6 [22.9–33.3]	0.043	23.2 [21.4–27.4]	26.4 [22.5–34.1]	0.003
Appendicular muscle mass (m^2)	6.7 [5.9–7.3]	7.8 [6.5–8.9]	<0.001	6.4 [5.85–7.1]	7.6 [6.3–8.5]	<0.001
Protein content	8.9 [8.1–10.0]	9.5 [8.25–11.6]	0.048	8.4 [7.5–9.4]	9.3 [8.25–11.6]	0.002
Minerals	3.1 [2.8–3.4]	3.9 [2.9–4.0]	0.03	3.0 [2.5–3.5]	3.6 [2.8–3.9]	0.044

According to the bioimpedancemetry data, the main group showed an increase in fat mass, percentage of fat mass, and visceral fat area compared with the control group, as well as a more pronounced decrease in skeletal muscle mass than in the control group and also content of protein and minerals. The appendicular mass scores were reduced in both men and women in the main group.

The next step was the evaluation of proinflammatory and oxidative stress markers in patients with and without sarcopenia (Table 4).

Table 4. Distribution of metabolic markers in patients with and without sarcopenia.

Metabolites	Main Group (F = M = 47)	Control Group (F = M = 28)	p
Fibroblast growth factor 21 ng/L	263.8 [251.4–274.8]	267 [246.5–273.5]	0.80
Nitrates, mmol/L	0.21 [0.21–0.355]	0.105 [0.07–0.14]	0.05
Malondialdehyde (MDA), µmol/L	290.32 [260.97–290.32]	147.42 [78.06–216.77]	0.76

When analyzing the metabolic parameters in the main group, there was an increase in nitrates in comparison with the control two times ($p = 0.05$). Fibroblast growth factor 21 and malondialdehyde values were not statistically significant.

In a subsequent analysis adjusted for multiple variables, there was a negative association of nitrate levels for weak grip strength ($p = 0.004$) and appendicular muscle mass ($p = 0.005$).

An additional analysis revealed that the complaint of pain in the lower extremities was more frequent in patients of the main group ($p = 0.023$), as well as constipation ($p = 0.008$) and pathology of thyroid gland ($p = 0.026$), and they were more frequently diagnosed with arterial hypertension ($p = 0.032$). At the same time, patients from the main group more frequently took vitamin D ($p = 0.014$).

So, as a result of the study, it was found that the groups did not differ according to the questionnaires. The dynamometry values for the main group were lower than those for the control group. The walking speed test did not allow us to objectively evaluate the functional ability of the muscles, because the walking time in the control group was longer than in the main group, both in men and in women. When conducting body composition, the main group recorded a higher weight and visceral fat content, as well as a decrease in appendicular and skeletal muscle mass, these changes were accompanied by a decrease in protein and minerals. Among the markers that differed significantly were nitrates, and it was this that was associated with decreased muscle strength and appendicular mass, which may indicate both a possible mechanism and a possible predictive marker, as well as malonic dialdehyde indices, which are significantly increased in the main group, but are not statistically significant.

4. Discussion

There is now evidence that sarcopenia can be diagnosed at a younger age, so in Poland, sarcopenia has been found in 4.5–5.1% at a young age (20–35 years) by appendicular mass [22]. In this regard, the relevance of assessing the signs or predicting factors for the development of sarcopenia at an age less than 65 years is of interest and will also allow the preclinical stage to identify the risk group and conduct rehabilitative measures.

Screening by questionnaires for depression and quality of life in patients with sarcopenia did not differ between the groups. This is probably because the participants were middle-aged patients who did not have significant clinical symptoms of sarcopenia yet. In a recent study the investigators assessed quality of life in patients with osteoporosis/osteopenia and sarcopenia, and the SF-36 questionnaire showed decreased quality of life; it should be considered that this study involved people over 65 years of age [23]. In a survey of elderly people aged 65 years and older living in South Korea, the relationship between reduced quality of life by the SarQoL questionnaire and nutritional risk was statistically significant [24]. Therefore, these questionnaires have little significance in persons with preclinical signs of sarcopenia, but they can be used in the older age group to assess disease progression and therapy efficacy.

Perhaps a more extensive questionnaire than the SARC-F is needed to assess nutritional status. For example, a study was conducted in Poland to evaluate the effectiveness of a version of the MRSA (Mini Sarcopenia Risk Assessment) questionnaire. It includes questions assessing age, weight loss in the last year, frequency of hospitalizations in the last year, physical activity level, frequency of food intake, and intake of dairy products and protein. As a result, PL-MSRA-5 is more effective than PL-MSRA-7 for sarcopenia risk assessment [25]. An analysis of a patient's nutritional status is very important because a lack of protein-containing foods leads to a progressive decline in muscle mass [26].

Although the sarcopenia screening questionnaire did not differ between groups and showed no risk of sarcopenia, muscle mass and muscle function were reduced. The diagnosis was confirmed by bioimpedanceometry; in middle-aged patients, in addition to changes in adipose tissue, altered skeletal muscle was registered, and the diagnosis of sarcopenia was confirmed by sarcopenia. Sarcopenic obesity is associated with low functional status and high mortality. The low prevalence of verification of the diagnosis seems to be due to the underestimation of sarcopenia in obese individuals; this can be avoided when using the body-mass-index assessment, where an isolated skeletal musculature assessment is performed, and the appendicular skeletal mass index. It should be noted that this condition occurs not only in middle age but also at a young age. The Danish study assessing sarcopenic obesity involved a group aged 20 to 59 years with a BMI ≥ 35 kg/m^2 and comorbidities or a BMI > 40 kg/m^2. The body composition was assessed by dual-energy X-ray absorptiometry (DEXA), and muscle function and strength were assessed by dynamometry and a functional test (standing up from a chair five times). As a result, low leg-muscle strength was found in 33% of participants, and the prevalence of sarcopenia ranged from 11.1% to 13.9%, with a higher prevalence in middle-aged women than in men [27]. Our study confirms these findings and, once again, proves the importance and timeliness of diagnosing a decrease in muscle mass and strength in middle-aged individuals.

Muscle mass showed a moderate correlation with hand-grip strength, which is partly explained by age-related fibrosis of some myocytes, as well as their replacement by adipose tissue [28]. These data are supported by high levels of fat mass in our study. Studies show that the degree of obesity is associated with greater muscle mass and absolute muscle strength when compared to non-obese people. However, when the body mass or muscle mass are normalized, people living with obesity have reduced muscle performance in comparison with individuals of normal weight. Therefore, a high-protein diet, in combination with exercise, should be used when losing weight in order to maintain lean body mass and prevent loss of muscle mass in the process of weight loss [29].

The muscle-weakness criterion and hand dynamometry scores of the EWGSOP2 algorithms are likely to identify different populations of older people as likely to have sarcopenia, given the same prevalence when either measure was used alone, but when both measures were used simultaneously, the prevalence of sarcopenia was much higher. The decrease in bone mass in the main group can be explained by an excessive amount of visceral fat, which is associated with increased proinflammatory activity of adipocytes and insulin resistance, which eventually leads to changes in the protein structure of the bones [30]. The results of our study contradict data obtained by colleagues in Spain, where the combined prevalence of sarcopenic obesity and osteoporosis was 0% [31]. This is due to the fact that, in this study, only the BMI was taken into account; bioimpedance measurements were not performed. Protein deficiency in the group of patients with sarcopenia may be of an alimentary nature in the sense that it is associated with an unbalanced diet due to excessive intake of carbohydrates and fats; it could also be of an endogenous origin due to the predominance of catabolic processes, due to the activation of proinflammatory markers. The absence of differences in fibroblast growth factor in the main and control groups is explained by the multifocal property of this metabolic regulator in middle-aged and elderly people; its increase is probably associated with a compensatory decrease in insulin resistance, as well as correction of dyslipidemia due to activation of lipolysis, b-oxidation in the liver [28]. In a study conducted in South Korea in elderly people aged 70 to 84 years, a decrease in plasma FGF21 levels was observed in participants with decreased muscle strength than in participants with normal muscle strength. At the same time, there was an increase in FGF21 in the group with decreased muscle strength than in the control group, which confirms our results [32]. This may be due to the fact that the participants in our study were middle-aged.

When conducting a review of the literature review, there are not enough publications on the study of nitrates in sarcopenia, but it was found that the decreased expression of inhibitor of nitric oxide synthase (iNOS) in the early stage of myocyte damage leads to disruption of satellite cell accumulation and muscle regeneration [33]. It can be assumed that their increase in the main group manifests itself as a response to fibrosis, since nitric oxide acts as a neurotransmitter, improving blood circulation, as well as cellular respiration processes [34]. Indeed, low nitrate levels have been reported in older adults, and dietary expansion showed the potential benefit of a nitrate-rich diet on muscle strength and physical function in a large cohort of older women [35]. Among the supplements tested, nitrates have received ample evidence to support their acute beneficial effects on muscle strength [36]. In addition, vasodilators increase levels of vitamin D, which is known to maintain mineral homeostasis, as well as improve muscle function [34]. There is great interest in assessing muscle mass and strength and nitric oxide levels in patients taking vitamin D supplements. A placebo-controlled study conducted in 2020 found improvements in grip strength, decreased time to get up from stool, and decreased body fat in the main group taking supplements for 12 weeks [37].

Currently, malondialdehyde is considered to be a marker of oxidative stress, which is one of the links in the pathogenesis of sarcopenia [36]. Previously, reliable data on its increase in coronary heart disease, stroke, and liver damage were obtained [37]. Perhaps their increase is concomitantly associated with excess body weight, since there is evidence of increased malondialdehyde in persons with sarcopenic obesity [38], and in our work, we observed excess body weight in both the main and the control groups. As a result, changes in high-density lipoprotein levels and malondialdehyde–low-density-lipoprotein ratios were significantly and independently associated with changes in muscle strength [39]. Antioxidants (dark chocolate and astaxanthin) were found to reduce oxidative LDL and malondialdehyde levels for a month and increase nitric oxide levels, helping prevent muscle mass loss [40].

It was found that combined aerobic and strength training during body weight loss can reduce the levels of proinflammatory markers IL-6 and TNF-α, due to a decrease in visceral fat and improved protein synthesis and myocyte cell membrane strength [41]. Extended studies are needed to further investigate the mechanisms by which physical activity affects chronic inflammatory processes and pro-inflammatory markers.

The pathophysiology of sarcopenia resembles that of other prototypical geriatric conditions for which a multifactorial etiology is at play, involving many of the biological hallmarks of aging (i.e., genomic and epigenetic instability, loss of proteostasis, mitochondrial dysfunction, telomere shortening, dysregulated nutrient signaling, stem-cell exhaustion, cellular senescence, and altered intercellular signaling). The currently available biomarkers of biological aging might not capture the multitude of intrinsic and extrinsic factors underlying the decline in physical function that characterizes sarcopenia.

The sample size was a limitation of the study, but material is being recruited for an epidemiologic evaluation of the potential of bioimpedance and metabolic markers in the early preclinical screening of probable sarcopenia and will be expanded. In addition, an older cohort is needed in the supplement to evaluate the content of predictive markers in confirmed sarcopenia and to provide a diagnostic algorithm; recruitment is ongoing and will be considered in future publications.

5. Conclusions

Anxiety, depression, and quality-of-life assessments show no change in middle-aged patients. Thus, for the primary screening of muscle mass reduction, it is objective to use bioimpedancemetry и dynamometry. These techniques will allow for the timely identification of patients from the risk group, which will allow early preventive and rehabilitative measures to be carried out. In addition, the use of bioimpedance as a method of assessing the dynamics of weight loss in overweight patients will make it possible to select a training program aimed at preserving muscle mass. Evaluation of the ratio of protein, minerals, and fluids in the body may be relevant for the development of an individual nutrition program. Early screening of the disease at the presarcopenia stage and preventive measures will reduce the number of patients with severe forms of sarcopenia, thereby increasing the quality of life and life expectancy of older people.

Because of the current high prevalence of carbohydrate metabolism disorders (type 2 diabetes mellitus and obesity), further study of the role of metabolic markers in sarcopenic obese individuals in a broader population is required. Further results on the study of metabolic markers may clarify new pathogenetic features associated with the development of sarcopenia. This will allow for the identification of new points for drug exposure, as well as the confirmation of statistical significance in a wider population, along with the use a panel of biomarkers for the predictive diagnosis of sarcopenia. I=The implementation of a multivariate predictive diagnostic methodology for sarcopenia will provide a way to stratify the risk of muscle mass loss, facilitate identification of a deteriorating condition, and provide monitoring of treatment effectiveness. In addition, such a marker as nitrates was not previously underestimated in the cross-section of decrease and loss of muscle mass and strength, which requires more in-depth study and will, in the future, probably open new fundamental ways of development of sarcopenia in middle age. Nitrates should be studied in more depth not only from the standpoint of sarcopenia, but also for predictive diagnosis in middle-aged individuals.

Author Contributions: Conceptualization, methodology, writing—review and editing, data curation, formal analysis, and software, Y.G.S., M.V.M.; formal analysis, curation of patients, writing—original draft preparation, and writing—review and editing, E.A.K.; conceptualization and methodology, D.A.K.; curation of patients, administration, and record keeping, O.A.O.; laboratory analysis, L.V.S. All authors have read and agreed to the published version of the manuscript.

Funding: This research was funded by Grant of the Russian Science "Early diagnosis of sarcopenia based on the metabolic profile", 22-25-00632 dated 10 January 2022.

Institutional Review Board Statement: The study was performed in accordance with Good Clinical Practice and the principles of the Declaration of Helsinki. The study protocol was approved by the ethical committee of Siberian State Medical University No. 8888 dated 29 November 2021.

Informed Consent Statement: Informed consent was obtained from all subjects involved in the study.

Data Availability Statement: Not applicable.

Conflicts of Interest: The authors declare no conflict of interest.

References

1. United Nations News Service Section. *UN News Centre Opening Remarks at Press Event on Day of Seven Billion*; UN News Service Section: New York, NY, USA, 2011.
2. Grigorieva, I.I.; Raskina, T.A.; Letaeva, M.V.; Malyshenko, O.S.; Averkieva, Y.V.; Masenko, V.L.; Kokov, A.N. Sarcopenia: Features of pathogenesis and diagnosis. *Fundam. Clin. Med.* **2019**, *4*, 105–116. [CrossRef]
3. Shafiee, G.; Keshtkar, A.; Soltani, A.; Ahadi, Z.; Larijani, B.; Heshmat, R. Prevalence of sarcopenia in the world: A systematic review and meta- analysis of general population studies. *J. Diabetes Metab. Disord.* **2017**, *16*, 21. [CrossRef] [PubMed]
4. Cruz-Jentoft, A.J.; Bahat, G.; Bauer, J.; Boirie, Y.; Bruyère, O.; Cederholm, T.; Cooper, C.; Landi, F.; Rolland, Y.; Sayer, A.A.; et al. Writing Group for the European Working Group on Sarcopenia in Older People 2 (EWGSOP2), and the Extended Group for EWGSOP2. Sarcopenia: Revised European consensus on definition and diagnosis. *Age Ageing* **2019**, *48*, 16–31. [CrossRef] [PubMed]
5. Bogat, S.V. The prevalence of sarcopenia in patients of older age groups. *Gerontology* **2014**, *3*, 305–310. (In Russian)
6. Bischoff-Ferrari, H.A.; Orav, J.E.; Kanis, J.A.; Rizzoli, R.; Schlögl, M.; Staehelin, H.B.; Willett, W.C.; Dawson-Hughes, B. Comparative performance of current definitions of sarcopenia against the prospective incidence of falls among community-dwelling seniors age 65 and older. *Osteoporos. Int.* **2015**, *26*, 2793–2802. [CrossRef]
7. Misnikova, I.V.; Kovaleva, Y.A.; Klimina, N.A. Sarkopenic obesity. *Russ. Med. J.* **2017**, *25*, 24–29. (In Russian)
8. Nipp, R.D.; Fuchs, G.; El-Jawahri, A.; Mario, J.; Troschel, F.M.; Greer, J.A.; Gallagher, E.R.; Jackson, V.A.; Kambadakone, A.; Hong, T.S.; et al. Sarcopenia is Associated with Quality of Life and Depression in Patients with Advanced Cancer. *Oncologist* **2018**, *23*, 97–104. [CrossRef]
9. Morville, T.; Sahl, R.E.; Trammell, S.A.; Svenningsen, J.S.; Gillum, M.P.; Helge, J.W.; Clemmensen, C. Divergent effects of resistance and endurance exercise on plasma bile acids, FGF19, and FGF21 in humans. *JCI Insight* **2018**, *3*, e122737. [CrossRef]
10. Sanchis-Gomar, F.; Pareja-Galeano, H.; Santos-Lozano, A.; Garatachea, N.; Fiuza-Luces, C.; Venturini, L.; Ricevuti, G.; Lucia, A.; Emanuele, E. A preliminary candidate approach identifies the combination of chemerin, fetuin-A, and fibroblast growth factors 19 and 21 as a potential biomarker panel of successful aging. *Age* **2015**, *37*, 42. [CrossRef]
11. Yamakage, H.; Tanaka, M.; Inoue, T.; Odori, S.; Kusakabe, T.; Satoh-Asahara, N. Effects of dapagliflozin on the serum levels of fibroblast growth factor 21 and myokines and muscle mass in Japanese patients with type 2 diabetes: A randomized, controlled trial. *J. Diabetes Investig.* **2020**, *11*, 653–661. [CrossRef]
12. Zeng, Y.; Nie, C.; Min, J.; Liu, X.; Li, M.; Chen, H.; Xu, H.; Wang, M.; Ni, T.; Li, Y.; et al. Novel loci and pathways significantly associated with longevity. *Sci Rep.* **2016**, *6*, 21243. [CrossRef] [PubMed]
13. Di Marco, S.; Mazroui, R.; Dallaire, P.; Chittur, S.; Tenenbaum, S.A.; Radzioch, D.; Marette, A.; Gallouzi, I.-E. NF-κB-mediated MyoD decay during muscle wasting requires nitric oxide synthase mRNA stabilization, HuR protein, and nitric oxide release. *Mol. Cell. Biol.* **2005**, *25*, 6533–6545. [CrossRef] [PubMed]
14. Hall, D.T.; Ma, J.F.; Marco, S.D.; Di Marco, S.; Gallouzi, I.-E. Inducible nitric oxide synthase (iNOS) in muscle wasting syndrome, sarcopenia, and cachexia. *Aging* **2011**, *3*, 702–715. [CrossRef] [PubMed]

15. Coggan, A.R.; Racette, S.B.; Thies, D.; Peterson, L.R.; Stratford, R.E., Jr. Simultaneous Pharmacokinetic Analysis of Nitrate and its Reduced Metabolite, Nitrite, Following Ingestion of Inorganic Nitrate in a Mixed Patient Population. *Pharm. Res.* **2020**, *37*, 235. [CrossRef] [PubMed]
16. Barrera, G.; Pizzimenti, S.; Daga, M.; Dianzani, C.; Arcaro, A.; Cetrangolo, G.P.; Giordano, G.; Cucci, M.A.; Graf, M.; Gentile, F. Lipid Peroxidation-Derived Aldehydes, 4-Hydroxynonenal and Malondialdehyde in Aging-Related Disorders. *Antioxidants* **2018**, *7*, 102. [CrossRef]
17. Standley, R.A.; Distefano, G.; Pereira, S.L.; Tian, M.; Kelly, O.J.; Coen, P.M.; Deutz, N.E.P.; Wolfe, R.R.; Goodpaster, B.H. Effects of β-hydroxy-β-methylbutyrate on skeletal muscle mitochondrial content and dynamics, and lipids after 10 days of bed rest in older adults. *J. Appl. Physiol.* **2017**, *123*, 1092–1100. [CrossRef]
18. Lu, Y.; Niti, M.; Yap, K.B.; Tan, C.T.Y.; Nyunt, M.S.Z.; Feng, L.; Tan, B.Y.; Chan, G.; Khoo, S.A.; Chan, S.M.; et al. Effects of multi-domain lifestyle interventions on sarcopenia measures and blood biomarkers: Secondary analysis of a randomized controlled trial of community-dwelling pre-frail and frail older adults. *Aging* **2021**, *13*, 9330–9347. [CrossRef]
19. Krzymińska-Siemaszko, R.; Fryzowicz, A.; Czepulis, N.; Kaluźniak-Szymanowska, A.; Dworak, L.B.; Wieczorowska-Tobis, K. The impact of the age range of young healthy reference population on the cut-off points for low muscle mass necessary for the diagnosis of sarcopenia. *Eur. Rev. Med. Pharmacol. Sci.* **2019**, *23*, 4321–4332. [CrossRef]
20. Chen, L.-K.; Woo, J.; Assantachai, P.; Auyeung, T.-W.; Chou, M.-Y.; Iijima, K.; Jang, H.C.; Kang, L.; Kim, M.; Kim, S.; et al. Asian Working Group for Sarcopenia: 2019 Consensus Update on Sarcopenia Diagnosis and Treatment. *J. Am. Med. Dir. Assoc.* **2020**, *21*, 300–307.e2. [CrossRef]
21. Shahar, S.; Kamaruddin, N.S.; Badrasawi, M.; Sakian, N.I.; Manaf, Z.A.; Yassin, Z.; Joseph, L. Effectiveness of exercise and protein supplementation intervention on body composition, functional fitness, and oxidative stress among elderly Malays with sarcopenia. *Clin. Interv. Aging* **2013**, *8*, 1365–1375. [CrossRef]
22. Soysal, P.; Smith, L.; Isik, A.T. Validation of population-based cut-offs for low muscle mass and strength. *Eur. Geriatr. Med.* **2020**, *11*, 713–714. [CrossRef] [PubMed]
23. Zhang, J.X.; Li, J.; Chen, C.; Yin, T.; Wang, Q.A.; Li, X.X.; Wang, F.X.; Zhao, J.H.; Zhao, Y.; Zhang, Y.H. Reference values of skeletal muscle mass, fat mass and fat-to-muscle ratio for rural middle age and older adults in western China. *Arch. Gerontol. Geriatr.* **2021**, *95*, 104389. [CrossRef] [PubMed]
24. Kim, Y.; Park, K.S.; Yoo, J.I. Associations between the quality of life in sarcopenia measured with the SarQoL® and nutritional status. *Health Qual. Life Outcomes* **2021**, *19*, 28. [CrossRef] [PubMed]
25. Krzymińska-Siemaszko, R.; Deskur-Śmielecka, E.; Styszyński, A.; Wieczorowska-Tobis, K. Polish Translation and Validation of the Mini Sarcopenia Risk Assessment (MSRA) Questionnaire to Assess Nutritional and Non-Nutritional Risk Factors of Sarcopenia in Older Adults. *Nutrients* **2021**, *13*, 1061. [CrossRef] [PubMed]
26. Vandewoude, M.F.J.; Alish, C.J.; Sauer, A.C.; Hegazi, R.A. Malnutrition-sarcopenia syndrome: Is this the future of nutrition screening and assessment for older adults? *J. Aging Res.* **2012**, *2012*, 651570. [CrossRef]
27. Suetta, C.; Haddock, B.; Alcazar, J.; Noerst, T.; Hansen, O.M.; Ludvig, H.; Kamper, R.S.; Schnohr, P.; Prescott, E.; Andersen, L.L.; et al. The Copenhagen Sarcopenia Study: Lean mass, strength, power, and physical function in a Danish cohort aged 20–93 years. *J. Cachexia Sarcopenia Muscle* **2019**, *10*, 1316–1329. [CrossRef] [PubMed]
28. Geerinck, A.; Bruyère, O.; Locquet, M.; Reginster, J.Y.; Beaudart, C. Evaluation of the Responsiveness of the SarQoL® Questionnaire, a Patient-Reported Outcome Measure Specific to Sarcopenia. *Adv. Ther.* **2018**, *35*, 1842–1858. [CrossRef]
29. Verreijen, A.M.; Engberink, M.F.; Memelink, R.G.; van der Plas, S.E.; Visser, M.; Weijs, P.J. Effect of a high protein diet and/or resistance exercise on the preservation of fat free mass during weight loss in overweight and obese older adults: A randomized controlled trial. *Nutr. J.* **2017**, *16*, 10. [CrossRef]
30. Yamaguchi, T. Updates on Lifestyle-Related Diseases and Bone Metabolism. The metabolic syndrome and bone metabolism. *Clin. Calcium* **2014**, *24*, 1599–1604.
31. Hernández-Martínez, P.; Olmos, J.M.; Llorca, J.; Hernández, J.L.; González-Macías, J. Sarcopenic osteoporosis, sarcopenic obesity, and sarcopenic osteoporotic obesity in the Camargo cohort (Cantabria, Spain). *Arch. Osteoporos.* **2022**, *17*, 105. [CrossRef]
32. Roh, E.; Hwang, S.Y.; Yoo, H.J.; Baik, S.H.; Cho, B.; Park, Y.S.; Kim, H.J.; Lee, S.-G.; Kim, B.J.; Jang, H.C.; et al. Association of plasma FGF21 levels with muscle mass and muscle strength in a national multicentre cohort study: Korean Frailty and Aging Cohort Study. *Age Ageing* **2021**, *50*, 1971–1978. [CrossRef] [PubMed]
33. Kawashima, M.; Miyakawa, M.; Sugiyama, M.; Miyoshi, M.; Arakawa, T. Unloading during skeletal muscle regeneration retards iNOS-expressing macrophage recruitment and perturbs satellite cell accumulation. *Histochem. Cell Biol.* **2020**, *154*, 355–367. [CrossRef] [PubMed]
34. Bulatova, I.A.; Shchekotova, A.P.; Krivtsov, A.V.; Ulitina, P.V.; Larionova, G.G.; Paducheva, S.V. Significance of malondialdehyde and glutathione transferase in assessing liver damage and monitoring therapy in chronic hepatitis. *Fundam. Res.* **2014**, *4*, 246–251.
35. Sim, M.; Lewis, J.R.; Blekkenhorst, L.C.; Bondonno, C.P.; Devine, A.; Zhu, K.; Peeling, P.; Prince, R.L.; Hodgson, J.M. Dietary nitrate intake is associated with muscle function in older women. *J. Cachexia Sarcopenia Muscle* **2019**, *10*, 601–610. [CrossRef]
36. Valenzuela, P.L.; Morales, J.S.; Emanuele, E.; Pareja-Galeano, H.; Lucia, A. Supplements with purported effects on muscle mass and strength. *Eur. J. Nutr.* **2019**, *58*, 2983–3008. [CrossRef]
37. Córdova, A.; Caballero-García, A.; Noriega-González, D.; Bello, H.J.; Pons, A.; Roche, E. Nitric-Oxide-Inducing Factors on Vitamin D Changes in Older People Susceptible to Suffer from Sarcopenia. *Int. J. Environ. Res. Public Health* **2022**, *19*, 5938. [CrossRef]

38. Pin, F.; Beltrà, M.; Garcia-Castillo, L.; Pardini, B.; Birolo, G.; Matullo, G.; Penna, F.; Guttridge, D.; Costelli, P. Extracellular vesicles derived from tumor cells as a trigger of energy crisis in the skeletal muscle. *J. Cachexia Sarcopenia Muscle* **2022**, *13*, 481–494. [CrossRef]
39. Kawamoto, R.; Kohara, K.; Katoh, T.; Kusunoki, T.; Ohtsuka, N.; Abe, M.; Kumagi, T.; Miki, T. Changes in oxidized low-density lipoprotein cholesterol are associated with changes in handgrip strength in Japanese community-dwelling persons. *Endocrine* **2015**, *48*, 871–877. [CrossRef]
40. Petyaev, I.M.; Klochkov, V.A.; Chalyk, N.E.; Pristensky, D.V.; Chernyshova, M.P.; Kyle, N.H.; Bashmakov, Y.K. Markers of Hypoxia and Oxidative Stress in Aging Volunteers Ingesting Lycosomal Formulation of Dark Chocolate Containing Astaxanthin. *J. Nutr. Health Aging* **2018**, *22*, 1092–1098. [CrossRef]
41. Wang, S.; Zhou, H.; Zhao, C.; He, H. Effect of Exercise Training on Body Composition and Inflammatory Cytokine Levels in Overweight and Obese Individuals: A Systematic Review and Network Meta-Analysis. *Front. Immunol.* **2022**, *13*, 921085. [CrossRef]

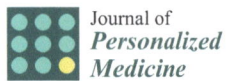 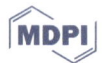

Article

The Profile of Glucose Lowering Therapy in Persons with Type 2 Diabetes Mellitus in an Aging Russian Population

Sofia Malyutina *, Elena Mazurenko *, Ekaterina Mazdorova, Marina Shapkina, Ekaterina Avdeeva, Svetlana Mustafina, Galina Simonova and Andrey Ryabikov

Research Institute of Internal and Preventive Medicine—Branch of the Institute of Cytology and Genetics, Siberian Branch of Russian Academy of Sciences, 630089 Novosibirsk, Russia
* Correspondence: smalyutina@hotmail.com (S.M.); poltorackayaes@gmail.com (E.M.); Tel.: +7-(952)-945-72-11 (E.M.)

Abstract: We aimed to analyze the profile of glucose lowering therapy (GLT) in persons with diabetes mellitus type 2 (DM2) in an aging Russian population. A random population sample (n = 3898, men/women, 55–84) was examined in Novosibirsk, during 2015–2018 (HAPIEE Project). The design of the present work is a cross-sectional study. DM2 was defined in those with a history of DM2 receiving GLT, or at a level of fasting plasma glucose (FPG) $\geq$7.0 mmol/L. The entire DM2 group was included in the analysis (n = 803); of these, 476 persons were taking GLT and were included in the analysis at stage 2. Regular GLT medication intake for 12 months was coded with ATC. In studied sample, the prevalence of DM2 was 20.8%. Among subjects with DM2, 59% of individuals received GLT, 32% did not. Glycemic control (FPG < 7.0 mmol/L) was achieved in every fifth participant with DM2 (35% in those receiving GLT). In frequency of GLT use, biguanides ranked in first place (75%), sulfonylurea derivatives in second (35%), insulins in third (12%), and iDPP-4 in fourth (5%). Among those receiving GLT, 24% used combined oral therapy, and 6% used insulin-combined therapy. In conclusion, in a population sample aged 55–84 examined in 2015–2018, glycemic control was achieved in every fifth participant with DM2, and in every third participant receiving GLT. The proportion of participants using new GLT drugs was small, and there was a lack of HbA1c monitoring for intensive glycemic control.

Keywords: diabetes mellitus type 2; glucose lowering therapy; glycemic control; HAPIEE cohort; population

Citation: Malyutina, S.; Mazurenko, E.; Mazdorova, E.; Shapkina, M.; Avdeeva, E.; Mustafina, S.; Simonova, G.; Ryabikov, A. The Profile of Glucose Lowering Therapy in Persons with Type 2 Diabetes Mellitus in an Aging Russian Population. *J. Pers. Med.* **2022**, *12*, 1689. https://doi.org/10.3390/jpm12101689

Academic Editor: Emilio González-Jiménez

Received: 30 August 2022
Accepted: 6 October 2022
Published: 10 October 2022

Publisher's Note: MDPI stays neutral with regard to jurisdictional claims in published maps and institutional affiliations.

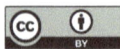

Copyright: © 2022 by the authors. Licensee MDPI, Basel, Switzerland. This article is an open access article distributed under the terms and conditions of the Creative Commons Attribution (CC BY) license (https://creativecommons.org/licenses/by/4.0/).

1. Introduction

Diabetes mellitus (DM) is a global problem, due to an annual increase in its prevalence in the world. According to the latest data, the global number of patients with type 2 diabetes (DM2) has reached 463 million people [1]. In the Russian Federation (RF), a similar situation has been observed, and, according to the Russian Diabetes Register, this figure had reached 4.58 million people (3.1% of the population) by 1 January 2019 [2]. According to our early data, DM2 was found in 11.4% of subjects in a population sample aged 45–69 years in Novosibirsk [3,4].

The financial burden for people with diabetes and for society as a whole is growing due to lifelong daily care, glycemic control, treatment of diabetes complications and hospitalizations, as well as by indirect costs associated with reduced quality of life and disability.

The most dangerous consequences of DM2 include vascular complications—nephropathy, retinopathy, lesion of coronary, cerebral and lower extremities arteries. These complications are the main cause of disability and mortality in patients with DM2. Among the methods of evidence-based medicine that have demonstrated the highest effectiveness in reducing the risk of diabetic complications, the achievement of targeted glycemic control is the most essential [5].

Early achievement of stable glycemic control is a key component of effective management of patients with DM2 [6–8]. A prospective study, UKPDS, demonstrated that absolute reduction in glycated hemoglobin (HbA1c) by 1.0% was associated with a 21%, 14% and 37% reduction in the risk of diabetes-related death, myocardial infarction and microvascular complications, respectively [6].

Based on these data, most clinical guidelines recommend a target level of HbA1c <7.0% or ≤6.5%, depending on additional factors such as age, duration of diabetes, comorbidities, and risk of hypoglycemia [9–11]. When a patient's HbA1c level is above the target level for more than 6 months following the last update of therapy, an intensification of treatment is recommended [11,12]. Despite established guidelines and the availability of modern glucose-lowering medications, there is evidence of poor achievement of glycemic targets and untimely intensification of therapy [13,14].

The achievement of target levels of HbA1c was assessed in the EUROASPIRE I–V [15] and NHANES [16] studies. According to the summarized data, about 50% of patients with DM2 did not reach the target levels of HbA1c. The 3-year project DISCOVER, which studied 15,992 subjects aged >18 years with DM2 who received standard medical care as determined by their treating physicians in 38 countries including Russia, confirmed this fact [17]. In particular, stable high levels of HbA1c were observed in patients with DM2 at the beginning of their second-line therapy: about one half of patients had HbA1c levels >8.0% and more than a quarter had HbA1c levels >9.0%. Overall, <20% of patients had an HbA1c < 7.0% [17]. In the NHANES study, the percentage of subjects with diabetes who achieved glycemic control (HbA1c < 7%) decreased from 57.4% (in the period 2007–2010) to 50.5% (in the period 2015–2018) [18]. According to the Russian Diabetes Register in 2017, the distribution of DM2 patients by HbA1c level was as follows: HbA1c < 7, 52.2%; from 7% to 7.9, 29.0%; from 8% to 8.9, 9.9%; and ≥9.0, 8.8% of patients [19].

Knowledge on the effectiveness of glucose-lowering therapy (GLT) in the Russian population has mainly been obtained from clinical trials; there are a lack of population studies in different regions and age ranges. In ageing, the size of the DM2 problem is rising. Therefore, in connection with changing approaches to the treatment of diabetes, permanent monitoring is relevant.

The aim of this study was to analyze the profile of GLT in persons with DM2 aged 55–84 years in a Russian population sample (Novosibirsk).

Early findings on drug therapy for atrial fibrillation, antihypertensive and lipid-lowering therapy in the studied population have previously been reported [20–22]. The present paper continues a systematic series of works on the pharmacotherapy of cardiometabolic diseases in the modern Russian population, using a population-based urban sample of older age persons in Novosibirsk.

2. Material and Methods

2.1. Participants

The study was performed on the material of a population cohort examined in Novosibirsk (the Russian arm of the multicenter project "Determinants of cardiovascular diseases in Central and Eastern Europe: cohort study", the HAPIEE Project) [23]. A random sample of men and women aged 45–69 was drawn from residents of two districts typical of Novosibirsk in terms of infrastructure, demographic indicators and the level of population migration. The sample was formed on the basis of electoral lists using a table of random numbers and stratified by 5-year age groups; the design and protocol of the project have been published previously [23]. The design of the present work is a cross-sectional study. At baseline 9360 people were examined in 2003/05 (98% Caucasians, 61% response), the cohort was re-examined twice in 2006/08 and 2015/18. The present study focused on a sample of the third wave (n = 3898, age 55–84, response 60.1%). The analysis included 3896 people with the full required data set. The study was approved by the Ethics Committee of Research Institute of Internal and Preventive Medicine—Branch of the Institute of Cytology and Genetics, SB RAS. All participants signed an informed consent.

2.2. Study Questionnaire

The details of protocol and methods of the study have been published previously [23]. In brief, the protocol included the epidemiological assessment of cardiovascular diseases (CVD) and their risk factors using standardized questionnaires (medical history of hypertension and diabetes and their treatment, history of CVD and other chronic diseases, smoking, alcohol consumption, socio-demographic characteristics) and objective measurements (anthropometry, blood pressure measurement, electrocardiography, lipid and blood glucose levels).

A person who smoked at least 1 cigarette a day was considered a smoker. Alcohol consumption was assessed using the Graduated Frequency Questionnaire (GFR) and 5 groups were distinguished according to the frequency of consumption: non-drinkers, less than 1 time per month, 1–3 times per month, 1–4 times per week, 5 or more times per week.

2.3. Objective Measurements

Blood pressure (BP) levels were measured three times using an Omron M-5 tonometer on the right arm in a sitting position after a 5 min rest, with 2 min intervals between measurements. The mean value of three measurements of the office BP was used in analysis. Hypertension (HT) was defined according to the ESC/ESH criteria, 2018 [24], at systolic (SBP) or diastolic (DBP) BP levels $\geq$140/90 mmHg and/or taking antihypertensive drugs within the last 2 weeks.

Waist–hip ratio (WHR) and body mass index (BMI) were calculated using the formula:

$$\text{BMI (kg/m}^2\text{)} = \text{body weight (kg)}/\text{height}^2 \text{ (m}^2\text{)} \quad (1)$$

$$\text{WHR (units)} = \text{waist circumference}/\text{hip circumference} \quad (2)$$

A 12 lead ECG was recorded on electrocardiograph Cardiax (IMEDLtd., Budapest, Hungary) and assessed using the Minnesota code (MC).

Blood samples were collected at fasting stage; levels of total cholesterol (TC), triglycerides (TG), high-density lipoprotein cholesterol (HDL-C), and glucose in blood serum were measured by the enzymatic method on a KoneLab 300i autoanalyzer (Thermo Fisher Scientific, Waltham, MA, USA). The level of low-density lipoprotein cholesterol (LDL-C) was calculated using the Friedewald formula. The conversion of fasting blood serum glucose into fasting plasma glucose (FPG) was performed according to the formula of the European Association for the Study of Diabetes, 2007 [25]:

$$\text{FPG (mmol/L)} = -0.137 + 1.047 \times \text{serum glucose concentration (mmol/L)} \quad (3)$$

DM2 was established by having a history of DM2 with treatment and/or a FPG level $\geq$7 mmol/L [26]. All individuals with DM2 history or first ever revealed DM2, were included in the analysis of hypoglycemic therapy.

Coronary heart disease (CHD) was defined by epidemiological criteria: a positive score of the Rose Angina questionnaire or ischemic ECG changes (MC classes 1, 4, and 5) [27,28], or a medical history of myocardial infarction (MI), acute coronary syndrome, or coronary revascularization (confirmed by hospitalization). A composite CVD category was defined in the presence of CHD, based on above specified criteria or a history of stroke/transient ischemic attack (confirmed by hospitalization information).

The regular intake of hypoglycemic drugs was evaluated as a daily intake for the last 12 months without taking into account the dosage of the drug substance. Medicinal products were coded according to the Anatomical Therapeutic Chemical Classification System (ATC) [29]. The following drugs were included in the analysis: insulins (code A10A), biguanides (code A10BA), sulfonylurea drugs (SU, code A10BB), alpha-glucosidase inhibitors (iAG, code A10BF), thiazolidinediones (glitazones) (TZD, code A10BG), inhibitors DPP-4 (iDPP-4, code A10BH), glucagon-like peptide-1 receptor agonists (aGLP1, code A10BJ), inhibitors of sodium glucose cotransporter type 2 (gliflozins) (iSGLT-2, code A10BK), glinides (meglitinides) (code A10BX), and other drugs. Coding was performed by three specialists (cardiologists and endocrinologists). Reproducibility was assessed in a 10% subgroup by a double-blind fashion, and the Kappa agreement coefficient was 0.84.

A total of 3896 people were examined. At stage 1, the analysis included 803 persons with DM2. Of these, 476 persons were taking GLT and were included in the analysis at stage 2. The proportion of people who reported specific GLT was more than half—322 people. Next, we analyzed the proportion of glycemic control among all individuals with DM2 (including newly diagnosed) and among those taking GLT.

2.4. Statistical Analysis

Statistical analysis was carried out using the SPSS package v.13.0. Data are presented as means and standard deviation, M (SD), or as proportions, n (%). The frequency of the trait in the groups was compared using the χ^2-Pearson test and the non-parametric Mantel–Hansel and Cochrane tests; ANOVA (analysis of variance) was used for quantitative comparisons. The Mann–Whitney test was used for abnormal distribution. Hypothesis testing was performed at a 95% confidence level for two-tailed tests.

3. Results

The general characteristics of the study sample aged 55–84, are presented in Table 1.

Table 1. General characteristics of the studied population sample (men and women 55–84 years old, Novosibirsk, n = 3896).

Risk Factors	General Sample	Men	Women	p *
		Mean (SD)/n (%)		
Examined, n	3896	1499 (38.42)	2397 (61.58)	
Age, years	69.29 (6.89)	69.04 (6.95)	69.46 (6.85)	0.061
SBP, mmHg	145.72 (21.31)	146.88 (20.64)	145.0 (21.69)	0.007
DBP, mmHg	83.63 (11.37)	85.79 (11.82)	82.28 (10.87)	<0.001
Heart rate, b/min	71.75 (11.41)	71.34 (12.16)	72.01 (10.91)	0.084
BMI, kg/m^2	29.47 (5.49)	27.76 (4.59)	30.55 (5.73)	<0.001
WHR, unit	0.90 (0.08)	0.95 (0.07)	0.87 (0.07)	<0.001
TC, mmol/L	5.46 (1.19)	5.17 (1.14)	5.65 (1.19)	<0.001
LDL-C, mmol/L	3.46 (1.06)	3.28 (0.99)	3.58 (1.08)	<0.001
HDLC, mmol/L	1.32 (0.39)	1.24 (0.38)	1.38 (0.38)	<0.001
TG, mmol/L	1.49 (0.92)	1.44 (0.89)	1.52 (0.94)	<0.005
FPG, mmol/L	6.34 (1.81)	6.41 (1.84)	6.29 (1.8)	0.041
HT, n (%)	3137 (80.9)	1162 (78.0)	1975 (82.6)	<0.001
Treatment of HT (among subjects with HT), n (%)	2399 (77.4)	723 (62.8)	1676 (86.1)	<0.001
DM2, n (%)	803 (20.8)	299 (20.1)	504 (21.2)	0.463
Treatment of DM2 (among subjects with DM2), n%	476 (59.3)	143 (47.8)	333 (66.1)	<0.001
CHD, n (%)	573 (14.9)	261 (17.5)	312 (13.2)	<0.001
CVD, n (%)	769 (19.9)	337 (22.6)	432 (18.2)	0.001
Menopause, n (%)	(-)	(-)	1924 (81.5)	(-)
Smoking, n (%)				
Smokers	714 (18.6)	572 (38.5)	142 (6.0)	<0.001
Former smokers	515 (13.4)	410 (27.6)	105 (4.4)	
Non-smokers	2619 (68.1)	504 (33.9)	2115 (89.5)	
Frequency of alcohol intake, n (%)				
2–4 times/week	47 (1.2)	40 (2.7)	7 (0.3)	<0.001
Once a week	413 (10.7)	326 (21.9)	87 (3.7)	
1–3 times/month	835 (21.7)	444 (29.9)	391 (16.6)	
Less than once a month	1609 (41.8)	413 (27.8)	1196 (50.6)	
Non-drinkers	944 (24.5)	263 (17.7)	681 (28.8)	

Table 1. Cont.

Risk Factors	General Sample	Men	Women	p *
		Mean (SD)/n (%)		
Education, n (%)				
Primary	246 (6.3)	86 (5.7)	160 (6.7)	
Professional	1063 (27.3)	335 (22.3)	728 (30.4)	<0.001
Secondary	1252 (32.1)	478 (31.9)	774 (32.3)	
University	1335 (34.3)	600 (40.0)	735 (30.7)	
Marital status, n (%)				
Single	1535 (39.9)	230 (15.5)	1305 (55.1)	<0.001
Married	2319 (60.2)	1258 (84.5)	1061 (44.9)	

Note: * p comparison by sex, for categorical variables—non-parametric Mann–Whitney test, for quantitative variables—Pearson's χ^2 test. SBP/DBP—systolic/diastolic blood pressure, HR—heart rate, BMI—body mass index, WHR—ratio of waist circumference/hip circumference, FPG—fasting plasma glucose, TC—total cholesterol, TG—triglycerides, HDL-C—high-density lipoprotein cholesterol, LDL-C—low-density lipoprotein cholesterol, HT—hypertension, DM2—diabetes mellitus type 2, CHD—coronary heart disease, CVD—cardiovascular diseases.

In the studied sample, the average age of the respondents was 69.3 years (SD 6.89) and was similar in men and women. The distribution of the participants by 10-year groups was 32.1% for the age of 55–64 years, 40% for the age of 65–74, and somewhat less (27.2%) for the group 75 years of age and older. Women, compared with men, had higher BMI and blood lipid values, a higher frequency of HT and antihypertensive therapy, and a similar prevalence of DM2 with a higher frequency of taking GLT; more often women had a low level of education and the status of "single." Compared with women, men had higher levels of BP, WHR and FPG, a higher prevalence of CHD and CVD, and smoking and alcohol consumption was more common.

The prevalence of DM2 in the population sample aged 55–84 years was 20.8%, and was similar in men and women (20.1% and 21.2%, respectively, $p = 0.463$). Among subjects with DM2, 59.3% received GLT, women more often than men (66.1% vs. 47.8%, respectively, $p < 0.001$), Table 2. About 32% of subjects with DM2, including newly diagnosed diabetes, did not receive GLT, and another 8.8% did not provide information on GLT.

Table 2. The frequency of use of GLT and blood glucose control in persons with DM2 (population sample, 55–84 years old, $n = 3896$).

Parameters	General Sample	Men	Women	p_{m-w}
Examined, n	3896	1499	2397	
DM2, n (%)	803 (20.8)	299 (20.1)	504 (21.2)	0.463
GLT among persons with DM2 (total), n (%)	476 (59.3)	143 (47.8)	333 (66.1)	
Not receiving GLT, n (%)	256 (31.9)	112 (37.5)	144 (28.6)	<0.001
No data on receiving GLT, n (%)	71 (8.8)	44 (14.7)	27 (5.4)	
Proportion of GLT with specified drugs, n (%)	322 (67.6)	87 (60.8)	235 (70.6)	0.037
Proportion of undifferentiated GLT, n (%)	154 (32.4)	56 (39.2)	98 (29.4)	
Effective control of blood glucose in subjects with DM 2 (total), n (%) $n = 803$	166 (20.7)	38 (12.7)	128 (25.4)	<0.001
Effective control of blood glucose (in those receiving GLT), n (%) $n = 476$	166 (34.9)	38 (26.6)	128 (38.4)	0.013
Effective control of blood glucose (in those who specified GLT drug, n (%) $n = 322$	102 (33.2)	21 (24.1)	81 (34.5)	0.184
Effective blood glucose control (in those with undifferentiated GLT), n (%) $n = 154$	64 (42.2)	17 (30.4)	47 (48.0)	0.068

Note: —p comparison by sex, Pearson's χ^2 test. GLT—glucose-lowering therapy, DM2—diabetes mellitus type 2.

FPG control < 7.0 mmol/L was achieved in every fifth participant with DM2 and in 35% of those taking GLT, Table 3, Figure 1. Participants who reported the name of a specific drug had control of glucose levels in about the same proportion (33%). Overall, women monitored their blood glucose levels more often than men.

Table 3. The profile of drug classes of GLT in persons with DM2 (population sample, 55–84 years old).

Classes of GLT in Persons Who Specified Medicinal Products, n = 322	Total	Men	Women	p m-w
GLT, n	322	87	235	
Insulins, total, n (%)	38 (11.8)	12 (16.1)	24 (10.2)	0.146
Biguanides, n (%)	242 (75.2)	60 (69.0)	182 (77.4)	0.118
Sulfonylureas, n (%)	114 (35.4)	35 (40.2)	79 (33.6)	0.271
Heterocyclic sulfonamides, n (%)	0 (0.0)	0 (0.0)	0 (0.0)	–
Alpha-glucosidase inhibitors, n (%)	0 (0.0)	0 (0.0)	0 (0.0)	–
Thiazolidinediones, n (%)	0 (0.0)	0 (0.0)	0 (0.0)	–
iDPP-4, n (%)	15 (4.7)	9 (10.3)	6 (2.6)	0.003
aGLP1, n (%)	0 (0.0)	0 (0.0)	0 (0.0)	–
iSGLT-2, n (%)	0 (0.0)	0 (0.0)	0 (0.0)	–
Combined oral drugs, n (%)	76 (23.6)	26 (28.9)	50 (21.8)	0.042
Combined GLT, total, n (%)	95 (29.5)	35 (40.2)	60 (25.5)	0.010

Note: —p comparison by sex, Pearson's χ² test. GLT—glucose-lowering therapy, DM2—diabetes mellitus type 2, iDPP-4—dipeptidyl peptidase-4 inhibitors, aGLP1—analogues of glucagon-like peptide-1 receptors, iSGLT-2—inhibitors of sodium-glucose cotransporter type 2.

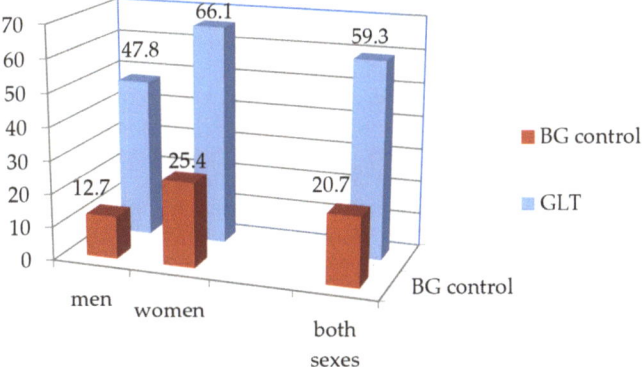

Figure 1. Frequency of glucose-lowering therapy (GLT) and blood glucose control (BG control) among people with type 2 diabetes, n = 803 (population sample, 55–84 years old).

In frequency of GLT use, biguanides ranked first place (75%), sulfonylurea derivatives in second place (35%), insulins in third place (12%), and DPP4 inhibitors in fourth place (5%). Combination GLT drugs were used by about one-third of individuals with DM2 (24% oral, another 6% in combination with insulin). One third of individuals with DM2 (including those newly diagnosed) did not receive GLT, which significantly affects the insufficient control of DM in the population.

4. Discussion

The prevalence of DM2 in the Novosibirsk population sample aged 55–84 years was 20.8%. Among persons with DM2, including newly diagnosed disease, 35% did not receive GLT. The target values of glycemia (FPG < 7.0%) were achieved in 20.7% of the group with DM2 and in 31.9% among those taking GLT. HbA1c levels were not assessed in this population study. Women effectively controlled glycemia more often than men.

In our study, in the entire DM2 group, we identified 35% of individuals with newly diagnosed diabetes who had not previously received GLT, which potentially contributes to a strong prediction of future CVD. The worsened prognosis is supported by the findings of a negative effect of prior hyperglycemia on coronary circulation, by an increased likelihood of having more severe and extensive CHD, and by the poorer profile of cardiometabolic risk factors in newly revealed DM2, compared with those with known diabetes [30,31].

It has also been reported that among patients with ST-elevation MI (STEMI) undergoing percutaneous coronary intervention (PCI), those with overt or newly diagnosed diabetes have a similar in-hospital and 3-year mortality rate, though mortality is lower in patients with pre-diabetes or no dysglycemia [32]. Patients with increased FPG or newly diagnosed diabetes following MI have an increased incidence of major adverse cardiac events (MACE) with the negative outcomes [33].

Plasma glucose measurement plays an important role in predicting adverse events, especially in subjects with previously unknown DM2 [34]. Given the above, more attention should be paid to individuals with newly diagnosed DM who should be screened for complications, particularly among those with a history of CV events.

The frequency of GLT use in our sample was expectedly lower compared with the EUROASPIRE-V study, which analyzed a sample of patients after a coronary event [15]. In the EUROASPIRE I–V study, 29% of all patients reported having DM2; of them, GLT was taken as follows: insulin, 32%; oral GLT, 74%; and 16% of the examined patients did not assess their blood glucose levels after discharge [15].

Our results were closer to the findings of a retrospective analysis of medical and pharmacological data on GLT use in the United States (more than 1.6 million, age 18–75+) [35], where the proportion of patients with diabetes who did not take GLT in the period 2006–2013 ranged from 25.7 to 24.1%.

The level of glycemic control among those receiving therapy in our sample was 35% (<7.0 mmol/L) and was approximately two times lower than the achieved control by the target HbA1c < 7.0% in the general EUROASPIRE-V cohort (54%) [15], and 1.5 times lower than in the Russian portion of the EUROASPIRE-V cohort (47%) [36]. At the same time, in the NHANES study, 2009–2014 [37], the results were close to our data. In particular, in the NHANES study, 2009–2014, the prevalence of intensive glycemic control was studied, taking into account the factors contributing to the achievement of the target level of HbA1C < 7.0%, such as duration of diabetes, smoking, comorbidities, disability, depression and taking the definite drugs, as well as socio-demographic factors. After adjusting, it was found that in the adjusted model, the frequency of intensive control was 23.5%, 32.5%, and 35.6%, for persons aged 50–64, 65–74, and 75+ years, respectively, with no significant difference by sex [37]. Lipska KJ et al., 2017, similarly, showed that less than half of the youngest patients (48.0%), but more than 60% of the oldest patients (61.6%) achieved the level of HbA1c < 7.0% [37]. Thus, older people have been shown to be treated more aggressively than young people to achieve HbA1c < 7.0% despite the presence of comorbidities and other factors.

In the Tromso study, which included 27,281 women and men aged 40–84 years, there was a linear increase in the prevalence of diabetes from 1994 to 2016. The overall prevalence of diabetes, including HbA1c ≥ 6.5%, increased from 3.2% to 5.9% in women and from 3.7% to 7.9% in men. According to the latest survey, the treatment goal (HbA1c ≤7.0% or <7.5%) was achieved in 43.8% of women and 38.5% of men using antidiabetic drugs, compared with 83.6% and 76.1% of women and men, respectively, who did not take antidiabetic drugs [38]. The authors found that target achievement was lower among patients using antidiabetics compared with non-users, which could be explained by less severe disease among non-users (i.e., diet-regulated diabetes).

According to the Russian DM Register, in 2017, the number of people who reached the level of HbA1c < 7.0% was 52.2% [20], which was higher, compared with our study, according to the other criterion of FGP < 7 mmol/L.

In the profile of hypoglycemic therapy in the Novosibirsk sample, about 90% of individuals treated for DM2 took oral agents, and 12% received insulin. The proportion of oral therapy in our study was higher, and insulin therapy two times lower, than in the general EUROASPIRE-V cohort where insulin therapy and oral GLT were 32% and 74%, respectively [15]. In the Russian sample of EUROASPIRE-V, the frequency of insulin therapy was close to ours, at 14.9%, and the proportion of oral therapy was lower, at 72.4% [36].

In our study, two-thirds of patients with DM2 received monotherapy, 30% took combined therapy, including near 24% who received oral drugs combination. These figures are close to the data from the Federal Russian Register, which showed that in the structure of DM2 therapy in the RF in 2017, the prescription of oral GLT prevailed (75.2% of patients), mainly in the form of monotherapy (46.8% of patients); 25.6% of patients received a combination of two drugs, and 2.8% a combination of three drugs. The number of patients with DM2 on insulin therapy in 2017 was 18.6%, of which 10.8% received insulin therapy combined with oral GLT, and 7.8% were on insulin monotherapy [19]. Among the oral agents in our study, metformin was predominantly used (75.2%), SU derivatives were in second place (35.4%), about 5% of people with DM2 took iDPP-4. TZD group, aGLP-1 and iSGLT-2 were not taken by the participants of the examined sample. Similar data with a slightly lower proportion of metformin use were shown by the Russian DM Register, where the most commonly prescribed drugs in monotherapy were metformin, 57.3%, and SU, 41.2%; in third place by prescription in monotherapy was iDPP-4, 1.0%. The remaining classes of glucose-lowering medications accounted for less than 1% of monotherapy: glinides, 0.5%; iSGLT-2, 0.1%; TZD group, aGLP-1 and iAG—less than 0.01%. The most frequent combinations of two glucose-lowering medications were metformin and SU (92.58%), and metformin and iDPP-4 (5.63%) [19].

In DIGAMI 2, metformin was not associated with lower CVD mortality, but it conferred a reduced risk of non-fatal MI or stroke in the short-term follow-up [39], and lower mortality rates and risk of death from neoplasms in the long-term period [40]. Metformin is considered cardioprotective, since treatment with this agent is associated with a lower risk of mortality (compared with sulfonylurea or insulin therapy) in patients with diabetes and heart failure or MI, and with a decreased risk of non-fatal MI or stroke in patients with diabetes and MI [39]. For example, although some studies found no increased risk of adverse outcomes in patients receiving sulfonylurea before an index event [41], other studies found that patients with diabetes and MI on sulfonylurea, at the time of admission for a CV event had higher CV risk compared with those receiving metformin [42]. According to a large-scale CVD-REAL study (300,000 patients with DM2 from national registers), in clinical practice in Europe and the United States in the structure of GLT for the period of 2015–2017, metformin was prescribed in 78.7%, SU derivatives in 38.7%, iDPP-4 in 33.3%, TZD in 8.9%, aGLP-1 in 20.3%, and insulin in 29.3%, of patients [43].

Lipska KJ et al., 2017, reported a retrospective study based on the U.S. Pharmacological Service, which analyzed the data for 1,657,610 individuals with DM2 (age 18–75+) from 2006 to 2013. During the study period, the use of metformin (from 47.6 to 53.5%), iDDP-4 (from 0.5 to 14.9%), aGLP-1 (from 3.3 to 5.0%) and insulin (from 17.1 to 23.0%) increased, but the proportion of SU (from 38.8 to 30.8%) and TZD (from 28.5 to 5.6%) (all $p < 0.001$) decreased. Increased insulin use was caused primarily by contribution of basal insulin analogs (10.9 to 19.3%; $p < 0.001$) and rapid-acting insulin analogs (6.7 to 11.6%; $p < 0.001$) while the use of human insulin products actually decreased (from 11.6% to 5.6%; $p < 0.001$). The proportion of diabetic patients who did not intake any GLT, decreased slightly (from 25.7% to 24.1%; $p < 0.001$). Considering the complexity of treatment, the use of oral monotherapy increased slightly (from 24.3 to 26.4%) and the use of multiple (two or more) oral agents decreased (from 33.0 to 26.5%), while the use of insulin alone and in combination with oral agents increased (from 6.0 to 8.5%, and from 11.1 to 14.6%, respectively; all values $p < 0.001$) [35].

Similar trends were observed in the Russian Federation, in 2013–2017. The prescription of metformin increased to 68.3% and insulin to 19.8%, and the share of SU decreased to 53.6% [19].

While alogliptin and lixenatide have shown safety in the EXAMINE study in the earlier phase after ACS, empagliflozin (EMPA-REG [44], liraglutide (LEADER [45]), and semaglutide (SUSTAIN-6 [46]) may offer an opportunity for effective secondary prevention of cardiovascular disease. In our region, the percentage of people receiving this therapy is extremely small, which yields a poor level of secondary prevention of CVD in patients with type 2 diabetes.

A recent analysis of patients in the U.S.A. showed no improvement in overall glycemic control and noted an increase in the proportion of patients with HbA1c $\geq$ 9.0% (from 9.9 to 12.2%; $p < 0.001$) between 2006 and 2013, despite the increased use of newer and more expensive glucose-lowering drugs among these patients [35]. These data, combined with our present results, highlight the urgent need to re-evaluate existing therapies for patients with DM2 in order to improve glycemic control.

In the group with effective glucose control, the frequency of metformin use as expected, was higher compared with the group with ineffective control. We found differences neither by the frequency of combined therapy nor by the average number of drugs depending on the effectiveness of glycemic control, in our sample.

5. Study Limitations

The present study had a number of limitations. In a population-based screening, we were not able to assess the level of HbA1c, and the level of blood glucose was measured at one visit, which may have affected the identification of DM2. However, this limitation was minimized by the standardized blood sampling procedure (8 h of fasting, the same personnel and storage protocol) and the performance of analyses according to a unified protocol on one autoanalyzer KoneLab 300i device (Thermo Fisher Scientific Inc., Waltham, MA, USA) using the same Thermo Fisher kits in a certified IIPM—Branch of IC&G SB RAS laboratory.

The antihyperglycemic profile was analyzed on the basis of self-assessment, which may have been a source of inaccuracy. However, about 70% of those receiving GLT named specific drugs; ATC coding was performed by three certified specialists (cardiologists and an endocrinologist); and in the 10% group, reproducibility was controlled with a double-blind approach (coefficient of agreement 0.84); this made it possible to eliminate significant errors in the results. Additionally, the present analysis did not include data on other drugs or comorbidities. The focus of the paper was SLT in a population-based sample of DM2, while the interaction between mentioned conditions and profile of DM2 treatment and glucose control, requires a specific analysis, and is not in the scope of current paper. Furthermore, non-inclusion of other diseases and drugs for the present analysis is unlikely to affect the estimates of coverage by GLT, drug profile and frequency of glucose control among persons with DM2 in a studied population.

Another potential limitation was that we were not able to take into account the regimen and dosage of drugs in a population epidemiological study, but this did not affect the assessment of the frequency of use and the profile of GLT, or the revealed fact of insufficient glycemic control in general. In addition, the applied epidemiological approach provided comparability with a number of population studies, including long-term studies for dynamic evaluation.

The results of the analysis are limited to the Novosibirsk sample and cannot be extrapolated to other Russian regions. At the same time, a typical urban population was studied, which had a country-specific epidemiological profile and medical care practices, as well as mortality rates close to the average Russian mortality rates, and the results allow us to state the insufficiency of GLT on the example of a certain Russian population.

The analysis was carried out in a sample of predominantly elderly people, which limits the generalization of the results, but given the highest incidence of DM2 in older age, the results informatively reflect the profile of GLT in a more susceptible part of the population.

Altogether, this study has several strengths. In general, GLT in the Russian Federation has been investigated by the Federal Register of Diabetes [19]. Data from 2016–2017 on key cardiometabolic factors in the secondary prevention of CVD, including DM2, have recently been discussed on the basis of the Russian sample of EUROASPIRE-V for patients after a coronary event [31]. As an advantage of the present study, we continued monitoring in the Siberian region and provided new knowledge on the assessment of the GLT profile and DM2 control in a non-selective Russian population. The analysis revealed a significant prevalence of undiagnosed DM2 and insufficient glycemic control. In addition, these findings were based on a large sample, for the first time establishing the magnitude of a lack in glucose control at a population level in Russia. In the management of DM2, the proportion of new glucose-lowering medications was shown to be small, and HbA1c monitoring was insufficient for appropriate glycemic control, which has a public health implication to define directions and strengthen efforts for diabetes control.

6. Conclusions

In a population sample of men and women 55–84 years old, examined in a typical Russian city in 2015–2018, the frequency of DM2 was about 21%. Glycemic control was achieved in every fifth participant with DM2 (fasting plasma glucose < 7.0 mmol/L) and in every third participant receiving GLT. Overall, women monitored their blood glucose levels better than men. In the GLT profile in terms of frequency of use, biguanides ranked first place, sulfonylurea derivatives ranked second place, insulins ranked third place, and iDPP-4 ranked fourth place. Combined GLT was used by about one third of individuals with DM2 (24%—oral, and another 6% in combination with insulin). One third of persons with DM2 (including those newly diagnosed) did not receive GLT, which significantly affects the insufficient control of diabetes mellitus in the population.

Author Contributions: Conceptualization, A.R., S.M. (Sofia Malyutina) and E.M. (Elena Mazurenko); data curation, S.M. (Sofia Malyutina) and E.M. (Elena Mazurenko)); formal analysis—S.M. (Sofia Malyutina), E.M. (Elena Mazurenko) and A.R.; funding acquisition, A.R., S.M. (Sofia Malyutina); investigation, E.M. (Ekaterina Mazdorova), M.S., E.A., E.M. (Elena Mazurenko) (and S.M. (Sofia Malyutina); methodology, S.M. (Sofia Malyutina), E.M. (Elena Mazurenko)), E.M. (Ekaterina Mazdorova), M.S. and E.A.; project administration, A.R.; resources—A.R., S.M. (Sofia Malyutina); software, S.M. (Sofia Malyutina); supervision, A.R.; validation, E.M. (Elena Mazurenko), E.M. (Ekaterina Mazdorova), M.S., E.A., S.M. (Svetlana Mustafina) and G.S.; visualization, S.M. (Sofia Malyutina), E.M. (Elena Mazurenko) and A.R.; writing—original draft preparation, S.M. (Sofia Malyutina), E.M. (Elena Mazurenko), A.R.; writing—review and editing, S.M. (Sofia Malyutina), E.M. (Elena Mazurenko), E.M. (Ekaterina Mazdorova), M.S., E.A., S.M. (Svetlana Mustafina), G.S. and A.R. All authors have read and agreed to the published version of the manuscript.

Funding: This study was supported by the Russian Science Foundation, Grant No. 20-15-00371.

Institutional Review Board Statement: The study was conducted according to the guidelines of the Declaration of Helsinki and approved by the Ethics Committee of the Federal State Budgetary Institution "Research Institute of Internal and Preventive Medicine", Siberian Branch of the Russian Academy of Sciences (renamed in 2017: Research Institute of Internal and Preventive Medicine—Branch of the Institute of Cytology and Genetics, Siberian Branch of the Russian Academy of Sciences) Protocol No. 1 as of 14 March 2002 and Protocol No. 12 from 8 December 2020. The study did not involve animals.

Informed Consent Statement: Informed consent was obtained from all subjects involved in the study.

Data Availability Statement: The data presented in this study are available in tabulated form on request. The data are not publicly available due to ethical restrictions and project regulations.

Acknowledgments: The authors acknowledge the core HAPIEE Project for access to baseline cohort and an opportunity to develop a long-term study. We are grateful to E. Verevkin and L. Sherbakova for preparation of the database.

Conflicts of Interest: The authors declare no conflict of interest.

References

1. *IDF Diabetes Atlas*, 9th ed.; International Diabetes Federation: Brussels, Belgium, 2019; Available online: https://www.diabetesatlas.org/en/ (accessed on 5 October 2022).
2. Dedov, I.I.; Shestakova, M.V.; Vikulova, O.K.; Isakov, M.; Zheleznyakova, A.V. Atlas of Diabetes Register in Russian Federation, status 2018. *Diabetes Mellit.* **2019**, *22*, 4–61. [CrossRef]

3. Nikitin, Y.P.; Voevoda, M.I.; Simonova, G.I. Diabetes mellitus and metabolic syndrome in Siberia and in the far east. *Ann. Russ. Acad. Med. Sci.* **2012**, *67*, 66–74. [CrossRef]
4. Mustafina, S.V.; Rymar, O.D.; Malyutina, S.K.; Denisova, D.V.; Shcherbakova, L.V.; Voevoda, M.I. Prevalence of diabetes in the adult population of Novosibirsk. *Diabetes Mellit.* **2017**, *20*, 329–334. [CrossRef]
5. Vikulova, O.K.; Zheleznyakova, A.V.; Isakov, M.A.; Serkov, A.A.; Shestakova, M.V.; Dedov, I.I. Dynamic monitoring of HbA1c in Russian regions: Data comparison of mobile medical center (Diamodul) and national diabetes register of Russian Federation. *Diabetes Mellit.* **2020**, *23*, 104–112. [CrossRef]
6. Stratton, I.M.; Adler, A.I.; Neil, H.A.; Matthews, D.R.; Manley, S.E.; Cull, C.A.; Hadden, D.; Turner, R.C.; Holman, R.R. Association of glycaemia with macrovascular and microvascular complications of type 2 diabetes (UKPDS 35): Prospective observational study. *BMJ* **2000**, *321*, 405–412. [CrossRef]
7. Inzucchi, S.E.; Bergenstal, R.M.; Buse, J.B.; Diamant, M.; Ferrannini, E.; Nauck, M.A.; Peters, A.; Tsapas, A.; Wender, R.; Matthews, D.R. Management of hyperglycaemia in type 2 diabetes, 2015: A patient-centred approach. Update to a position statement of the American Diabetes Association and the European Association for the Study of Diabetes. *Diabetologia* **2015**, *58*, 429–442. [CrossRef]
8. Chinese Diabetes Society. Chinese guideline for type 2 diabetes prevention (2013). *Chin. J. Diabetes* **2014**, *22*, 2–42.
9. American Diabetes Association. Standards of medical care in diabetes—2017. *Diabetes Care* **2017**, *40* (Suppl. S1), S1–S132.
10. Garber, A.J.; Abrahamson, M.J.; Barzilay, J.I.; Blonde, L.; Bloomgarden, Z.T.; Bush, M.A.; Dagogo-Jack, S.; Davidson, M.B.; Einhorn, D.; Garber, J.R.; et al. AACE/ACE comprehensive diabetes management algorithm 2015. *Endocr. Pract.* **2015**, *21*, 438–447. [CrossRef]
11. Buse, J.B.; Wexler, D.J.; Tsapas, A.; Rossing, P.; Mingrone, G.; Mathieu, C.; D'Alessio, D.A.; Davies, M.J. 2019 update to: Management of hyperglycaemia in type 2 diabetes, 2018. A consensus report by the American Diabetes Association (ADA) and the European Association for the Study of Diabetes (EASD). *Diabetologia* **2020**, *63*, 221–228. [CrossRef] [PubMed]
12. Dedov, I.; Shestakova, M.; Mayorov, A.; Vikulova, O.; Gagik, G.; Kuraeva, T.; Peterkova, V.; Smirnova, O.; Starostina, E.; Surkova, E.; et al. Standards of specialized diabetes care. *Diabetes Mellit.* **2019**, *22*, 1–144. [CrossRef]
13. Juarez, D.T.; Ma, C.; Kumasaka, A.; Shimada, R.; Davis, J. Failure to reach target glycated A1C levels among patients with diabetes who are adherent to their antidiabetic medication. *Popul. Health Manag.* **2014**, *17*, 218–223. [CrossRef] [PubMed]
14. Khunti, K.; Gomes, M.B.; Pocock, S.; Shestakova, M.V.; Pintat, S.; Fenici, P.; Hammar, N.; Medina, J. Therapeutic inertia in the treatment of hyperglycaemia in patients with type 2 diabetes: A systematic review. *Diabetes Obes. Metab.* **2018**, *20*, 427–437. [CrossRef] [PubMed]
15. Kotseva, K.; De Backer, G.; De Bacquer, D.; Ryden, L.; Hoes, A.; Grobbee, D.; Maggioni, A.; Marques-Vidal, P.; Jennings, C.; Abreu, A.; et al. Lifestyle and impact on cardiovascular risk factor control in coronary patients across 27 countries: Results from the European Society of Cardiology ESC-EORP EUROASPIRE V registry. *Eur. J. Prev. Cardiol.* **2019**, *26*, 824–835. [CrossRef]
16. Selvin, E.; Parrinello, C.M.; Sacks, D.B.; Coresh, J. Trends in prevalence and control of diabetes in the United States, 1988–1994 and 1999–2010. *Ann. Intern. Med.* **2014**, *160*, 517–525. [CrossRef] [PubMed]
17. Khunti, K.; Chen, H.; Cid-Ruzafa, J.; Fenici, P.; Gomes, M.B.; Hammar, N.; Ji, L.; Kosiborod, M.; Pocock, S.; Shestakova, M.V.; et al. Glycaemic control in patients with type 2 diabetesinitiating second-line therapy: Results from the global DISCOVER study programme. *Diabetes Obes. Metab.* **2020**, *22*, 66–78. [CrossRef] [PubMed]
18. Fang, M.; Wang, D.; Coresh, J.; Selvin, E. Trends in Diabetes Treatment and Control in U.S. Adults, 1999–2018. *N. Engl. J. Med.* **2021**, *384*, 2219–2228. [CrossRef]
19. Dedov, I.I.; Shestakova, M.V.; Vikulova, O.K.; Zheleznyakova, A.A.; Isakov, M.A. Diabetes mellitus in Russian Federation: Prevalence, morbidity, mortality, parameters of glycaemic control and structure of hypoglycaemic therapy according to the Federal Diabetes Register, status 2017. *Diabetes Mellit.* **2018**, *21*, 144–159. [CrossRef]
20. Malyutina, S.K.; Shapkina, M.Y.; Ryabikov, A.N.; Mazdorova, E.V.; Avdeeva, E.M.; Shcherbakova, L.V.; Bobak, M.; Hubacek, J.A.; Nikitin, Y.P. Characteristics of main drug therapy types in subjects with atrial fibrillation in population. *Cardiovasc. Ther. Prev.* **2018**, *17*, 43–48. [CrossRef]
21. Malyutina, S.K.; Mazdorova, E.V.; Shapkina, M.Y.; Avdeeva, E.M.; Maslacov, N.A.; Simonova, G.I.; Bobak, M.; Nikitin, Y.P.; Ryabikov, A.N. The profile of drug treatment in subjects aged over 50 years with hypertension in an urban Russian population. *Kardiologiia* **2020**, *60*, 21–29. [CrossRef]
22. Malyutina, S.K.; Mazdorova, E.V.; Shapkina, M.Y.; Avdeeva, E.M.; Simonova, G.I.; Hubacek, J.A.; Bobak, M.; Nikitin, Y.P.; Ryabikov, A.N. The frequency and profile of drug treatment in subjects with dyslipidemias and cardiometabolic diseases in an urban Russian population older then 55 years. *Kardiologiia* **2021**, *61*, 49–58. [CrossRef] [PubMed]
23. Peasey, A.; Bobak, M.; Kubinova, R.; Malyutina, S.; Pajak, A.; Tamosiunas, A.; Pikhart, H.; Nicholson, A.; Marmot, M. Determinants of cardiovascular disease and other non-communicable diseases in Central and Eastern Europe: Rationale and design of the HAPIEE study. *BMC Public Health* **2006**, *6*, 255. [CrossRef] [PubMed]
24. Williams, B.; Mancia, G.; Spiering, W.; Agabiti Rosei, E.; Azizi, M.; Burnier, M.; Clement, D.L.; Coca, A.; De Simone, G.; Dominiczak, A.; et al. 2018 ESC/ESH Guidelines for the management of arterial hypertension. The Task Force for the management of arterial hypertension of the European Society of Cardiology (ESC) and the European Society of Hypertension (ESH). *J. Hypertens.* **2018**, *36*, 1953–2041. [CrossRef]

25. Rydén, L.; Standl, E.; Bartnik, M.; van den Berghe, G.; Betteridge, J.; de Boer, M.; Cosentino, F.; Jönsson, B.; Laakso, M.; Malmberg, K.; et al. Guidelines on diabetes, pre-diabetes, and cardiovascular diseases: Executive summary: The Task Force on Diabetes and Cardiovascular Diseases of the European Society of Cardiology (ESC) and of the European Association for the Study of Diabetes (EASD). *Eur. Heart J.* **2007**, *28*, 88–136. [CrossRef]
26. Authors/Task Force Members; Rydén, L.; Grant, P.J.; Anker, S.D.; Berne, C.; Cosentino, F.; Danchin, N.; Deaton, C.; Escaned, J.; Hammes, H.; et al. ESC Guidelines on diabetes, pre-diabetes, and cardiovascular diseases developed in collaboration with the EASD: The Task Force on diabetes, pre-diabetes, and cardiovascular diseases of the European Society of Cardiology (ESC) and developed in collaboration with the European Association for the Study of Diabetes (EASD). *Eur. Heart J.* **2013**, *34*, 3035–3087. [CrossRef]
27. Rose, G.A.; Blackburn, H.; Gillim, R.F.; Prineas, R.J. *Cardiovascular Survey Methods*, 2nd ed.; WHO: Geneva, Switzerland, 1984; p. 223. ISBN 9242400564.
28. Kalinina, A.M.; Shalnova, S.A.; Gambaryan, M.G.; Eganyan, R.A.; Muromtseva, G.A.; Bochkareva, E.V.; Kim, I.V. *Epidemiological Methods for Identifying the Main Chronic Non-Communicable Diseases and Risk Factors during Mass Population Surveys. Methodical Guide*; Boytsov, S.A.-M., Ed.; GNICPM: Russia, 2015; 96p, Available online: http://www.gnicpm.ru (accessed on 5 October 2022).
29. WHO Collaborating Centre for Drug Statistics Methodology. Guidelines for ATC Classification and DDD Assignment. 2019. Available online: https://www.whocc.no/atc_ddd_index_and_guidelines/atc_ddd_index/ (accessed on 5 October 2022).
30. Ohara, C.; Inoue, K.; Kashima, S.; Inoue, M.; Akimoto, K. Undiagnosed diabetes has poorer profiles for cardiovascular and metabolic markers than known diabetes: The Yuport Medical Checkup Center Study. *Diabetes Res. Clin. Pract.* **2013**, *101*, e7–e10. [CrossRef]
31. Phan, K.; Mitchell, P.; Liew, G.; Plant, A.J.; Wang, S.B.; Xu, J.; Chiha, J.; Thiagalingam, A.; Burlutsky, G.; Gopinath, B. Severity of coronary artery disease and retinal microvascular signs in patients with diagnosed versus undiagnosed diabetes: Cross-sectional study. *J. Thorac. Dis.* **2016**, *8*, 1532–1539. [CrossRef] [PubMed]
32. Aggarwal, B.; Shah, G.K.; Randhawa, M.; Ellis, S.G.; Lincoff, A.M.; Menon, V. Utility of glycated hemoglobin for assessment of glucose metabolism in patients with ST-segment elevation myocardial infarction. *Am. J. Cardiol.* **2016**, *117*, 749–753. [CrossRef]
33. George, A.; Bhatia, R.T.; Buchanan, G.L.; Whiteside, A.; Moisey, R.S.; Beer, S.F.; Chattopadhyay, S.; Sathyapalan, T.; John, J. Impaired glucose tolerance or newly diagnosed diabetes mellitus diagnosed during admission adversely affects prognosis after myocardial infarction: An observational study. *PLoS ONE* **2015**, *10*, e0142045. [CrossRef]
34. Avogaro, A.; Bonora, E.; Consoli, A.; Del Prato, S.; Genovese, S.; Giorgino, F. Glucose-lowering therapy and cardiovascular outcomes in patients with type 2 diabetes mellitus and acute coronary syndrome. *Diabetes Vasc. Dis. Res.* **2019**, *16*, 399–414. [CrossRef] [PubMed]
35. Lipska, K.J.; Yao, X.; Herrin, J.; McCoy, R.G.; Ross, J.S.; Steinman, M.A.; Inzucchi, S.E.; Gill, T.M.; Krumholz, H.M.; Shah, N.D. Trends in Drug Utilization, Glycemic Control, and Rates of Severe Hypoglycemia, 2006–2013. *Diabetes Care* **2017**, *40*, 468–475. [CrossRef]
36. Pogosova, N.V.; Oganov, R.G.; Boytsov, S.A.; Ausheva, A.K.; Sokolova, O.Y.; Kursakov, A.A.; Osipova, I.V.; Antropova, O.N.; Pozdnyakov, Y.M.; Salbieva, A.O.; et al. Secondary prevention in patients with coronary artery disease in Russia and Europe: Results from the Russian part of the EUROASPIRE V survey. *Cardiovasc. Ther. Prev.* **2020**, *19*, 2739. [CrossRef]
37. Casagrande, S.; Cowie, C.C.; Fradkin, J.E. Intensive glycemic control in younger and older U.S. adults with type 2 diabetes. *J. Diabetes Complicat.* **2017**, *31*, 1299–1304, Erratum in *J. Diabetes Complicat.* **2019**, *33*, 406. [CrossRef]
38. Langholz, P.L.; Wilsgaard, T.; Njølstad, I.; Jorde, R.; Hopstock, L.A. Trends in known and undiagnosed diabetes, HbA1c levels, cardiometabolic risk factors and diabetes treatment target achievement in repeated cross-sectional surveys: The population-based Tromsø Study 1994–2016. *BMJ Open* **2021**, *11*, e041846. [CrossRef] [PubMed]
39. Mellbin, L.G.; Malmberg, K.; Norhammar, A.; Wedel, H.; Rydén, L.; DIGAMI 2 Investigators. The impact of glucose lowering treatment on long-term prognosis in patients with type 2 diabetes and myocardial infarction: A report from the DIGAMI 2 trial. *Eur. Heart J.* **2008**, *29*, 166–176. [CrossRef]
40. Mellbin, L.G.; Malmberg, K.; Norhammar, A.; Wedel, H.; Rydén, L.; DIGAMI 2 Investigators. Prognostic implications of glucose-lowering treatment in patients with acute myocardial infarction and diabetes: Experiences from an extended follow-up of the Diabetes Mellitus Insulin-Glucose Infusion in Acute Myocardial Infarction (DIGAMI) 2 Study. *Diabetologia* **2011**, *54*, 1308–1317. [CrossRef]
41. Zeller, M.; Danchin, N.; Simon, D.; Vahanian, A.; Lorgis, L.; Cottin, Y.; Berland, J.; Gueret, P.; Wyart, P.; Deturck, R.; et al. Impact of type of preadmission sulfonylureas on mortality and cardiovascular outcomes in diabetic patients with acute myocardial infarction. *J. Clin. Endocrinol. Metab.* **2010**, *95*, 4993–5002. [CrossRef]
42. Jørgensen, C.H.; Gislason, G.H.; Andersson, C.; Ahlehoff, O.; Charlot, M.; Schramm, T.K.; Vaag, A.; Abildstrøm, S.Z.; Torp-Pedersen, C.; Hansen, P.R. Effects of oral glucose-lowering drugs on long term outcomes in patients with diabetes mellitus following myocardial infarction not treated with emergent percutaneous coronary intervention—A retrospective nationwide cohort study. *Cardiovasc. Diabetol.* **2010**, *9*, 54. [CrossRef]
43. Kosiborod, M.; Cavender, M.A.; Fu, A.Z.; Wilding, J.; Khunti, K.; Holl, R.W.; Norhammar, A.; Birkeland, K.I.; Jørgensen, M.E.; Thuresson, M.; et al. Lower Risk of HeartFailure and Death in Patients Initiated on Sodium-Glucose Cotransporter-2 Inhibitors Versus Other Glucose-Lowering Drugs: The CVD-REAL Study (Comparative Effectiveness of Cardiovascular Outcomes in New Users of Sodium-Glucose Cotransporter-2 Inhibitors). *Circulation* **2017**, *136*, 249–259. [CrossRef] [PubMed]

44. Zinman, B.; Wanner, C.; Lachin, J.M.; Fitchett, D.; Bluhmki, E.; Hantel, S.; Mattheus, M.; Devins, T.; Johansen, O.E.; Woerle, H.J.; et al. Empagliflozin, Cardiovascular Outcomes, and Mortality in Type 2 Diabetes. *N. Engl. J. Med.* **2015**, *373*, 2117–2128. [CrossRef] [PubMed]
45. Marso, S.P.; Daniels, G.H.; Brown-Frandsen, K.; Kristensen, P.; Mann, J.F.; Nauck, M.A.; Nissen, S.E.; Pocock, S.; Poulter, N.R.; Ravn, L.S.; et al. Liraglutide and cardiovascular outcomes in type 2 diabetes. *N. Eng. J. Med.* **2016**, *375*, 311–322. [CrossRef]
46. Marso, S.P.; Bain, S.C.; Consoli, A.; Eliaschewitz, F.G.; Jódar, E.; Leiter, L.A.; Lingvay, I.; Rosenstock, J.; Seufert, J.; Warren, M.L.; et al. Semaglutide and cardiovascular outcomes in patients with type 2 diabetes. *N. Eng. J. Med.* **2016**, *375*, 1834–1844. [CrossRef] [PubMed]

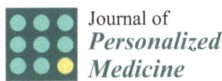

Systematic Review

Stomatognathic System Changes in Obese Patients Undergoing Bariatric Surgery: A Systematic Review

Gerson Fabián Gualdrón-Bobadilla [1], Anggie Paola Briceño-Martínez [1], Víctor Caicedo-Téllez [1], Ginna Pérez-Reyes [1], Carlos Silva-Paredes [2], Rina Ortiz-Benavides [3], Mary Carlota Bernal [4], Diego Rivera-Porras [5,*] and Valmore Bermúdez [6]

1. Facultad de Salud, Universidad de Pamplona, Pamplona 543050, Colombia
2. Facultad de Medicina, Universidad del Zulia, Maracaibo 4002, Venezuela
3. Facultad de Medicine, Universidad Católica de Cuenca, Cuenca 010109, Ecuador
4. Facultad de Ingenierías, Universidad Simón Bolívar, Cúcuta 540001, Colombia
5. Facultad de Ciencias Jurídicas y Sociales, Universidad Simón Bolívar, Cúcuta 540001, Colombia
6. Facultad de Ciencias de la Salud, Universidad Simón Bolívar, Barranquilla 080022, Colombia
* Correspondence: d.rivera@unisimonbolivar.edu.co

Abstract: Background: Obesity is a multifactorial chronic disease involving multiple organs, devices, and systems involving important changes in the stomatognathic system, such as in the orofacial muscles, temporomandibular joint, cheeks, nose, jaw, maxilla, oral cavity, lips, teeth, tongue, hard/soft palate, larynx, and pharynx. Patients with obesity indicated for bariatric surgery reportedly presented with abnormalities in the structures and function of the stomatognathic apparatus. This occurs through the accumulation of adipose tissue in the oral cavity and pharyngeal and laryngeal regions. Therefore, this systematic review aimed to elucidate the changes occurring in the stomatognathic system of patients with obesity after undergoing bariatric surgery. Method: Information was searched based on the equations developed with the descriptors obtained in DECS and MESH using the PRISMA methodology. Studies published between 2010 and October 2021 in databases including PubMed, ProQuest, Scielo, Dialnet, EBSCO, and Springer Link were considered. Results: Eighty articles met the inclusion criteria after evaluating the articles, thereby allowing for the determination of the morphophysiological correlation of the stomatognathic system with the population studied. At the morphological or structural level, changes were observed in the face, nose, cheeks, maxilla, jaw, lips, oral cavity, teeth, tongue, palate, temporomandibular joint, neck, muscles, head, shoulders, larynx, and pharynx. At the morphological level, the main changes occurred in, and the most information was obtained from, the labial structures, teeth, muscles, pharynx, and larynx. Physiological changes were in breathing, phonation, chewing, and swallowing, thereby revealing the imbalance in basic and vital functions. Conclusions: Analyzing the changes and structures of obese patients and candidates for bariatric surgery revealed that, in the preoperative period, the evidence is clear owing to the presence of a wide range of information. However, the information is more limited regarding the postoperative period; thus, further research focusing on characterization of the system postoperatively is warranted.

Keywords: obesity; bariatric surgery; stomatognathic system; physiology

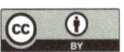

1. Introduction

The stomatognathic system is an integrated and coordinated morpho-functional unit comprising skeletal, muscular, angiological, nervous, glandular, and dental structures organized around the occipito-atloidal, atlantoaxial, cervical vertebral, temporomandibular, dento-dental in occlusion, and dentoalveolar joints, which are organically ligated and functionally related to the digestive, respiratory, phonological, and facial aesthetic expression systems. Consequently, this system is associated with the senses of taste, touch, balance, and orientation. It intervenes in functions of suction, oral digestion (mastication, salivation, tasting, and degradation of carbohydrates), swallowing, verbal communication (phonological modulation, articulation of sounds, speech, and whistles), oral sexuality (smiling, laughing, orofacial gesticulation, and kissing, among other aesthetic-affective manifestations), alternate breathing, and vital defense (coughing, expectorating, sneezing, yawning, sighing, and exhalation and vomiting), which are considered essential for an individual's survival [1].

Obesity has become a 21st century problem, as well as one of the fastest growing health problems worldwide [2,3]. Currently, it is one of the most important and concerning public health conditions, which is why it has become a priority [4]. According to the Center for Disease Control and Prevention, obesity is defined as "weight above what is adequate or considered healthy given the height of each subject". Concurrently, it defines it as a chronic disease requiring timely medical care, thereby limiting the activities of daily living. Its main characteristic is excessive accumulation of body fat that has harmful effects on health. However, it is considered a treatable disease [3,5,6].

According to statistics from the World Health Organization (WHO), in 2005, 1.6 billion people aged > 15 years were classified as overweight and 400 million were classified as obese [7]. Currently, there are approximately 1200 million people in the world with problems related to overweight and obesity [8]. This constitutes evidence of high levels of prevalence of the disease, which affects approximately 23% of the adult population of Latin America and the Caribbean, or ~140 million people [9].

However, the Colombian Ministry of Health and Social Protection (MinSalud) estimates that the prevalence of overweight people in Colombia is approximately 56.4% and, thus, it is considered a public health problem for the country. Based on data provided by the same entity, it is predicted that, by the year 2030, 1 out of 2 adults will be obese, and 1 in 4 adults will have severe obesity [10,11]. However, obesity is a preventable disease, and it can be addressed through multidisciplinary intervention, which includes allowing the interaction of several professionals during treatment, involving diet, physical exercise, and pharmacological treatment [12]. However, the combination of eating, sports, and medicinal habits is sometimes not effective or successful. Therefore, patients resort to extreme alternatives, such as bariatric surgery, since it provides an effective solution to the problem in order to reduce food intake and nutrient absorption. This is despite the fact that the procedure includes invasive surgical intervention in the digestive system [2,13]. It is necessary to clarify that not everyone is an ideal candidate for the procedure, even though bariatric surgery is a reliable method for long-term weight loss. Candidates must at least be adults, with a body mass index (BMI) $\geq 40 \text{ kg/m}^2$ or with a BMI between 35 and 39.9 kg/m^2 and a severe associated comorbidity [12,13].

Historically, bariatric surgery emerged in the United States in the 1950s. It was the pioneering country in the American continent, followed by Brazil, the second country in the world to perform more bariatric surgeries, with approximately 80,000 surgeries per year [4,14]. For this approach, it must be highlighted that a suitable bariatric technique must primarily be very safe; i.e., with a morbidity of <10% and a mortality of <1%. Second, such a technique must be able to cause the loss of at least 50% of the additional weight, which must be maintained for a period of approximately 5 years, thereby improving the patient's quality of life. It should be noted that there are three techniques for performing these interventions (malabsorptive, restrictive, and mixed) [15]. The restrictive technique consists of reducing the capacity of the stomach and preventing the passage of food. However, over time, this technique forces patients to undergo a reintervention. The malabsorptive technique reduces the capacity of the stomach by half, producing crossover with the intestine, so that there is a malabsorption of nutrients from food, forcing the patient into restrictive control after surgery. The mixed technique has a restrictive and somewhat malabsorptive character, which allows it to be a well-tolerated procedure, without the patient presenting long-term complications or requiring reintervention [16]. Another technique used to address this problem is sleeve gastrectomy (SG) (the malabsorptive type), and it has been the most commonly performed technique in the world, and in Colombia, since 2004, followed by the Roux-en-Y gastric bypass (RYGB) (the mixed type) [17].

In conclusion, it is important to highlight that, despite the many benefits of making use of this procedure, there are also various changes and anomalies in the structures and functioning of the different systems, including the stomatognathic system [18,19]. The literature and the investigated studies make it clear that these anomalies severely compromise the entire stomatognathic system due to the accumulation of adipose tissue in the oral cavity and in the pharyngeal and laryngeal regions [19], with the adiposity of these regions being the etiology responsible for the changes in these large and important structures of the patient, thus compromising morphology and physiology [20]. Considering the arguments and findings previously revealed, the following research question arises: how are the stomatognathic systems of obese patients, and those of obese patients with bariatric surgery, characterized?

2. Materials and Methods

This review was performed following the parameters proposed by the PRISMA methodology. For this, the databases were identified, and thesauruses were defined in the search for information. The studies were also selected based on inclusion and exclusion criteria that facilitated the assessment of the studies' quality and reliability and that, eventually, allowed answering the research question posed [21–23].

The PICO tool was used to construct the research question. This tool was employed owing to the fact that it is used to improve the specificity and conceptual clarity of the clinical problems to be studied, as well as to perform searches with greater quality and precision, which allows for the collection of pertinent and accurate data to answer the problem question [24,25].

2.1. Research Question

In accordance with the theme established for the research, the components of the PICO strategy shown in Table 1 were established, resulting in the following research question: how are the stomatognathic systems of obese patients, and those of obese patients with bariatric surgery, characterized?

Table 1. Research Question.

Component	Description
P: Patient or problem of interest (Population)	Obese patient and post-bariatric surgery
I: Intervention	Assessment of the stomatognathic system
C: Comparison	Stomatognathic system
O: Outcome	Alterations or changes in anatomical and functional structures

2.1.1. Inclusion Criteria

1. Overweight subjects, those with obesity or morbid obesity, or those who had undergone bariatric surgery
2. A publication time window of 10 years;
3. Articles focused on the evaluation of aspects related to the distal airways, upper airways, lower airways, stomatognathic system (morphology and physiology), respiratory system, masticatory system, and swallowing mechanics;
4. Studies conducted with humans;
5. Full-text articles;
6. Free-access articles and current DOIs.

2.1.2. Exclusion Criteria
1. Articles with DOIs that were not current within the databases for download;
2. Research with a time window of >10 years;
3. Articles that were not related to human beings;
4. Grey literature, such as theses, white books, research and project reports, annual or activity reports, conference proceedings, preprints, working papers, newsletters, technical reports, recommendations and technical standards, patents, technical notes, data and statistics, presentations, field notes, laboratory research books, abstracts, academic courseware, lecture notes, and evaluations, were excluded.

2.2. Sources of Information

The key terms were selected from the Descriptors in Health Sciences (DECS) and the Medical Subject Headings (MESH) (see Table 2).

Table 2. DECS and MESH descriptors.

Source	Keyword	Related Terms
DECS	Distal airways	No records found
MESH	Distal airways	No records found
DECS	Obesity	No records found
MESH	Obesity	Morbid obesity, excess adipose tissue, abnormal weight gain
DECS	Overweight	No records found
MESH	Overweight	Excess weight, increased body fat, increased adipose tissue
DECS	Bariatric surgery	No records found
MESH	Bariatric surgery	Weight reduction, metabolic surgery, bariatric surgical procedure, stomach stapling, gastroenterostomy, gastric bypass, gastroplasty, jejunoileal bypass, lobectomy, lipoabdominoplasty
DECS	Upper respiratory tract	No records found
MESH	Upper respiratory tract	Respiratory system, respiratory tract, upper respiratory tract
DECS	Lower respiratory tract	No records found
MESH	Lower respiratory tract	No records found
DECS	Respiratory system	No records found
MESH	Respiratory system	Airways, respiratory function
DECS	Masticatory system	No records found
MESH	Masticatory system	Stomatognathic system
DECS	Masticatory apparatus	No records found
MESH	Masticatory apparatus	No records found
DECS	Masticatory dynamic	No records found
MESH	Masticatory dynamic	No records found
DECS	Swallowing disorder	No records found
MESH	Swallowing disorder	Swallowing disorder, difficulty swallowing, dysphagia
DECS	Swallowing reflex	No records found
MESH	Swallowing reflex	No records found
DECS	Swallowing physiology	No records found
MESH	Swallowing physiology	No records found

Table 2. *Cont.*

Source	Keyword	Related Terms
DECS	Swallowing biomechanics	No records found
MESH	Swallowing biomechanics	No records found
DECS	Dysphagia	No records found
MESH	Dysphagia	Swallowing disorder, neuromuscular disorder, or mechanical obstruction
DECS	Aspiration	No records found
MESH	Aspiration	Pneumonia, respiratory aspiration
DECS	Myofunctional disorder	No records found
MESH	Myofunctional disorder	No records found
DECS	Orofacial disorder	No records found
MESH	Orofacial disorder	No records found
DECS	Swallowing	No records found
MESH	Swallowing	Swallow
DECS	Masticatory alteration	No records found
MESH	Masticatory alteration	No records found
DECS	Orofacial motor skills	No records found
MESH	Orofacial motor skills	No records found
DECS	Myofunctional therapy	No records found
MESH	Myofunctional therapy	Orofacial myotherapy, orofacial myologies
DECS	Stomatognathic system	No records found
MESH	Stomatognathic system	No records found
DECS	Breathing	No records found
MESH	Breathing	Breath work
DECS	Suction	No records found
MESH	Suction	No records found
DECS	Speech	No records found
MESH	Speech	Verbal communication
DECS	Phonation	No records found
MESH	Phonation	Sound production
DECS	Chewing	No records found
MESH	Chewing	No records found

Source: Information obtained from DECS and MESH.

2.2.1. Search Strategies

A search strategy was developed with the aid of trained institutional professional librarians from la Universidad Simón Bolívar, Colombia, and la Universidad de Pamplona, Colombia.

Subsequently, the search equations were designed with the terms found. These equations were created using the logical operators AND/OR/NOT and symbols such as "" and (). The information search was conducted in PubMed, ProQuest, Scielo, Dialnet, EBSCO, and Springer Link in the English language (see Table 3).

Table 3. Search equations.

Database	Search Algorithm
PubMed, ProQuest, Scielo, Dialnet, EBSCO, and Springer Link	("Bariatric Surgery") AND ("Disorders") AND ("Myofunctional")
	("Bariatric Surgery") AND ("Disorders") AND ("Myofunctional" OR "Orofacial") OR ("Disorder Physiology") AND ("Obesity")
	("Alteration") AND ("Masticatory System") AND ("bariatric surgery" OR "Obese")
	("Deglutition") AND ("bariatric surgery" OR "Obese")
	("Orofacial Motor Skills") AND ("Physiology")
	("Myofunctional Therapy" OR "Stomatognathic System") AND ("Physiology")
	("Orofacial") AND ("Disorder") AND ("bariatric surgery") AND ("Respiration" OR "Suction" OR "Swallowing" OR "Speech" OR "Phonation")
	("Orofacial" OR "Bariatric Surgery") AND ("Breathing")
	("Orofacial") AND ("Disorder") AND ("Bariatric Surgery") AND ("Suction")
	("Disorder") AND ("Bariatric Surgery") AND ("Swallowing")
	("Bariatric Surgery") AND ("Speech")
	("Disorder") AND ("Bariatric Surgery") AND ("Phonation")
	("Orofacial") AND ("Disorder") AND ("Obesity") AND ("Breathing")
	("Orofacial") AND ("Disorder") AND ("Obesity") AND ("Suction")
	("Orofacial") AND ("Obesity") AND ("Swallowing")
	("Orofacial") AND ("Disorder") AND ("Obesity") AND ("Speech")
	("Orofacial") AND ("Disorder") AND ("Obesity") AND ("Phonation")
	("Distal Airways") AND ("Obesity")
	("Distal Airways") AND ("Overweight")
	("Distal Airways") AND ("Obesity") AND ("Bariatric Surgery")
	("Distal Airways") AND ("Overweight") AND ("Bariatric Surgery")
	("Upper Airways") AND ("Obesity")
	("Upper Respiratory Tract") AND ("Overweight")
	("Upper Airway") AND ("Overweight") AND ("Bariatric Surgery")
	("Lower Respiratory Tract") AND ("Obesity")
	("Lower Respiratory") AND ("Overweight")
	("Lower Respiratory Tract") AND ("Obesity") AND ("Bariatric Surgery")
	("Respiratory System") AND ("Obesity")
	("Masticatory System") AND ("Obesity")
	("Masticatory Apparatus") AND ("Obesity")
	("Masticatory Dynamics") AND ("Obesity")
	("Swallowing Disorder") AND ("Obesity")
	("Swallowing Reflex") AND ("Obesity")
	("Swallowing Physiology") AND ("Obesity")
	("Swallowing Biomechanics") AND ("Obesity")
	("Dysphagia") AND ("Obesity")
	("Aspiration") AND ("Obesity")

2.2.2. Characteristics of the Studies

Initially, the interventions and the respective descriptions of the treatment therapy were classified. Likewise, these interventions were compared from the perspective of the control and experimental groups—based on the characteristics of the therapies—including the model, the technique (if applicable), whether they involved group or individual interventions, the characteristics of the sessions (number of sessions and frequency and duration of each session), the effectiveness and benefit of therapies, the intervention protocol, randomization, and the characteristics of the participants.

Additionally, the characteristics of the therapists and evaluators of the results, the follow-up in time after the interventions, and the findings of the studies were identified. In cases of missing or unclear data, emails were sent requesting the additional information.

2.3. Selection and Analysis

Initially, a preliminary selection of studies based on a review of inclusion criteria, population characteristics, type of study, and year was taken into consideration. Subsequently, a registration table was filled out independently in Excel, prepared by the authors, in which the key elements of each of the selected studies were specified. The process used in the identification, screening, eligibility, and inclusion of articles is briefly described, following the structure proposed by the PRISMA statement [26].

3. Results

The eligibility criteria were determined following the order established in the methodology by developing each of the phases of the PRISMA flowchart (Figure 1).

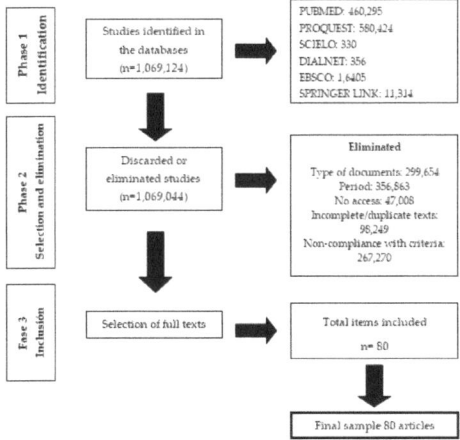

Figure 1. PRISM diagram.

3.1. Identification Phase

The search was performed in the databases PubMed, ProQuest, Scielo, Dialnet, EBSCO, and Springer Link, according to the crosses of variables constructed from DECS and MESH keywords. Then, the following filters were applied: type of document, time window, full or duplicate text, articles without access, and non-compliance with criteria. Finally, articles were selected to obtain the final sample of 80 articles that were used in this investigation (See Table 4).

Table 4. Filters applied.

Database	Total Articles	Type of Document	Period	Incomplete and/or Duplicate Texts	No Access	Non-Compliance with Criteria	Selected Articles
PUBMED	460,295	29,752	330,324	79,016	20,345	832	26
PROQUEST	580,424	259,904	18,580	18,667	24,348	258,901	24
SCIELO	330	120	36	32	15	111	16
DIALNET	356	43	43	1	0	266	3
EBSCO	16,405	5280	4012	3	0	7105	5
SPRINGER LINK	11,314	4555	3868	530	2300	55	6
TOTAL	1,069,124	299,654	356,863	98,249	47,008	267,270	80

3.2. Selection and Elimination Phase

The initial selection of the research articles was carried out through the preliminary reading of the titles, summaries, and, later, the introduction, allowing the identification of the most relevant articles regarding the subject under investigation, with a total of 80 selected articles. The results for each variable crossing in English are listed below (see Table 5) for the six PubMed, ProQuest, Scielo, Dialnet, EBSCO, and Springer Link databases.

Table 5. Results of the English language crosses in the databases.

Matches/Databases	PUBMED	PROQUEST	SCIELO	DIALNET	EBSCO	SPRINGER LINK
Obesity + Bariatric Surgery	7	8	3	1	1	1
Obesity + Stomatognathic System	6	6	5	2	1	2
Obesity + Physiology	9	6	8	0	3	3
Obesity + Upper Airway	2	2	0	0	0	0
Obesity + Lower Airway	2	2	0	0	0	0
Total	26	24	16	3	5	6

In the first search, 17 crosses were made in English between the different variables, resulting in 26 articles from PubMed, 24 from ProQuest, 16 from Scielo, 3 from Dialnet, 5 from EBSCO, and 6 from Springer Link, for a total of 80 items.

3.3. Inclusion Phase

The selection proceeded after reading the titles and the summaries of the articles, and they were analyzed in their entirety with a complete read-through, applying criteria that allowed a selection that, thus, made it possible to obtain those that clearly answered the question posed initially. The selection corresponded to a final sample of 80 articles (See Table 6).

Table 6. Study selection.

N	Database	Title	Author	Year	URL
1	DIALNET	Standardized care plan in bariatric surgery [27]	Mesa García, C; Muñoz Del Castillo, M.	2016	https://dialnet-unirioja-es.unipamplona.basesdedatosezproxy.com/servlet/articulo?codigo=7801587 (accessed on 23 November 2021)
2	DIALNET	Formulation of criteria to record tongue position in patients with atypical swallowing [28]	Pachon Salem, L. E.	2016	https://dialnet.unirioja.es/descarga/articulo/6045809.pdf (accessed on 23 November 2021)
3	DIALNET	Structural and Functional Alterations of the Stomatognathic System: Speech-Language Management [29]	Pérez Serey, J; Hernández Mosqueira, C; Fuenzalida Cabezas, R.	2021	https://arete.ibero.edu.co/article/view/art.17105 (accessed on 23 November 2021)

Table 6. *Cont.*

N	Database	Title	Author	Year	URL
4	EBSCO	Myofunctional and electromyographic characteristics of obese adolescent children [30]	Bolzan Berlese, D; Copetti, F; Maciel Weimmann, A; Fantinel Ferreira, P; Bonfanti Haeffner, L.	2013	https://web-s-ebscohost-com.ezproxy.uniminuto.edu/ehost/detail/detail?vid=0&sid=97de324b-fcf4-47c4-a413-4b7a6cde6c62%40redis&bdata=Jmxhbmc9ZXMmc2l0ZT1laG9zdC1saXZlJlnNjb3BlPXNpdGU%3d#AN=90594980&db=a9h (accessed on 04 December 2021)
5	EBSCO	Pulmonary Function and Obesity [31]	Carpio, C., Santiago, A., García De Lorenzo, A; Álvarez-Sala, R	2014	https://scielo.isciii.es/scielo.php?script=sci_arttext&pid=S0212-16112014001200009 (accessed on 04 December 2021)
6	EBSCO	Characterization of sleep disorders, snoring, and alterations of the stomatognathic system of obese candidates for bariatric surgery [20]	Mores, R; Delgado, S. E; Martins, N. F; Anderle, P; Da Silva Longaray, C; Pasqualeto, V. M; Batista Berbert, M. C.	2017	http://www.rbone.com.br/index.php/rbone/article/view/447 (accessed on 04 December 2021)
7	EBSCO	Maximum phonation time in people with obesity not undergoing or undergoing bariatric surgery [11]	Fonseca, A; Salgado, W; Dantas, R.	2019	https://www.hindawi.com/journals/jobe/2019/5903621/ (accessed on 04 December 2021)
8	EBSCO	Obesity, bariatric surgery, and the impact on oral health: A review of the literature [32]	Mosquim, V; Aparecido Foratori, J. G; Saory Hissano, W; Wang, L; Sales Peres, S.	2019	https://pesquisa.bvsalud.org/portal/resource/pt/biblio-1051047 (accessed on 04 December 2021)
9	PROQUEST	Impaired swallowing reflex in patients with obstructive sleep apnea syndrome [33]	Teramoto, S; Sudo, F; Matsuse, T; Ohga, E.	1999	https://www.proquest.com/docview/200498630/9EDD348CC9A4A96PQ/2?accountid=48797&forcedol=true (accessed on 17 December 2021)
10	PROQUEST	The stomatognathic system and body scheme [1]	Barreto, J. F	1999	https://www.redalyc.org/pdf/283/28330405.pdf (accessed on 17 December 2021)
11	PROQUEST	Obesity and the lungs: 2 · Obesity and sleep-disordered breathing [34]	Crummy, F; Piper, A. J; Naughton, M. T	2008	https://www.proquest.com/docview/1781775154/FFC00B28C8B14725PQ/73?accountid=48797&forcedol=true&forcedol=true (accessed on 17 December 2021)
12	PROQUEST	The effect of dental status on changes in chewing in obese patients after bariatric surgery [35]	Godlewski, A. E; Veyrune, J; Ciangura, C; Chaussain, C.	2011	https://www.proquest.com/docview/1306252768/9EDD348CC9A4A96PQ/4?accountid=48797&forcedol=true (accessed on 17 December 2021)
13	PROQUEST	Habitual snoring and atopic status: Correlations with respiratory function and tooth occlusion [36]	Zicari, A. M; Marzo, G; Rugiano, A; Celani, C; Carbone, M. P.	2012	https://www.proquest.com/docview/1197719038/8A83C372D8DF4F3DPQ/9 (accessed on 17 December 2021)
14	PROQUEST	Impairment of the distal airway in normally reactive obese women [37]	Marin, G; Gamez, A. S; Molinari, N; Kacimi, D; Vachier, I.	2013	https://www.proquest.com/docview/1434621519/2E1BA5ED485B4119PQ/4?accountid=48797 (accessed on 17 December 2021)
15	PROQUEST	Airway dysfunction in obesity: The response to voluntary restoration of end-expiratory lung volume [38]	Oppenheimer, Beno W; Berger, Kenneth I; Segal, Leopoldo N; Stabile, A; Coles, K.	2014	https://www.proquest.com/docview/1494399689/2E1BA5ED485B4119PQ/2?accountid=48797 (accessed on 17 December 2021)
16	PROQUEST	Perioperative respiratory care in obese patients undergoing bariatric surgery: Implications for clinical practice [39]	Pouwels, S; Smeenk, F. W; Manschot, L; Lascaris, B; Nienhuijs, S; Bouwman, R. A; Buise, M. P.	2016	https://www.sciencedirect.com/science/article/pii/S0954611116301287 (accessed on 17 December 2021)
17	PROQUEST	Therapeutic strategies for the management of dry mouth with emphasis on electrostimulation as a treatment option [40]	Tulek, A; Mulic, A; Hogset, M; Utheim, T. P; Sehic, A.	2021	https://www.hindawi.com/journals/ijd/2021/6043488/ (accessed on 17 December 2021)

Table 6. *Cont.*

N	Database	Title	Author	Year	URL
18	PROQUEST	Pulmonary vascular congestion: A mechanism for distal pulmonary unit dysfunction in obesity [41]	Oppenheimer, Beno W; Berger, Kenneth I; Saleem, Alí; Segal, Leopoldo N; Donnino, R.	2016	https://www.proquest.com/docview/1777735040/2E1BA5ED485B4119PQ/1?accountid=48797&forcedol=true (accessed on 17 December 2021)
19	PROQUEST	Comparison of Interview to Questionnaire for Assessment of Eating Disorders after Bariatric Surgery [4]	Globus, I; Kissileff, H. R; Hamm, J. D; Herzog, M; Mitchell, J. E; Latzer, Y.	2021	https://www.mdpi.com/2077-0383/10/6/1174 (accessed on 17 December 2021)
20	PROQUEST	Food insecurity as a determinant of obesity in humans: The insurance hypothesis [3]	Ortiga, D; Andrews, C; Bateson, M.	2017	https://www.proquest.com/docview/1988264531/144D2D2995EF403FPQ/471 (accessed on 17 December 2021)
21	PROQUEST	The impact of bariatric surgery on sleep-disordered breathing parameters from overnight polysomnography and home sleep apnea testing [13]	Mashaqi, S; Steffen, K; Crosby, R; Garcia, L; Cureus, P.	2018	https://www.proquest.com/docview/2080487482/8E81C0CD3DA94C5EPQ/198 (accessed on 17 December 2021)
22	PROQUEST	Perceived oral health in patients after bariatric surgery using measures of quality of life related to oral health [2]	Karlsson, L; Carlsson, J; Jenneborg, K; Kjaeldgaard, M.	2018	https://www.proquest.com/docview/2266411926/8E81C0CD3DA94C5EPQ/155 (accessed on 17 December 2021)
23	PROQUEST	Obstructive Sleep Apnea: A Focus on Myofunctional Therapy [42]	Felicio, C. M; Da Silva Dias, F; Voi Trawitzki, L.	2018	https://www.proquest.com/docview/2229610711/ECF01209F16B4AFCPQ/12 (accessed on 17 December 2021)
24	PROQUEST	Why is primary obesity a disease? [7]	De Lorenzo, A; Gratteri, S; Gualtieri, P; Cammarano, A; Bertucci, P.	2019	https://www.proquest.com/resultsol/144D2D2995EF403FPQ/28#scrollTo (accessed on 17 December 2021)
25	PROQUEST	Binge eating disorder and related features in candidates for bariatric surgery [43]	Cella, S., Fei, L; D'Amico, R; Giardiello, C; Allaria, A; Cotrufo, P.	2019	https://www.proquest.com/docview/2244691685/8E81C0CD3DA94C5EPQ/67 (accessed on 17 December 2021)
26	PROQUEST	Obesity, a risk factor in COVID-19 [5]	Cadea, E.	2021	https://www.minsalud.gov.co/Paginas/Obesidad-un-factor-de-riesgo-en-el-covid-19.aspx (accessed on 17 December 2021)
27	PROQUEST	Dysphagia symptoms in obstructive sleep apnea: Prevalence and clinical correlates [44]	Pizzorni, N; Radovanovic, D; Pecis, M; Lorusso, R; Annoni, F; Bartorelli, A; Santus, P.	2021	https://www.proquest.com/docview/2528901432/CDDFC8E76B784FF0PQ/20 (accessed on 17 December 2021)
28	PROQUEST	Obesity in the world [8]	Malo-Serrano, M; Castillo, N; Pajita, D.	2017	http://www.scielo.org.pe/scielo.php?pid=S1025-55832017000200011&script=sci_arttext (accessed on 17 December 2021)
29	PROQUEST	Social support for people with morbid obesity in a bariatric surgery program: A qualitative descriptive study [45]	Torrente-Sánchez et al.	2021	https://www.proquest.com/docview/2544977715/8E81C0CD3DA94C5EPQ/ (accessed on 17 December 2021)
30	PROQUEST	The development of eating and eating disorders after bariatric surgery: A systematic review and meta-analysis [14]	Victor Taba, J; Oliveira Suzuki, M; Sayuri do Nascimento, F; Ryuchi Iuamoto, L; Hsing, W. T; Zumerkorn Pipek, L; Andraus, W.	2021	https://www.proquest.com/docview/2554777851/8E81C0CD3DA94C5EPQ/28 (accessed on 17 December 2021)
31	PROQUEST	Design and Conduct of Systematic Reviews: A training guide for Early Literacy (EL) researchers [21]	Red Para La Lectoescritura Inicial De Centroamérica Y El Caribe–Redlei-	2021	https://red-lei.org/wp-content/uploads/2021/03/Directrices-de-Revisiones-Sistematicas.pdf (accessed on 17 December 2021)

Table 6. *Cont.*

N	Database	Title	Author	Year	URL
32	PROQUEST	Imbalanced coagulation in the airways of Type 2-high asthma with comorbid obesity [46]	Womble, J. T; McQuade, V. L; Ihrie, M. D; Ingram, J. L.	2021	https://www.ncbi.nlm.nih.gov/pmc/articles/PMC8364356/ (accessed on 17 December 2021)
33	PUBMED	Obesity and the pulmonologist [47]	Deane, S; Thomson, A.	2006	https://adc.bmj.com/content/91/2/188.short (accessed on 13 January 2022)
34	PUBMED	Altered respiratory physiology in obesity [48]	Parameswaran, K; Todd, D. C; Soth, M.	2006	https://www.hindawi.com/journals/crj/2006/834786/ (accessed on 13 January 2022)
35	PUBMED	Obesity and respiratory diseases [49]	Zammit, C; Liddicoat, H; Moonsie, I; Makker, H.	2006	https://pubmed.ncbi.nlm.nih.gov/21116339/ (accessed on13 January 2022)
36	PUBMED	Altered respiratory physiology in obesity for the anesthesiologist-critical physician [50]	Porhomayon, J; Papadakos, P; Singh, A; Nader, N. D.	2011	https://pubmed.ncbi.nlm.nih.gov/23439281/ (accessed on 13 January 2022)
37	PUBMED	The stomatognathic system [51]	Mizraji, M; Freese, A. M; Bianchi, R.	2012	https://pesquisa.bvsalud.org/portal/resource/pt/lil-706324 (accessed on 13 January 2022)
38	PUBMED	Fundamental frequency, maximum phonation time, and vocal complaints in morbidly obese women [52]	Rocha de Souza, L. B; Medeiros Pereira, R; Marques dos Santos, M; Almeida Godoy, C. M.	2014	https://www.ncbi.nlm.nih.gov/pmc/articles/PMC4675479/ (accessed on 13 January 2022)
39	PUBMED	PICO tool for the formulation and search of clinically relevant questions in evidence-based psycho-oncology [24].	Landa-Ramírez, E; Arredondo, A.	2014	https://www.seom.org/seomcms/images/stories/recursos/05%20PSICOVOL11N2-3w.pdf (accessed on 13 January 2022)
40	PUBMED	Gastrointestinal symptoms in morbid obesity–the presence of dysphagia [53]	Huseini, M; Wood, G. C; Seiler, J; Argyropoulos, G; Irving, B. A; Gerhard, G. S; Rolston, D. D.	2014	https://pubmed.ncbi.nlm.nih.gov/25593922/ (accessed on 13 January 2022)
41	PUBMED	Speech, hearing, and language science therapy in bariatric surgery for the elderly: A case report [54]	Braude Canterji, M; Miranda Correa, S. P; Vargas, G. S; Ruttkay Pereira, J. L; Finard, S. A.	2015	https://www.scielo.br/j/abcd/a/zXYmf9QDgCCspDc5wyYdwHn/?lang=pt (accessed on 13 January 2022)
42	PUBMED	Respiratory management of obese patients undergoing surgery [55]	Hodgson, L. E; Murphy, P. B; Hart, N.	2015	https://www.ncbi.nlm.nih.gov/pmc/articles/PMC4454851/ (accessed on 14 January 2022)
43	PUBMED	Dysphagia after vertical sleeve gastrectomy: An evaluation of risk factors and evaluation of endoscopic intervention [56]	Nath, A; Yewale, S; Tran, T; Brebbia, J. S; Shope, T. R; Koch, T. R.	2016	https://pubmed.ncbi.nlm.nih.gov/28058017/ (accessed on 14 January 2022)
44	PUBMED	Monitoring of respiration and oxygen saturation in patients during the first night after elective bariatric surgery: A cohort study [57]	Wickerts, L; Forsberg, S; Bouvier, F; Jakobsson, J.	2017	https://pubmed.ncbi.nlm.nih.gov/28794858/ (accessed on 14 January 2022)
45	PUBMED	The pathogenesis of obesity: A scientific statement from an endocrine society [58]	Schwartz, M. W; Seeley, R. J; Zeltser, L. M; Drewnowski, A; Ravussin, E; Redman, L. M; Leibel, R. L.	2017	https://www.ncbi.nlm.nih.gov/pmc/articles/PMC5546881/ (accessed on 14 January 2022)
46	PUBMED	Positive airway pressure vs. inspiratory load exercises focused on pulmonary and respiratory muscle functions in the postoperative period of bariatric surgery [59]	Simões da Rocha, M. R; Souza, S; Moraes da Costa, C; Bertelli Merino, D. F; de Lima Montebelo, M. I; Rasera-Júnior; Pazzianotto-Forti, E. M.	2018	https://pubmed.ncbi.nlm.nih.gov/29972391/ (accessed on 13 January 2022)

Table 6. Cont.

N	Database	Title	Author	Year	URL
47	PUBMED	Obesity, obstructive sleep apnea, and type 2 diabetes mellitus: Epidemiologic and pathophysiologic data [60]	Jehan, S; Myers, A. K; Zizi, F; Pandi-Perumal, S. R; Jean-Louis, G; McFarlane, S. I.	2018	https://www.ncbi.nlm.nih.gov/pmc/articles/PMC6112821/ (accessed on 15 January 2022)
48	PUBMED	Perioperative treatment of sleep-disordered breathing and outcomes in bariatric patients [61]	Meurgey, J. H; Brown, R; Woroszyl-Chrusciel, A; Steier, J.	2018	https://pubmed.ncbi.nlm.nih.gov/29445538/ (accessed on 13 January 2022)
49	PUBMED	Evaluation and management of obesity hypoventilation syndrome: An official clinical practice guideline of the American Thoracic Society [62]	Mokhlesi, B; Masa, J. F; Brozek, J. L; Gurubhagavatula, I; Murphy, P. B; Piper, A. J; Teodorescu, M.	2018	https://pubmed.ncbi.nlm.nih.gov/31368798/ (accessed on 13 January 2022)
50	PUBMED	Breathing matters [17]	Del Negro, C. A; Funk, G. D; Feldman, J. L.	2018	https://pubmed.ncbi.nlm.nih.gov/29740175/#affiliation-3 (accessed on 13 January 2022)
51	PUBMED	Duration and stability of metabolically healthy obesity over 30 years [6]	Camhi, S. M; Must, A; Gona, P. N; Hankinson, A; Odegaard, A; Reis, J; Carnethon, M. R.	2019	https://www.nature.com/articles/s41366-018-0197-8 (accessed on 13 January 2022)
52	PUBMED	Respiratory mechanics of patients with morbid obesity [63]	Sant'Anna, M. D; Ferreira Carvalhal, R; Bastos de Oliveira, F. D; Araújo Zin, W; Lopes, A. J; Lugon, J. R; Silva Guimarães, F.	2019	https://pubmed.ncbi.nlm.nih.gov/31644708/ (accessed on 13 January 2022)
53	PUBMED	Esophageal pathophysiologic changes and adenocarcinoma after bariatric surgery: A systematic review and meta-analysis [64]	Jaruvongvanich, V; Matar, R; Ravi, K; Murad, M. H; Vantanasiri, K; Wongjarupong, N; Dayyeh, B. K. A.	2020	https://www.ncbi.nlm.nih.gov/pmc/articles/PMC7447443/ (accessed on 13 January 2022)
54	PUBMED	Perception of dyspnea during inspiratory resistive load testing in obese subjects awaiting bariatric surgery [12]	Tomasini, K; Ziegler, B; Sanches, P. R. S; da Silva Junior, D. P; Thomé, P. R; Dalcin, P. D. T. R.	2020	https://pubmed.ncbi.nlm.nih.gov/32415112/ (accessed on 13 January 2022)
55	PUBMED	Orofacial functions and forces in healthy young and adult males and females [65]	Dantas Giglio, L; Felício, C. M. D; Voi Trawitzki, L. V.	2020	https://pubmed.ncbi.nlm.nih.gov/33174985/ (accessed on 13 January 2022)
56	PUBMED	Obesity, bariatric surgery, and periodontal disease: An update of the literature [66]	Franco, R; Barlattani Jr, A; Perrone, M. A; Basili, M; Miranda, M; Costacurta, M; Bollero, P.	2020	https://www.europeanreview.org/article/21196 (accessed on 13 January 2022)
57	PUBMED	Altered airway mechanics in the context of obesity and asthma [9]	Bates, J. H; Peters, U; Daphtary, N; MacLean, E. S; Hodgdon, K; Kaminsky, D. A; Dixon, A. E.	2021	https://pubmed.ncbi.nlm.nih.gov/33119471/ (accessed on 13 January 2022)
58	PUBMED	Pre-habilitation for bariatric surgery: A pilot study and randomized controlled trial protocol [67]	García-Delgado, Y; López-Madrazo-Hernández, M. J; Alvarado-Martel, D; Miranda-Calderín, G; Ugarte-Lopetegui, A; González-Medina, R. A; Wägner, A. M.	2021	https://pubmed.ncbi.nlm.nih.gov/34578781/ (accessed on 13 January 2022)
59	SCIELO	Bariatric surgery [16]	Maluenda, G. F.	2012	https://www.sciencedirect.com/science/article/pii/S0716864012702961 (accessed on 30 January 2022)

Table 6. Cont.

N	Database	Title	Author	Year	URL
60	SCIELO	Myofunctional characteristics of obese mouth-nose breathers [68]	Bolzan Berlese, D; Ferreira Fontana, P. F; Botton, L; Maciel Weimnann, A. R; Bonfanti Haeffner, L. S.	2012	https://www.scielo.br/j/rsbf/a/NtJSY7LfJzPWyzRTsyN4cYL/?lang=pt (accessed on 30 January 2022)
61	SCIELO	Masticatory profile of morbidly obese subjects undergoing gastroplasty [69]	Marques Gonçalves, R. D. F; Zimberg Chehter, E.	2012	https://www.scielo.br/j/rcefac/a/cDMcdK4TtTt5WhQzpLR6pzD/?lang=pt (accessed on 30 January 2022)
62	SCIELO	The need for speech therapy assessment in the protocol of patients who are candidates for bariatric surgery [70]	Guerra Silva, A. S; Camargo Tanigute, C; Tessitore, A.	2014	https://www.scielo.br/j/rcefac/a/bHk9QNgbvFyXmw65QDJbzcD/?lang=pt (accessed on 30 January 2022)
63	SCIELO	Binge eating disorder [71]	Pinto de Azevedo, A. P; dos Santos, C. C; Cardoso da Fonseca, D.	2004	https://www.scielo.br/j/rpc/a/Mbjb77bcDLvBc4HPNgkT7Yn/?lang=pt (accessed on 30 January 2022)
64	SCIELO	Obesity, a risk factor in the COVID-19 pandemic [10]	de León Ramírez, L. L; de León Ramírez, L; Ramírez, J. A. B.	2021	http://www.revholcien.sld.cu/index.php/holcien/article/view/43 (accessed on 30 January 2022)
65	SCIELO	Chewing and swallowing in obese children and adolescents [19]	Souza, N. C. D; Ferreira Guedes, Z. C.	2016	https://www.scielo.br/j/rcefac/a/HypwyzNNyb9txHVPv5RX9mJ/?lang=pt (accessed on 30 January 2022)
66	SCIELO	Speech therapy intervention in morbidly obese patients undergoing the Fobi-Capella gastroplasty method [72]	Marques Gonçalves, R. D; Zimberg, E.	2016	https://www.scielo.br/j/abcd/a/crM36KrQZBYR3W5d4RtrTfm/?lang=en (accessed on 30 January 2022)
67	SCIELO	Oropharyngeal dysphagia: Multidisciplinary solutions [73]	Álvarez Hernández, J.	2018	https://senpe.com/libros/01_DISFAGIA_INTERACTIVO.pdf (accessed on 30 January 2022)
68	SCIELO	Physiology of exercise in orofacial motricity: Knowledge of the subject [74]	Xavier Torres, G. M; Hernández Alvez, C.	2019	https://www.scielo.br/j/rcefac/a/dpdn39WnSLkbj5D3hhvhhqP/?lang=en (accessed on 30 January 2022)
69	SCIELO	Chewing and swallowing in obese individuals referred for bariatric surgery/gastroplasty: A pilot study [18]	Andrade Rocha, A. C; Oliveira De Souza, N; Davison Mangilli Toni, C.	2019	https://www.scielo.br/j/rcefac/a/5K4ZGD3QJr8PdhyLg6fpVQB/?lang=en (accessed on 30 January 2022)
70	SCIELO	Tooth wear and tooth loss in morbidly obese patients after bariatric surgery [75]	Duarte Aznar, F; Aznar, F. D; Lauris, J. R; Adami Chaim, E; Cazzo, E; Sales Peres, S. H. D. C.	2019	https://www.scielo.br/j/abcd/a/xdF3p8Fjb3vWrF9r9mbDvVw/?lang=en (accessed on 30 January 2022)
71	SCIELO	Contributions of emotional overload, emotion dysregulation, and impulsivity to eating patterns in obese patients with binge eating disorder who seek bariatric surgery [15]	Benzerouk, F; Djerada, Z; Bertin, E; Barrière, S; Gierski, F; Kaladjian, A.	2020	https://www.mdpi.com/2072-6643/12/10/3099 (accessed on 30 January 2022)
72	SCIELO	Alimentary and bariatric surgery: Social representations of obese individuals [76]	Silva Gebara, T; Mocelin Polli, G; Wanderbroocke, A. C.	2021	https://www.scielo.br/j/pcp/a/6XkTBNs9MYqSPkkGnh3VJ5G/abstract/?format=html&lang=en (accessed on 02 February 2022)
73	SCIELO	Functional esophageal disorders in the preoperative evaluation of bariatric surgery [77]	Oliveira Lemme, E; Cerqueira Alvariz, A; Cotta Pereira, G.	2021	https://www.scielo.br/j/ag/a/Wh3kSvt3xqCQY7WRnZHFDjg/abstract/?lang=pt (accessed on 02 February 2022)

Table 6. Cont.

N	Database	Title	Author	Year	URL
74	SCIELO	The relationship of sensory processing and the stomatognathic system in children who breathe through the mouth [78]	Dantas Lima, A. C. D; Costa Albuquerque, R; Andrade Cunha, D. A; Dantas Lima, C; Henrique Lima, S. J; Justino Silva, H.	2022	https://www.scielo.br/j/codas/a/yRRKqnrSx59xCdXFyT6hjCg/?lang=pt (accessed on 02 February 2022)
75	SPRINGER LINK	Obesity: Systemic and pulmonary complications, biochemical abnormalities, and impaired lung function [79]	Mafort, T. T; Rufino, R; Costa, C. H; Lopes, A. J.	2016	https://mrmjournal.biomedcentral.com/articles/10.1186/s40248-016-0066-z (accessed on 02 February 2022)
76	SPRINGER LINK	Obstructive sleep apnea and lung function in severely obese patients prior to and after bariatric surgery: A randomized clinical trial [80]	Aguiar, I. C; Freitas, W. R; Santos, I. R; Apostolico, N; Nacif, S. R; Urbano, J. J; Oliveira, L. V.	2014	https://mrmjournal.biomedcentral.com/articles/10.1186/2049-6958-9-43 (accessed on 02 February 2022)
77	SPRINGER LINK	Can myofunctional therapy increase tongue tone and reduce symptoms in children with sleep-disordered breathing? [81]	Villa, M. P; Evangelisti, M; Martella, S; Barreto, M; Del Pozzo, M.	2017	https://link.springer.com/article/10.1007/s11325-017-1489-2 (accessed on 02 February 2022)
78	SPRINGER LINK	Laryngopharyngeal reflux and dysphagia in patients with obstructive sleep apnea: Is there an association? [82]	Caparroz, F; Campanholo, M; Stefanini, R; Vidigal, T; Haddad, L; Bittencourt, L. R; Haddad, F.	2019	https://link.springer.com/article/10.1007/s11325-019-01844-0 (accessed on 02 February 2022)
79	SPRINGER LINK	Silent gastroesophageal reflux disease in morbidly obese patients prior to primary metabolic surgery [83]	Kristo, I; Paireder, M; Jomrich, G; Felsenreich, D. M; Fischer, M; Hennerbichler, F. P; Schoppmann, S. F.	2020	https://link.springer.com/article/10.1007/s11695-020-04959-6 (accessed on 02 February 2022)
80	SPRINGER LINK		Sandoval-Munoz, C. P; Haidar, Z. S	2021	https://link.springer.com/article/10.1186/s13005-021-00257-3 (accessed on 02 February 2022)

Table 7 shows the characterization of the stomatognathic system from its morphological changes.

Table 7. Characterization of the stomatognathic system (morphological changes).

Obese Patient	Structure	Post-Bariatric Patient
• Facial asymmetry with greater size in the middle and lower third of the face [18,30] • Asymmetry in lip corners in normal position and in smile [65,70]	Face	Theoretical information not evidenced
• Flattened and narrow nostrils (turbinate hypertrophy) [30,36,52] • Deviated septum [54]	Nose	Theoretical information not evidenced
• Tension with slight drop [18,70] • Hypertonia [18] • Hypotonia [30,54] • Dysfunction for inflating, retracting, and sucking [18]	Cheeks	Theoretical information not evidenced
• Atretic [30]	Maxillary	Theoretical information not evidenced

Table 7. *Cont.*

Obese Patient	Structure	Post-Bariatric Patient
• Impaired mobility [18,47] • Clockwise rotation of the mandibular angle [30]	Mandible	Theoretical information not evidenced
• Contraction during swallowing [18] • Dysfunction when protruding, retracting, and lateralizing on both sides [18] • Decreased tone [30,54,69,70] • Without lip seal [30,54] • Short upper lip and functioning hiccups [30] • Thick lower lip [15,29] • Dryness [30]	Lips	Theoretical information not evidenced
• Mallampati scale with Class III (only the soft palate and uvula are visualized) and Class IV (only the hard palate is visualized) results [20] • Dental caries [32] • Open bite [30] • Protrusion of upper teeth [66] • Erosion, attrition, abrasion, and fraction [58] • Loss of teeth [54]	Oral cavity Teeth	• Invariance of Class III and IV on the Mallampati scale [20] • Dental caries and dental erosion due to recurrent acidity in the oral cavity, with a higher prevalence in patients undergoing a Roux-en-Y gastric bypass [58] • Increased periodontal disease and hypersensitivity [2]
• Abnormal position (lowered or low) [18,20,70] • Volume increase [18,20] • Decreased tone (hypotonia) [30,54,69] • Increased tone (hypertonia) [52,69] • Difficulty performing praxis or movements [30,69] • Tongue covered or interposed anteriorly between the dental arches [35,54]	Tongue	Theoretical information is not evidenced
• Dysfunction in the width and height of the hard palate (deep ogival) [18,70] • Soft palate with reduced mobility [30] • Increased length of the soft palate [52]	Palate	Theoretical information not evidenced
• Presence of noise [18]	Temporomandibular articulation	Theoretical information not evidenced
• Increase in circumference [42]	Neck	Theoretical information not evidenced
• Presence of mental muscle tension during swallowing [18] • Presence of reduced tone in temporalis muscle [70] • Hypotonic orofacial musculature [30] • Mental muscle hyperfunction [30] • Excessive contraction of the orbicularis oris muscle [54]	Muscles	Theoretical information not evidenced
• Left leaning posture in hyperextension [70] • Hyperflexion [18]	Head	Theoretical information not evidenced
• Right shoulder higher than left [70]	Shoulders	Theoretical information not evidenced
• Narrowing due to accumulation of fat in the respiratory tract [20] • Thickening of the lateral walls with little possibility of seeing the posterior pharyngeal wall [11,20,52] • Mechanical obstruction of the nasopharynx (adenotonsillar hypertrophy) [36] • Pharyngeal collapse [81]	Larynx and pharynx	Theoretical information not evidenced

Table 8 presents the characterization of the stomatognathic system from its physiological changes.

Table 8. Characterization of the stomatognathic system (physiological changes).

Obese Patient	Function	Post-Bariatric Patient
<ul><li>Respiratory disorder with hypoventilation [13,57,62]</li><li>Obstructive sleep apnea [13,18,20,40,57,61,62,69,81]</li><li>Oral respiration [18,30,36]</li><li>Reduced olfactory ability due to chronic nasal obstruction [68]</li><li>Respiratory failure due to collapse of the upper airway [42,53]</li><li>Lung disease and asthma [20]</li><li>Decrease in the fundamental frequency due to obstruction of the air flow [52]</li><li>Diaphragmatic dysfunction [59]</li><li>Difficulty in phonorespiratory coordination [52]</li><li>Presence of snoring [36]</li><li>Presence of moderate dyspnea [12]</li><li>Hypoxia [57]</li><li>Oxygen desaturation [57]</li><li>Reduced functional residual capacity [61]</li></ul>	Respiration	<ul><li>Significant reduction in obstructive sleep apnea-hypopnea index >50% and -20 events per hour [13]</li><li>Mild respiratory disturbances [57]</li><li>Presence of obstructive sleep apnea syndrome [57]</li><li>Adult respiratory distress syndrome (ARDS) [57]</li></ul>
<ul><li>Escape during the emission of phonemes [70]</li><li>Impaired spontaneous speech due to mandibular deviation [70]</li><li>Short maximum phonation time [11]</li><li>Altered voice quality (strangled, hoarse, and gasping) [11,79]</li><li>Presence of hoarseness, murmurs, vocal instability, altered nervousness, and brilliance; in addition, strangulation of the voice at the end of the emission [11]</li><li>Vocal fatigue with voice failure [37,52]</li><li>Phonatory dysfunction due to dehydrated mucosa [40,56]</li></ul>	Phonation	No significant improvement in MPT or maximum phonation time [11]
Masticatory dysfunction due to: <ul><li>Dental alterations [2]</li><li>Lack of bite force [18]</li><li>Chronic and mild unilateral preference [18,19,44]</li><li>Dehydrated mucosa [60]</li><li>No presence of grinding phase [18]</li><li>Hypotonicity of the lips and tongue [19]</li><li>Rapid masticatory pattern [70,72]</li><li>Taste reduction [80]</li><li>Alternate bilateral chewing [30]</li><li>Altered saliva production [40]</li></ul>	Mastication	Persistence of masticatory dysfunction
Swallowing dysfunction due to: <ul><li>Tension of facial muscles and altered posture [18]</li><li>At the level of consistencies, 50% alteration in solids and 25% alteration in liquids [18]</li><li>Dehydrated mucosa [40]</li><li>Adapted swallowing [30]</li><li>Low swallowing efficiency due to repeated swallowing of the bolus [18]</li><li>Hypotonicity of the lips and tongue [20]</li><li>Neural deterioration [83]</li><li>Multiple swallows due to cheek hypotonicity [19]</li><li>Difficulty in oral propulsion due to pharyngeal, nasal, or palatal obstruction [30]</li><li>Presence of food residues in the cavity [19,70]</li><li>Presence of large food bolus [70,72]</li><li>Gastroesophageal reflux [44,81,83]</li><li>Oropharyngeal dysphagia [84]</li><li>Esophagitis [83]</li><li>Swallowing dysfunction due to dehydrated mucosa [40]</li><li>Binge eating disorder [43,71]</li><li>Alteration in sense of taste and sensitivity of oral mucosa [77]</li><li>Nutcracker esophageal dysphagia [81]</li></ul>	Swallowing	<ul><li>Sensation of choking or stagnation [18,70]</li><li>Gastroesophageal reflux [2,18,70] after sleeve gastrectomy [83]</li><li>Binge eating disorder [43,71]</li><li>Acid reflux is increased in patients undergoing sleeve gastrectomy (SG) and decreased in patients undergoing Roux-en-Y gastric bypass (RYGB) [64]</li></ul>
Alteration of suction due to: <ul><li>Hypotonicity in cheeks [18]</li><li>Impaired mouth breathing [30]</li><li>Absence of lip seal with interposition of the tongue [54]</li></ul>	Suction	Theoretical information not evidenced

4. Discussion

The stomatognathic system (SS) is also called the masticatory apparatus (MA), and the word "stomatognathic" originates from the Greek "stoma" (mouth) and "gnathos" (jaw). The stomatognathic system refers to structures that are anatomically and functionally linked [51] to processes related to vital functions, such as breathing, sucking, chewing, and swallowing, and social functions, such as phonation and articulation [78], and these are integrated by different structures that allow the development of each function in a harmonious and balanced way [38,41]. First, there are bony structures, such as the skull, facial bones, hyoid bone, larynx, maxilla, mandible, and bony palate. There are also muscular structures, such as the muscles for mastication and facial expression and the muscles of the tongue, soft palate, pharynx, and neck, as well as other structures, such as the head, nose, oral cavity, teeth, and shoulders [29].

Based on the above, any change or alteration in any of the bodily structures can lead to its imbalance and this will simultaneously have an effect on the performance of its functions, thereby generating a negative influence on people's daily lives [48]. Currently, studies demonstrate that obesity is the etiology of these structural and physiological changes, given that obese patients present excessive accumulations of adipose tissue in regions that have direct effects [19,75]. To reduce the dysfunctions associated with obesity, these patients undergo surgical interventions, including bariatric surgery, which appears to have a positive impact. However, if a patient does not receive an intervention for existing alterations, the alterations reportedly persist and even worsen [39,50].

Within the investigated databases, it is possible to provide details on the characterization of the SSs of patients with obesity and post-bariatric surgery. In terms of the facial features, patients with obesity may present an asymmetry, with differences in measurements of the middle and lower thirds of the face [18,30], as well as in the corners of the lips in the habitual position and when the subjects smile [70]. A flattened nose, with a possible deviated septum and turbinate hypertrophy caused by the narrowing of the nostrils, may trigger these patients to become oral breathers and affect other SS functions [36,52]. Hypotonic cheeks, with slight sagging on one side and dysfunction in performing requested exercises, such as inflating, retracting, and sucking, may also be present [18]. However, other authors state that the cheek hypertonia of the patients included in their studies was attributable to continuous food intake, an argument contradicted by theory, as it has been determined that obese patients do not perform the chewing phase correctly and have preferences to swallow food whole [30,54].

Atretic maxilla is evidenced when the hard palate is arched or vaulted and the soft palate, for its part, is increased in length and reduced in mobility, as well as being characterized by mobility alterations in the mandible, with rotation of the mandibular angle [34], and repercussions related to the presence of noises from the temporomandibular joint. Lips show the presence of dryness and are contracted during the swallowing process. In the usual state, they do not present a lip seal, their tone is decreased [54,72], and they exhibit dysfunction when performing requested praxias (protruding, retracting, and lateralizing to both sides) [18]. The upper lip, for its part, is short and hypo-functional, and the lower lip is observed to have great volume [30].

Regarding the oral cavity, a study based on the Mallampati scale—which is useful for analyzing air obstructions that prevent its passage from the nose and mouth to the lower respiratory tract—reported that the results obtained by these patients were Class III (indicating visualization of only the soft palate and uvula) and Class IV (indicating visualization only of the hard palate) [20], states that may indicate the appearance of obstructive sleep apnea [34]. Authors emphasize that the results of this scale in the case of a post-bariatric patient will remain unchanged, since such changes only depend on the gradual loss and reduction of the BMI, as structures such as the larynx and pharynx in obese patients are affected through the accumulation of fat in the respiratory tract, thickening and narrowing the lateral walls and obstructing the nasopharyngeal mechanics (adenotonsillar hypertrophy), which is why pharyngeal collapse can occur [20,36,81].

Dental wear is the gradual loss of tooth substance without the involvement of the caries process or interference from the action of microorganisms or trauma. Changes in lifestyle, diet, and behavior play a fundamental role in this process. Patients with obesity usually consume unhealthy diets and, therefore, have an oral profile including loss of teeth [54], erosion, attrition, abrasion, and dental fraction [58], as well as other characteristics independent of their diet, such as dental caries, periodontitis [2,32,66], open bite, and upper teeth protrusion [30]. Patients undergoing RYGB present recurrent acidity in the oral cavity compared to those undergoing SG, affecting dental erosion, periodontal disease, and hypersensitivity [2,58].

The orofacial muscles are crucial for the performance of stomatognathic functions that are relevant to health and quality of life. Therefore, for example, problems may arise in chewing and in the manipulation and propulsion of the food bolus during swallowing if performance is affected [74]. In the case of patients with obesity, their musculatures will be perceived as hypotonic with hyperfunction of the mentalis muscle and tension during swallowing [30], excessive contraction of the orbicularis oris [54], and hypotonicity of the temporalis muscle [70]. Regarding the musculature of the tongue, some studies register an increased tone [52,70]; however, most studies agree that it is hypotonic [30,54,72]. In addition, an increase in volume and an abnormal position, called "cloaked or low tongue", or sometimes interposed between the dental arches [18,20,54], can be observed.

Finally, structures such as the head, neck, and shoulders are also highlighted within the information obtained from the studies, since functional harmony between them is necessary to ensure that each of the functions involved in the SS is correctly developed. When patients with obesity accumulate fat, the circumference of their neck increases, which is considered an anthropometric predictor of the severity of obstructive sleep apnea syndrome and of a possible collapse of the upper airway [42,52]. In addition, these patients adopt a head tilt and hyperflexion posture, with one shoulder more inclined relative to the other [30].

Undoubtedly, the results obtained reflect a broad characterization of the functions of the SS in obesity. Before bariatric surgery, patients with obesity suffer from respiratory disorders, such as alveolar hypoventilation and obstructive sleep apnea [63], apnea being a condition that has been reported on multiple occasions with a wide variety of evidence in scientific articles [13,18,20,44,57,60,82]. The respiratory mode of obese patients is oral because of the numerous structural changes; a chronic nasal obstruction is possibly maintained, thereby leading to attempts to restore the function that is vital for the patient's survival and, consequently, affecting physiological breathing [18,36]. Likewise, there is an insufficient ability to perceive odors from the environment [30]. In addition to this, the collapse in the structures that make up the upper airway [42] may lead to respiratory failure and other lung diseases, such as asthma [20]. When there is an obstruction of the flow of air coming from the pulmonary complex, the vibration of the vocal folds and the number of times per second in which they must vibrate are affected, which is known as a decreased fundamental frequency. Phonorespiratory incoordination occurs because of poor air support as a result of affected lung capacity, which leads to alterations in vocal mechanics [52].

Episodes of snoring are frequent and are the result of limitations related to and increases in respiratory effort, causing hypoventilation or slow breathing and generating sleep interruption, also known as apnea [36]. Likewise, patients experience moderate dyspnea or a feeling of shortness of breath [44], which can, in extreme circumstances, trigger hypoxia, decreased oxygen supply to various tissues, or low desaturation [57] and reduced residual lung capacity. This indicates inadequate chest expansion and can, therefore, affect normal respiratory function [76]. Obstructive sleep apnea persists even after bariatric surgery; however, the development of adult respiratory distress syndrome is also possible [61]. In contrast, some bibliographic bases show the existence of a significant reduction in the rate of obstructive sleep apnea and hypopnea by $\geq 50\%$ and of nocturnal episodes to <20 events per hour, which can be characterized as adequate or within a range of possible normality [57].

In the phonatory field, one study reports, through a speech evaluation, an air leak during the emission of phonemes, with mandibular deviation during spontaneous speech [70], as well as a short maximum phonation time, justified because ventilatory pressures are lower than expected during inspiration and expiration, causing a reduction in respiratory muscle strength, lung capacity, and respiratory reserve volume [11]. Obese patients present with fatigue and phonatory dysfunction because of the dehydration of the mucosa of the area, generating altered vocal qualities (strangled, hoarse, and gasping voice), the presence of murmurs, vocal instability, nervousness, and prosodic alteration of speech or vocal brightness [52]. However, these patients do not report significant improvements in the maximum phonation time after undergoing the surgical procedure [11].

The masticatory patterns of patients with obesity undergoing bariatric surgery are strongly affected. The characteristics are maintained before and after bariatric surgery, which means that the masticatory dysfunction does not change and is persistent. This dysfunction is caused by dental alterations, the cause of which is, theoretically, the high level of recurrent acidity in the oral cavity, which causes caries, erosion, or loss of teeth and dental hypersensitivity [2], as well as, simultaneously, a weak bite force. There is also a chronic unilateral preference [18,73] and mild mucosa in the dehydrated area [40], without a crushing phase, according to the food bolus [18], and hypotonicity, or low muscle tone, in the lips and tongue [28]. Chewing speed is also affected [69,70], and some patients show the ability to taste outside the normal parameters or decreased ability to taste [30] and low production of saliva or hyposalivation, which leads to difficulty in moistening and macerating food adequately and satisfactorily [40].

The swallowing function of patients with obesity, like the other vital functions, is also affected owing to the tension in the facial muscles and the abnormal position of the tongue during chewing (hooded or lowered tongue). The information that suggests that obese patients swallow repeatedly or abnormally is new, with alterations of 50% for swallowing solid consistencies and 25% for swallowing liquid consistencies [18]. The mucosa that converges in the process of swallowing food is dehydrated [4]. The swallowing pattern is classified as having low efficiency because of repeated swallowing of the bolus or multiple swallows [18]. These changes make it difficult to propel the food orally, in addition to the existence of pharyngeal, nasal, or palatal obstructions [30]. Patients may also show food residues in the oral cavity [70], a large food bolus construct [27,31], gastroesophageal reflux disease [32,44,83], and oropharyngeal dysphagia (OFD) [55], a symptom that refers to the difficulty in forming or moving the food bolus toward the pharyngeal wall or toward the esophagus and which is concurrently related to difficulty in oral propulsion. OFD causes alterations in safety (possible aspiration pneumonia) and efficacy (dehydration and malnutrition), thereby increasing the morbidity and mortality of individuals experiencing this condition and, consequently, deteriorating their quality of life [46,73]. Other features of the swallowing function in obese patients include esophagitis or inflammation, which damages the duct that extends from the throat to the stomach [83], and binge eating disorder or compulsive behavior through binge eating, where the main characteristic is loss of control over what is eaten [43,71]. The swallowing reflex is well coordinated with breathing patterns in normal humans. However, patients with obstructive sleep apnea syndrome may have a swallowing disorder that reflects abnormal nerve and muscle function in the suprapharynx [34].

Furthermore, the observation that patients with obesity have a nutcracker-shaped esophagus is frequently related to an anomaly or to hypercontractile motor disorder with characteristically high amplitude waves in the distal esophagus—the main symptoms being chest pain and dysphagia [81]. All the abovementioned alterations are categorized under the terms "swallowing dysfunction" and "adapted swallowing". Theory defines adapted or atypical swallowing as an alteration in the oral phase of swallowing that is characterized by the inadequate position of the tongue and other structures of the oral cavity and that appears when there is an alteration in the form and function of the same. This altered pattern is observed when the structures of the oral cavity have to adapt as a consequence of a structural or functional alteration [60]. Sensations of choking or stagnation [18], gastroesophageal reflux [2,18], and binge eating disorder [43,71] are alterations that, according to theory, continue to present even after the postoperative period, which indicates that swallowing dysfunction persists after bariatric surgery.

In addition, the reviewed studies show the mechanical effects of obesity on pulmonary physiology and the function of adipose tissue, this latter being an endocrine organ that produces systemic inflammation and affects central respiratory control [49]. Patients with morbid obesity show increased total, airway, peripheral, and tissue system resistance, even though they do not show limitations in expiratory flow or reduced respiratory muscle strength [63]. The already mentioned mechanical effects on the respiratory system can trigger dyspnea, wheezing, and cough, thereby becoming a morbidity of the respiratory system [47]. Major respiratory complications of obesity are considered to include increased ventilatory demand, increased effort in breathing, respiratory muscle inefficiency, and decreased respiratory compliance [48].

Changes in respiratory system compliance and lung volumes can negatively affect pulmonary gas exchange and lead to upper airway obstruction and sleep-disordered breathing. Therefore, the perioperative period should be carefully observed [82]. Among other things, decreased functional residual capacity, decreased expiratory reserve volume, decreased compliance, and increased resistance of the respiratory system imply breathing with low lung volume, promoting airway closure in dependent lung zones with consequent abnormalities in gas exchange, even though the capacity of the lungs to diffuse carbon monoxide is normal or increased [83].

Obesity is characterized by increased systemic and pulmonary blood volume (pulmonary vascular congestion). The concomitant abnormal diffusion of the alveolar membrane suggests subclinical interstitial edema. In this setting, functional abnormalities should encompass the entire distal lung, including the airways [38]. These abnormalities are caused by the reduction in lung volume at rest; however, airway inflammation, vascular congestion, and/or concomitant intrinsic airway disease may occur [41]. A study of obese women demonstrated that the airways are characterized by hyperreactivity. Bronchial hyperreactivity is an exaggerated response of the bronchial mucosa and is the cause of bronchospasm. Some of the agents that can trigger bronchial hyperreactivity are respiratory infections, substances present in the environment, such as pollen or smoke, and certain drugs [72].

Global dysfunction of the distal lung (alveolar membrane and distal airways) is associated with pulmonary vascular congestion and failure to reach the high-output state of obesity. Pulmonary vascular congestion and consequent fluid transudation and/or alterations in alveolar-capillary membrane structure can be considered as often unrecognized causes of airway dysfunction in obesity [41].

One study describes the phenotype of pulmonary dysfunction in obesity as reduced functional residual capacity (FRC) with airway narrowing, distal respiratory dysfunction, and bronchodilator response [38]. The repercussions of obesity on respiratory function are associated, above all, with the restrictive alteration caused by excess adipose tissue. Increased fat in the chest and abdomen can shift the elastic equilibrium point between the chest and lungs, thereby reducing FRC [42]. Obesity also significantly interferes with respiratory function by decreasing lung volume, particularly expiratory reserve volume, and FRC [84].

For this reason, bariatric surgery effectively reduces neck and waist circumference, increases peak ventilatory pressures, improves sleep architecture, and reduces sleep-disordered breathing, specifically obstructive sleep apnea, in patients with severe obesity [80].

5. Conclusions

There are compromises that negatively affect the harmonious and joint form of the morphological and physiological unit that is the stomatognathic system (SS) in patients with obesity, which are due to an imbalance caused by the concentrated accumulation of adipose tissue characteristic of a BMI ≥ 40 kg/m^2 or between 35 and 39.9 kg/m^2 above that established for normality according to an individual's height.

Breathing, chewing, and swallowing are the functions of the stomatognathic system in patients with obesity that provided the most information during the evidence search process. Most of the articles investigated coincided in specific information, which allowed the broad characterization of each of these functions and, in the same way, of those structural alterations that play a significant role in said functions. The most cited were lip dysfunction; cloaked tongue, or lingual and cheek hypotonia; lip hypotonia with no lip seal; the presence of periodontitis; dysfunction in the width and height of the hard palate; and, finally, thickening of the lateral walls of the pharynx.

Swallowing dysfunctions caused by gastroesophageal reflux may vary according to the bariatric procedure performed. If the patient undergoes RYGB, acid reflux will decrease, given the implications of the procedure, unlike if they undergo SG, which favors an increase in acid reflux in these patients and, simultaneously, the alteration of the stomatognathic system (SS) at the morphological level.

The information evidenced within the literature reflects the need to develop and implement multidisciplinary work with obese patients before and after they undergo bariatric surgery, given that the alterations of the stomatognathic system, if not treated in the preoperative period, may persist and even worse, thereby negatively impacting these patients' quality of life.

After performing an exhaustive search on the stomatognathic system in patients with obesity before and after surgery and analyzing all the information obtained on the structural and functional alterations of this system, we noted that there is ample and clear evidence regarding the condition of obese patients who are candidates for bariatric surgery. However, when considering post-bariatric patients in relation to the stomatognathic system, the information changes and shows great limitations. Certainly, in this case, the data obtained were scarce.

It is evident how interest in bariatric surgery has grown in recent years. The number of bariatric surgeons has been progressively increasing, along with the number of patients undergoing these surgeries, which highlights considerable positive impacts on weight loss, metabolic control, and self-esteem, among others. However, many other diseases in obese patients that compromise this population's quality of life, such as those of the SS, have been forgotten, and there is a lack of knowledge about the advantages of this surgery for the SS.

Considering the abovementioned information, the greatest contribution of this review would be to arouse interest in the evaluation of patients with obesity before and after surgery beyond weight control. A comprehensive and multidisciplinary evaluation should be performed that includes breathing, chewing, and swallowing as basic functions to be analyzed, thereby allowing patients to have a great opportunity to improve their quality of life.

Author Contributions: Conceptualization: G.F.G.-B., A.P.B.-M., V.C.-T. and G.P.-R.; Investigation: G.F.G.-B., A.P.B.-M., V.C.-T. and G.P.-R.; Methodology: C.S.-P., R.O.-B. and M.C.B.; Writing—original draft: G.F.G.-B., A.P.B.-M., V.C.-T., G.P.-R., C.S.-P., R.O.-B., M.C.B., D.R.-P. and V.B.; Writing—review and editing: G.F.G.-B., A.P.B.-M., V.C.-T., G.P.-R., C.S.-P., R.O.-B., M.C.B., D.R.-P. and V.B.; Funding acquisition: D.R.-P. and V.B. All authors have read and agreed to the published version of the manuscript.

Funding: (1) Ministerio de Ciencia, Tecnología e Innovación-Colombia and La Universidad Simón Bolívar-Colombia Joint Grant for strengthening health science, technology, and innovation for ongoing projects with young talent and regional impact. Call # 874-2020; Grant number (Contrato): No. 462, 2021. (2) Internal funds for research strengthening from Universidad Simón Bolívar, Vicerrectoría de Investigación, Extensión e Innovación, Barranquilla, Colombia.

Institutional Review Board Statement: Not applicable.

Informed Consent Statement: Not applicable.

Data Availability Statement: Not applicable.

Conflicts of Interest: The authors declare no conflict of interest.

References

1. Barreto, J.F. Sistema estomatognático y esquema corporal. *Colomb. Méd.* **1999**, *30*, 173–180.
2. Karlsson, L.; Carlsson, J.; Jenneborg, K.; Kjaeldgaard, M. Perceived oral health in patients after bariatric surgery using oral health-related quality of life measures. *Clin. Exp. Dent. Res.* **2018**, *4*, 230–240. [CrossRef] [PubMed]
3. Nettle, D.; Andrews, C.; Bateson, M. Food insecurity as a driver of obesity in humans: The insurance hypothesis. *Behav. Brain Sci.* **2017**, *40*, e105. [CrossRef] [PubMed]
4. Globus, I.; Kissileff, H.R.; Hamm, J.D.; Herzog, M.; Mitchell, J.E.; Latzer, Y. Comparison of interview to questionnaire for assessment of eating disorders after bariatric surgery. *J. Clin. Med.* **2021**, *10*, 1174. [CrossRef]
5. Cadena, E. *Obesidad un Factor de Riesgo en el COVID-19*; Ministerio de Salud y Protección Social: Bogotá, Colombia, 2021.
6. Camhi, S.M.; Must, A.; Gona, P.N.; Hankinson, A.; Odegaard, A.; Reis, J.; Gunderson, E.P.; Jacobs, D.R.; Carnethon, M.R. Duration and stability of metabolically healthy obesity over 30 years. *Int. J. Obes.* **2019**, *43*, 1803–1810. [CrossRef]
7. De Lorenzo, A.; Gratteri, S.; Gualtieri, P.; Cammarano, A.; Bertucci, P.; Di Renzo, L. Why primary obesity is a disease? *J. Transl. Med.* **2019**, *17*, 169. [CrossRef]
8. Malo Serrano, M.; Castillo, N.; Pajita, D. La obesidad en el mundo. *Anal. Fac. Med.* **2017**, *78*, 173–178. [CrossRef]
9. Bates, J.H.T.; Peters, U.; Daphtary, N.; MacLean, E.S.; Hodgdon, K.; Kaminsky, D.A.; Bhatawadekar, S.; Dixon, A.E. Altered airway mechanics in the context of obesity and asthma. *J. Appl. Physiol.* **2021**, *130*, 36–47. [CrossRef]
10. Valero, P.; Souki, A.; Arráiz Rodríguez, N.J.; Prieto Fuenmayor, C.; Cano-Ponce, C.; Acosta Martínez, J.; Chávez Castillo, M.; Sánchez, M.E.; Anderson Vásquez, H.E.; Plua Marcillo, W.; et al. *Aspectos Básicos en Obesidad*; Ediciones Universidad Simón Bolívar: Barranquilla, Colombia, 2018.
11. Fonseca, A.L.F.; Salgado, W.; Dantas, O. Maximum phonation time in people with obesity not submitted or submitted to bariatric surgery. *J. Obes.* **2019**, *2019*, 5903621. [CrossRef]
12. Tomasini, K.; Ziegler, B.; Sanchez, P.R.S.; da Silva Junior, D.P.; Thomé, P.R.; Dalcin, P.T.R. Dyspnea perception during the inspiratory resistive loads test in obese subjects waiting bariatric surgery. *Sci. Rep.* **2020**, *10*, 8023. [CrossRef]
13. Carpio, C.; Santiago, A.; García de Lorenzo, A.; Álvarez-Sala, R. Función pulmonar y obesidad. *Nutr. Hosp.* **2014**, *30*, 1054–1062. [PubMed]
14. Mashaqi, S.; Steffen, K.; Crosby, R.; Garcia, L. The impact of bariatric surgery on sleep disordered breathing parameters from overnight polysomnography and home sleep apnea test. *Cureus* **2018**, *10*, e2593. [CrossRef] [PubMed]
15. Victor Taba, J.; Oliveira Suzuki, M.; do Nascimento, F.S.; Ryuchi Iuamoto, L.; Hsing, W.T.; Zumerkorn Pipek, L.; Andraus, W. The development of feeding and eating disorders after bariatric surgery: A systematic review and meta-analysis. *Nutrients* **2021**, *13*, 2396. [CrossRef] [PubMed]
16. Benzerouk, F.; Djerada, Z.; Bertin, E.; Barrière, S.; Gierski, F.; Kaladjian, A. Contributions of emotional overload, emotion dysregulation, and impulsivity to eating patterns in obese patients with binge eating disorder and seeking bariatric surgery. *Nutrients* **2020**, *12*, 3099. [CrossRef]
17. Maluenda, G.F. Cirugía bariátrica. *Rev. Med. Clin. Condes* **2012**, *23*, 180–188.
18. Del Negro, C.A.; Funk, G.D.; Feldman, J.L. Breathing matters. *Nat. Rev. Neurosci.* **2021**, *19*, 351–367. [CrossRef]
19. Andrade Rocha, A.C.; De Souza Conceição, N.O.; Mangili Toni, L.D. Chewing and swallowing in obese individuals referred to bariatric surgery/gastroplasty—A pilot study. *Rev. CEFAC* **2021**, *221*, e8519.
20. Crummy, A.; Piper, A.; Naughton, M.T. Obesity and the lung: 2·Obesity and sleep-disordered breathing. *Thorax* **2008**, *63*, 38–746. [CrossRef]
21. Souza, N.; Guedes, Z.C.F. Mastigação e deglutição de crianças e adolescentes obesos. *Rev. CEFAC* **2016**, *18*, 1340–1347. [CrossRef]
22. Mores, R.; Delgado, S.E.; Martins, N.F.; Anderle, P.; Longaray, C.; Pasqualeto, V.M.; Berbert, M.B. Caracterização dos distúrbios de sono, ronco e alterações do sistema estomatognático de obesos candidatos à Cirurgia Bariátrica. *Rev. Bras. Obes. Nutr. Emagrecimento* **2017**, *11*, 64–74.
23. Red Para la Lectoescritura Inicial de Centroamérica y el Caribe. *Diseño y Realización de Revisiones Sistemáticas. Una Guía de Formación para Investigadores de Lectoescritura Inicial (LEI)*; Ediciones RedLEI: Guatemala, 2021; Available online: https://red-lei.org/wp-content/uploads/2021/03/Directrices-de-Revisiones-Sistematicas.pdf (accessed on 2 February 2022).
24. Beltrán, O.A. Revisiones sistemáticas de la literatura. *Rev. Colomb. Gastroenterol.* **2005**, *20*, 60–69.
25. Gonzalez de Dios, J.; Balaguer Santamaría, A. Valoración crítica de artículos científicos. Parte 2: Revisiones sistemáticas y metaanálisis. *FAPap Monogr.* **2021**, *6*, 14–26.
26. Landa-Ramírez, E.; Arredondo-Pantaleón, A. Herramienta Pico para la formulación y búsqueda de preguntas clínicamente relevantes en la psicooncología basada en la evidencia. *Psicooncología* **2014**, *11*, 259–270. [CrossRef]
27. Pergunta, D. Estrategia Pico para la construcción de la pregunta de investigación y la búsqueda de evidencias. *Rev. Latino Enfermagem.* **2007**, *15*. Available online: https://www.researchgate.net/publication/283522391_Estrategia_pico_para_la_construccion_de_la_pregunta_de_investigacion_y_la_bsqueda_de_evidencias (accessed on 2 February 2022).
28. Urrútia, G.; Bonfill, X. Declaración PRISMA: Una propuesta para mejorar la publicación de revisiones sistemáticas y metaanálisis. *Med. Clín.* **2012**, *135*, 507–511. [CrossRef]
29. García, C.M.; del Castillo, M.D.M. Plan de cuidados estandarizado en cirugía bariátrica. *NURE Investig. Rev. Cien. Enferm.* **2006**, *20*, 4.
30. Pachón Salem, L.E. Formulación de criterios para registrar posición lingual en pacientes con deglución atípica mediante Glumap. *Areté* **2016**, *16*, 109–120.

31. Fuenzalida, R.; Hernández-Mosqueira, C.; Serey, J.P. Alteraciones Estructurales y Funcionales del Sistema Estomatognático: Manejo fonoaudiológico. *Areté* **2017**, *17*, 29–35. [CrossRef]
32. Bolzan Berlese, D.; Copetti, F.; Maciel Weimmann, A.R.; Fabtinel Fontana, P.; Bonfanti Haeffner, L.S. Atividade dos Músculos Masseter e Temporal em Relação às Características Miofuncionais das Funções de Mastigação e deglutição em obesos. *Distúrbios Comun.* **2012**, *24*, 215–221.
33. Mosquim, V.; Foratoti Junior, G.A.; Saory Hissano, W.; Wang y, L.; de Carvalho Sales Peres, S.H. Obesidade, cirurgia bariátrica e O impactO na saúde bucal: RevisãO de literature. *Rev. Salusvita* **2019**, *38*, 117–132.
34. Teramoto, S.; Sudo, E.; Matsuse, T.; Ohga, E.; Ishii, T.; Ouch, Y.; Fukuchi, Y. Impaired swallowing reflex in patients with obstructive sleep apnea syndrome. *Chest* **1999**, *116*, 17–21. [CrossRef] [PubMed]
35. Godlewski, A.E.; Veyrune, J.L.; Nicolas, E.; Ciangura, C.A.; Chaussain, C.C.; Czernichow, S.; Basdevant, A.; Hennequin, M. Effect of dental status on changes in mastication in patients with obesity following bariatric surgery. *PLoS ONE* **2011**, *6*, e22324. [CrossRef] [PubMed]
36. Zicari, A.M.; Marzo, G.; Rugiano, A.; Celani, C.; Carbone, M.P.; Tecco, S.; Duse, M. Habitual snoring and atopic state: Correlations with respiratory function and teeth occlusion. *BMC Pediatrics* **2012**, *12*, 175. [CrossRef] [PubMed]
37. Marin, G.; Gamez, A.S.; Molinari, N.; Kacimi, D.; Vachier, I.; Paganin, F.; Chanez, P.; Bourdin, A. Distal airway impairment in obese normoreactive women. *BioMed Res. Int.* **2013**, *2013*, 707856. [CrossRef]
38. Oppenheimer, B.W.; Berger, K.I.; Segal, L.N.; Stabile, A.; Coles, K.D.; Parikh, M.; Goldring, R.M. Airway dysfunction in obesity: Response to voluntary restoration of end expiratory lung volume. *PLoS ONE* **2014**, *9*, e88015. [CrossRef]
39. Pouwels, S.; Smeenk, F.W.; Manschot, L.; Lascaris, B.; Nienhuijs, S.; Bouwman, R.A.; Buise, M.P. Perioperative respiratory care in obese patients undergoing bariatric surgery: Implications for clinical practice. *Respir. Med.* **2016**, *117*, 73–80. [CrossRef]
40. Tulek, A.; Mulic, A.; Hogset, M.; Utheim, T.P.; Sehic, A. Therapeutic strategies for dry mouth management with emphasis on electrostimulation as a treatment option. *Int. J. Dent.* **2021**, *2021*, 6043488. [CrossRef]
41. Oppenheimer, B.W.; Berger, K.I.; Ali, S.; Segal, L.N.; Donnino, R.; Katz, S.; Parikh, M.; Goldring, R.M. Pulmonary vascular congestion: A mechanism for distal lung unit dysfunction in obesity. *PLoS ONE* **2016**, *11*, e0152769. [CrossRef]
42. de Felício, C.M.; da Silva Dias, F.V.; Trawitzki, L.V.V. Obstructive sleep apnea: Focus on myofunctional therapy. *Nat. Sci. Sleep* **2018**, *10*, 271–286. [CrossRef]
43. Cella, S.; Fei, L.; D'Amico, R.; Giardiello, C.; Allaria, A.; Cotrufo, P. Binge eating disorder and related features in bariatric surgery candidates. *Open Med.* **2019**, *14*, 407–415. [CrossRef]
44. Pizzorni, N.; Radovanovic, D.; Pecis, M.; Lorusso, R.; Annoni, F.; Bartorelli, A.; Rizzi, M.; Schindler, A.; Santus, P. Dysphagia symptoms in obstructive sleep apnea: Prevalence and clinical correlates. *Respir. Res.* **2021**, *22*, 117. [CrossRef] [PubMed]
45. Torrente-Sánchez, M.J.; Ferer-Márquez, M.; Estébanez-Ferrero, B.; Jiménez-Lasserrotte, M.D.; Ruiz-Muelle, A.; Ventura-Miranda, M.I.; Dobarrio-Sanz, I.; Granero-Molina, J. Social support for people with morbid obesity in a bariatric surgery programme: A qualitative descriptive study. *Int. J. Environ. Res. Public Health* **2021**, *18*, 6530. [CrossRef] [PubMed]
46. Womble, J.T.; McQuade, V.L.; Ihrie, M.D.; Ingram, J.L. Imbalanced coagulation in the airway of Type-2 high asthma with comorbid obesity. *J. Asthma Allergy* **2021**, *14*, 967–980. [CrossRef] [PubMed]
47. Deane, S.; Thomson, A. Obesity and the pulmonologist. *Arch. Dis. Child.* **2006**, *91*, 188–191. [CrossRef]
48. Parameswaran, K.; Todd, D.C.; Soth, M. Altered respiratory physiology in obesity. *Can. Respir. J.* **2006**, *13*, 203–210. [CrossRef]
49. Zammit, C.; Liddicoat, H.; Moonsie, I.; Makker, H. Obesity and respiratory diseases. *Int. J. Gen. Med.* **2012**, *3*, 335–343.
50. Porhomayon, J.; Papadakos, P.; Singh, A.; Nader, N.D. Alteration in respiratory physiology in obesity for anesthesia-critical care physician. *HSR Proc. Intens. Care Cardiovasc. Anesth.* **2011**, *3*, 109–118.
51. Mizraji, M.; Freese, A.M.; Bianchi, R. Sistema estomatognático. *Actas Odontológicas* **2012**, *9*, 35–47.
52. Rocha de Souza, L.B.; Medeiros Pereira, R.; Marques Dos Santos, M.; Almeida Godoy, C.M. Fundamental frequency, phonation maximum time and vocal complaints in morbidly obese women. *Arq. Bras. Cir. Dig.* **2014**, *27*, 43–46. [CrossRef]
53. Huseini, M.; Wood, G.C.; Seiler, J.; Argyropoulos, G.; Irving, B.A.; Gerhard, G.S.; Benotti, P.; Still, C.; Rolston, D. Gastrointestinal symptoms in morbid obesity. *Front. Med.* **2014**, *1*, 49. [CrossRef]
54. Braude Canterji, M.; Miranda Correa, S.P.; Vargas, G.S.; Ruttkay Pereira, J.L.; Finard, S.A. Intervenção fonoaudiológica na cirurgia bariátrica do idoso: Relato De Caso. *Arq. Bras. Cir. Dig.* **2015**, *28*, 86–87.
55. Hodgson, L.E.; Murphy, P.B.; Hart, N. Respiratory management of the obese patient undergoing surgery. *J. Thorac. Dis.* **2015**, *7*, 943–952. [PubMed]
56. Nath, A.; Yewale, S.; Tran, T.; Brebbia, J.S.; Shope, T.R.; Koch, T.R. Dysphagia after vertical sleeve gastrectomy: Evaluation of risk factors and assessment of endoscopic intervention. *World J. Gastroenterol.* **2016**, *22*, 10371–10379. [CrossRef] [PubMed]
57. Wickerts, L.; Forsberg, S.; Bouvier, F.; Jakobsson, J. Monitoring respiration and oxygen saturation in patients during the first night after elective bariatric surgery: A cohort study. *F1000 Res.* **2017**, *6*, 735. [CrossRef]
58. Schwartz, M.W.; Seeley, R.J.; Zeltser, L.M.; Drewnowski, A.; Ravussin, E.; Redman, L.M.; Leibel, R.L. Obesity pathogenesis: An endocrine society scientific statement. *Endocr. Rev.* **2017**, *38*, 267–296. [CrossRef]
59. Simões da Rocha, M.R.; Souza, S.; Moraes da Costa, C.; Bertelli Merino, D.F.; de Lima Montebelo, M.I.; Pazzianotto-Forti, R.J. Airway positive pressure vs. exercises with inspiratory loading focused on pulmonary and respiratory muscular functions in the postoperative period of bariatric surgery. *Arq. Bras. Cir. Dig.* **2018**, *31*, e1363.

60. Jehan, S.; Myers, A.K.; Zizi, F.; Pandi-Perumal, S.R.; Jean-Louis, G.; McFarlane, S.I. Obesity, obstructive sleep apnea and type 2 diabetes mellitus: Epidemiology and pathophysiologic insights. *Sleep Med. Disord. Int. J.* **2018**, *2*, 52–58.
61. Meurgey, J.H.; Brown, R.; Woroszyl-Chrusciel, A.; Steier, J. Peri-operative treatment of sleep-disordered breathing and outcomes in bariatric patients. *J. Thorac. Dis.* **2018**, *10*, S144–S152. [CrossRef]
62. Mokhlesi, B.; Masa, J.F.; Brozek, J.L.; Gurubhagavatula, I.; Murphy, P.B.; Piper, A.J.; Tulaimat, A.; Afshar, M.; Balachandran, J.S.; Dweik, R.A.; et al. Evaluation and management of obesity hypoventilation syndrome. An official American Thoracic Society clinical practice guideline. *Am. J. Respir. Crit. Care Med.* **2019**, *200*, e6–e24. [CrossRef]
63. Sant'Anna, M.; Carvalhal, R.F.; Oliveira, F.; Zin, W.A.; Lopes, A.J.; Lugon, R.J.; Guimarães, F.S. Mecânica respiratória de pacientes com obesidade morbid. *J. Bras. Pneumol.* **2019**, *45*, e20180311. [CrossRef]
64. Jaruvongvanich, V.; Matar, R.; Ravi, K.; Murad, M.H.; Vantanasiri, K.; Wongjarupong, N.; Ungprasert, P.; Vargas, E.J.; Maselli, D.B.; Prokop, L.J.; et al. Esophageal pathophysiologic changes and adenocarcinoma after bariatric surgery: A systematic review and meta-analysis. *Clin. Transl. Gastroenterol.* **2020**, *11*, e00225. [CrossRef] [PubMed]
65. Dantas Giglio, L.; Felício, C.M.D.; Voi Trawitzki, L. Orofacial functions and forces in male and female healthy young and adults. *Codas* **2020**, *32*, e20190045. [CrossRef] [PubMed]
66. Franco, R.; Barlattani, A., Jr.; Perrone, M.A.; Basili, M.; Miranda, M.; Costacurta, M.; Gualtieri, P.; Pujia, A.; Merra, G.; Bollero, P. Obesity, bariatric surgery and periodontal disease: A literature update. *Eur. Rev. Med. Pharmacol. Sci.* **2020**, *24*, 5036–5045. [PubMed]
67. García-Delgado, Y.; López-Madrazo-Hernández, M.J.; Alvarado-Martel, D.; Miranda-Calderín, G.; Ugarte-Lopetegui, A.; González-Medina, R.A.; Wägner, A.M. Prehabilitation for Bariatric Surgery: A Randomized, Controlled Trial Protocol and Pilot Study. *Nutrients* **2021**, *13*, 2903. [CrossRef]
68. Berlese, D.B.; Fontana, P.F.F.; Botton, L.; Weimmann, A.R.M.; Haeffner, L.S. Características miofuncionais de obesos respiradores orais e nasais. *Rev. Codas* **2012**, *17*, 171–176. [CrossRef]
69. Marques Gonçalves, R.D.F.; Zimberg Chehter, E. Masticatory profile of morbidly obese patients undergoing gastroplasty/Perfil mastigatorio de obesos morbidos submetidos a gastroplastia. *Rev. CEFAC* **2012**, *14*, 489–498.
70. Silva, A.S.; Tanigute, C.C.; Tessitore, A. A necessidade da avaliação fonoaudiológica no protocolo de pacientes candidatos à cirurgia bariátrica. *Rev. CEFAC* **2014**, *16*, 1655–1668. [CrossRef]
71. Pd Azevedo, A.; Cd Santos, C.; Cd Fonseca, D. Transtorno da compulsão alimentar periódica. *Arch. Clin. Psychiatry* **2004**, *31*, 170–172. [CrossRef]
72. Gonçalves, M.; Zimberg, E. Speech therapy intervention in morbidly obese undergoing fobi-capell gastroplasty method. *ABCD. Arq. Bras. Cir. Dig.* **2016**, *29*, 43–47. [CrossRef]
73. Álvarez Hernández, J. *Disfagia Orofaríngea: Soluciones Multidisciplinares*; Hospital Universitario Príncipe de Asturias: Madrid, Spain, 2018.
74. Xavier Torres, G.M.; Hernandez Alvez, C. Physiology of exercise in orofacial motricity: Knowledge about the issue. *Rev. CEFAC* **2019**, *21*, e14318. [CrossRef]
75. Duarte Aznar, F.; Aznar, F.D.; Lauris, J.R.; Adami Chaim, E.; Cazzo, E.; Sales-Peres, S.H. Dental wear and tooth loss in morbid obese patients after bariatric surgery. *Arq. Bras. Cir. Dig.* **2019**, *32*, e1458. [CrossRef] [PubMed]
76. Silva Gebara, T.; Mocelin Polli, G.; Wanderbroocke, A.C. Eating and bariatric surgery: Social representations of obese people. *Psicol. Ciência Profissão* **2021**, *41*, e222795.
77. Lemme, E.M.O.; Alvariz, A.C.; Pereira, G.L. Esophageal functional disorders in the pre-operatory evaluation of bariatric surgery. *Arq. Gastroenterol.* **2021**, *58*, 190–194. [CrossRef] [PubMed]
78. Dantas Lima, A.C.D.; Costa Albuquerque, R.; Andrade Cunha, D.A.; Dantas Lima, C.; Henrique Lima, S.J.; Justino Silva, H. Relation of sensory processing and stomatognical system of oral respiratory children. *Codas* **2021**, *34*, e20200251.
79. Mafort, T.T.; Rufino, R.; Costa, C.H.; Lopes, A.J. Obesity: Systemic and pulmonary complications, biochemical abnormalities, and impairment of lung function. *Multidiscip. Respir. Med.* **2016**, *11*, 28. [CrossRef] [PubMed]
80. Aguiar, I.C.; Freitas, W.R.; Santos, I.R.; Apostolico, N.; Nacif, S.R.; Urbano, J.J.; Fonsêca, N.T.; Thuler, F.R.; Ilias, E.J.; Kassab, P.; et al. Obstructive sleep apnea and pulmonary function in patients with severe obesity before and after bariatric surgery: A randomized clinical trial. *Multidiscip. Respir. Med.* **2014**, *9*, 43. [CrossRef]
81. Villa, M.P.; Evangelisti, M.; Martella, S.; Barreto, M.; Del Pozzo, M. Can myofunctional therapy increase tongue tone and reduce symptoms in children with sleep-disordered breathing? *Sleep Breath* **2017**, *21*, 1025–1032. [CrossRef]
82. Caparroz, F.; Campanholo, M.; Stefanini, R.; Vidigal, T.; Haddad, L.; Bittencourt, L.R.; Tufik, S.; Haddad, F. Laryngopharyngeal reflux and dysphagia in patients with obstructive sleep apnea: Is there an association? *Sleep Breath* **2019**, *23*, 619–626. [CrossRef]
83. Kristo, I.; Paireder, M.; Jomrich, G.; Felsenreich, D.M.; Fischer, M.; Hennerbichler, F.P.; Langer, F.B.; Prager, G.; Schoppmann, S.F. Silent gastroesophageal reflux disease in patients with morbid obesity prior to primary metabolic surgery. *Obes. Surg.* **2020**, *30*, 4885–4891. [CrossRef]
84. Sandoval-Munoz, C.P.; Haidar, Z.S. Neuro-Muscular Dentistry: The "diamond' concept of electro-stimulation potential for stomato-gnathic and oro-dental conditions. *Head Face Med.* **2021**, *17*, 2. [CrossRef]

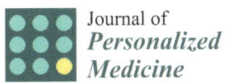

Review

Probiotics and Gut Microbiota in Obesity: Myths and Realities of a New Health Revolution

Xavier Eugenio León Aguilera [1], Alexander Manzano [2], Daniela Pirela [2] and Valmore Bermúdez [1,3,*]

1. Departamento de Post-Grado, Universidad Católica de Cuenca, Ciudad Cuenca 010109, Ecuador
2. Endocrine and Metabolic Diseases Research Center, School of Medicine, Universidad del Zulia, Maracaibo 4002, Venezuela
3. Facultad de Ciencias de la Salud, Universidad Simón Bolívar, Barranquilla 080022, Colombia
* Correspondence: v.bermudez@unisimonbolivar.edu.co

Abstract: Obesity and its comorbidities are humans' most prevalent cardio-metabolic diseases worldwide. Recent evidence has shown that chronic low-grade inflammation is a common feature in all highly prevalent chronic degenerative diseases. In this sense, the gut microbiota is a complete ecosystem involved in different processes like vitamin synthesis, metabolism regulation, and both appetite and immune system control. Thus, dysbiosis has been recognised as one of the many factors associated with obesity due to a predominance of *Firmicutes*, a decrease in *Bifidobacterium* in the gut, and a consequent short-chain fatty acids (SCFA) synthesis reduction leading to a reduction in incretins action and intestinal permeability increase. In this context, bacteria, bacterial endotoxins, and toxic bacterial by-products are translocated to the bloodstream, leading to systemic inflammation. This review focuses on gut microbiota composition and its role in obesity, as well as probiotics and prebiotics benefits in obesity.

Keywords: obesity; gut microbiota; short chain fatty acids; probiotics; prebiotics

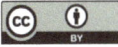

1. Introduction

Obesity is a chronic, complex, endocrine-metabolic disease that is a significant risk factor for numerous comorbidities [1]. Data from the National Health and Nutrition Examination Survey (NHANES) have shown that obesity prevalence in the United States increased from 30.5% in 1999–2000 to 42.4% in 2017–2018 [2], a fact that is conveyed in healthcare costs, not only in the USA but in many countries with Westernized lifestyles [3–5].

Some risk factors such as daily calories ingested, socioeconomic level, place of residence (urban or rural), sex, age, physical activity, diet quality, and behavioural disorders [6], among many others [7], drive obesity development throughout life in connection with genetic factors. Thus, scientific evidence has been accumulating regarding gut microbiota (dysbiosis) alterations can play a central role in the onset and further development of obesity, leading to coin the term "obese microbiota", as that microscopic community of the distal digestive tract that swifts away from its typical architecture [8]. In this vein, the gut microbiota refers to the microorganism population that usually inhabits the intestinal lumen, which plays a pivotal role in the physiology, pathophysiology, and evolution of multiple diseases such as diabetes mellitus [9], irritable bowel syndrome [10], Parkinson's disease [11], bronchial asthma [12], and even obesity [13], probably mediated by anti-inflammatory and immune response regulators metabolites [14,15]. Moreover, a significant proportion of individuals with obesity exhibit variations in their gut microbiota. There is scientific evidence enough to support that dysbiosis and inflammation play a pivotal role in many gastrointestinal and metabolic diseases, particularly obesity [16].

This review aims to briefly examine the intestinal microbiota structure, metabolism, and possible changes in obesity and the potential link with the endocrine-metabolic disorders usually associated with this condition. In addition, a critical analysis of first- and second-generation probiotics' usefulness in obesity management is presented, as well as promising innovations in dysbiosis therapy and their possible impact on obesity prevention and treatment.

2. Structure of the Human Gut Microbiota

The microbiota refers to the set of bacteria, fungi, and viruses found in different tissues that, although individual, have a common characteristic in most microorganisms for a particular host. Eubiosis occurs when microbiota microorganisms are functional compositional and ecologically in equilibrium with the host [17]. The human microbiota comprises nearly 10,000 microorganism species and sub-species [18], with the gut microbiome containing over nine million genes [19]. *Firmicutes, Bacteroidetes, Actinobacteria, Proteobacteria, Fusobacteria,* and *Verrucomicrobia* are the main microorganisms in the gut microbiota, with a clear predominance of *Firmicutes* and *Bacteroidetes* representing 90% of the human gut microbiota [20].

The *phylum Firmicutes* comprises Gram-positive endospores-forming bacteria and a genome with low DNA G + C content [21]. More than 200 genera, including *Lactobacillus, Bacillus, Clostridium, Enterococcus,* and *Ruminicoccus,* have rigid or semi-rigid walls, with Clostridium accounting for 95% of them [22]. The *phylum Actinobacteria,* which consists of Gram-positive, branched, non-motile, non-spore-forming microorganisms, is the least predominant at the intestinal level and is represented by the *genus Bifidobacterium* [23] and plays a vital role in the colonisation of the digestive tract of children born by vaginal delivery, conversely, it is significantly less in those born by cesarean section [24]. On the other hand, the *phylum Bacteroidetes* is composed of Gram-negative bacteria of *Bacteroides* and *Prevotella* genera [20], playing as primary polysaccharide processors [25] and whose final products are substrates for enzymes from other bacterial genera that eventually participate in the immune system regulation [26], intermediary metabolism [27] and intestinal–brain axis signalling [28–30]. Bacteria such as *Lactobacillus (Firmicutes)* and *Bifidobacterium (Actinobacteria)* hydrolyse and ferment very specific polysaccharides to produce the short-chain fatty acids (SCFA) acetate, butyrate, and propionate (Figure 1) [31]. In this regard, propionate is produced mainly by *Akkermansia muciniphila,* whereas butyrate is produced by *Faecalibacterium prausnitzii, Eubacterium hallii,* and *Eubacterium rectale* [32].

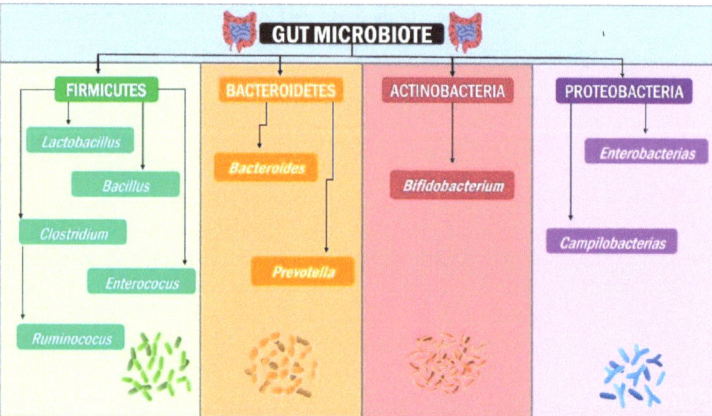

Figure 1. Gut microbiota composition: *Firmicutes, Bacteroidetes, Actinobacteria,* and *Proteobacteria* are the four "standard" *Phyla* in our gut intestinal microbiota. Each *phylum* comprises bacteria with diverse structures, metabolism, and functions.

3. Are the SCFA the Missing Link between Dysbiosis and Obesity?

SCFAs are G protein-coupled receptors (GPCRs) ligands, activating anti-inflammatory signaling cascades [33]. In addition, SCFA may also act by preserving intestinal integrity [34], reducing luminal pH [35,36], protecting intestinal lining, especially the luminal mucopolysaccharide layer [37], and regulating GAP and tight junction expression.

Although diffusion of short-chain fatty acids in their neutral (undissociated) form is an important absorption mechanism, anionic form uptake by transporter proteins is the main route for SCFA translocation across the cell membrane. Several transport systems have been described for SCFA transport in colonocytes: MCT1 (SLC16A1) and MCT4 (SLC16A3) are H+ coupled electroneutral transporter. MCT1 is expressed in the apical and basolateral membrane of the colonic epithelium, whereas MCT4 is specifically expressed in the basolateral membrane. SMCT1 (SLC5A8) is a Na+ a coupled electrogenic transporter [38], whilst SMCT2 (SLC5A12) is a Na+ a coupled transporter but electroneutral. SMCT1 and SMCT2 are expressed exclusively at the apical membrane [39,40]. Finally, an anion exchange mechanism coupled to bicarbonate efflux has been reported in the literature, but their identification and isolation have remained elusive. As a result of these mechanisms, SCFAs are efficiently absorbed across the colonocyte apical membrane in approximately 90–95% [41].

The downstream SCFA effects are mediated, at least in part, by histone deacetylase (HDAC) inhibition [42] downstream and thus decrease pro-inflammatory cytokine production. In addition, other essential functions of SCFA involve the peroxisome proliferator-activated receptor-alpha activation, increasing the substitution of old cells by renewed epithelial colonic cells [43] and the induction of IL-10 in T cells, as well as increasing the antibodies production through B cells differentiation into plasma cells [44] improving the adaptative immunity response [45]. In addition, factors such as SCFA speed, volume, and acetate/propionic/butyric ratio bring a complex interplay between fermentable diet polysaccharides, microbiome diversity and activity, and, eventually, the gut transit time.

It is well-known that fermentable carbohydrate consumption and SCFA administration produce a wide range of health benefits, including body composition improvement, increased insulin sensitivity, a low-risk lipid profile, body weight reduction, and cancer risk reduction as colon cancer. In the same vein, SCFA also plays an essential role in obesity pathophysiology by intermediary metabolism regulation and appetite control [46], at least, in part, by stimulating the incretins synthesis and secretion by entero-endocrine L cells, a specific butyrate-mediated effect [47,48]. Thus, an interesting group of scientific papers conducted in humans by Chambers et al. [49] using soluble fiber as inulin propionate-ester demonstrated an appetite and food intake attenuating effect mediated by propionate. Other studies from the same group have found equivalent results regarding food choice [50], improving pancreatic function and modulation of liver lipid metabolism. Moreover, oral propionate administration increases fat oxidation in humans regarding energetic metabolism regulation. Finally, in experimental models, propionate reduces food intake via the gut–brain axis in animals [51]. This evidence highlights an SCFA-rich diet's importance in managing obesity and associated diseases, including hypertension and other cardiovascular diseases. For instance, the butyrate induces renal prorenin receptors and renin expression, attenuating the angiotensin-II effects [52], and acetate and propionate regulate renin production via Olfr78 and a counter-regulation loop with FFAR3 [53] (Figure 2).

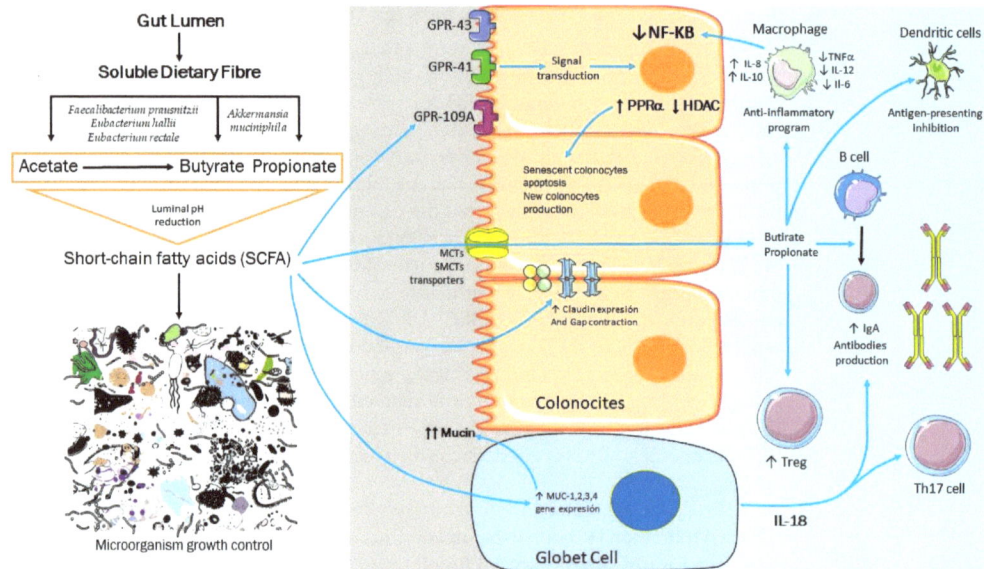

Figure 2. Main effects of short-chain fatty acids (SCFA) on microbiota and epithelium barrier. SCFA protect the intestinal barrier by lowering the levels of TNFα and interleukin (IL)-6, activating the G-protein coupled receptors (GPCR) to participate in PParα expression increase and the intestinal-mediated inflammatory and immune response by suppressing histone deacetylase (HDAC) and downregulating the expression of pro-inflammatory cytokines. Additionally, SCFA upregulates the gene expression of mucin family genes (MUC1–4) in the intestine, and the protons generated by SCFA dissociation produce an osmotic pressure imbalance in the bacteria. Furthermore, SCFA inhibits bacterial multiplication by interfering with DNA and protein synthesis.

4. Molecular Basis of Intestinal, Immunological, and Metabolic Homeostasis Control by Gut Microbiota

Dietary fiber is a sundry group of complex carbohydrates affecting human metabolism and gut microbiota [54]. Arabinoxylans (AX) are cell wall components that constitute a significant part of the dietary fiber fraction found in cereals and represent a significant fiber source in the human diet [55]. These heteroxylans, especially AX, deserve special attention with cellulose, β-1,3;1,4-glucan, arabinogalactan peptide, and lignin, as they are the major components of fiber in cereals [56].

Bifidobacteria metabolise non-digestible carbohydrates to produce acetate and lactate. Some studies have screened for genes encoding several putative AXOS-degrading enzymes in a wide Bifidobacteria variety species, but no clear correlation has been made regarding these polysaccharides' degradation [57,58]. The primary site for inulin fermentation is the ascending colon. In contrast, AXOS fermentation occurs in the transverse colon [59], and *Bifidobacterium*, *Bacteroides*, and *Roseburia* have been identified as the main fermenting species of these carbohydrates (Figure 3) [60].

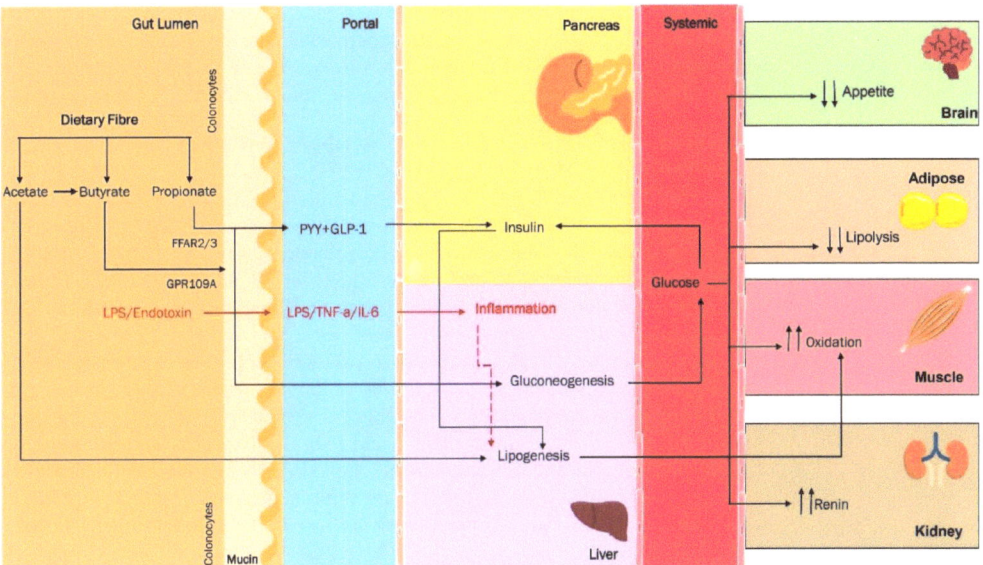

Figure 3. Dietary fibre and its effects on human metabolism and gut microbiota.

A high-fat diet has been established to increase Clostridia and Bifidobacteria gut population and decrease *Bacteroides*. However, there is also a significant influence on bile acid metabolism [61], highlighting its potential impact on dysbiosis, which might lead to changes in SCFA metabolism due to *Bifidobacteria* decrease.

5. Microbiota in Obesity: Cause, Effect, or Both?

Dysbiosis refers to the alteration of normal bacterial microbiota [62]. Several environmental factors affecting gut microbiota are closely associated with dysbiosis and obesity [63]. Overall, these factors increase *Firmicutes* species such as *Eubacterium rectale*, *Clostridium coccoides*, *Lactobacillus reuteri*, *Clostridium histolyticum*, and *Staphylococcus aureus* [64]. On the other hand, a significant decrease in the relative abundance of several Bacteroidetes taxa members such as *Faecalibacterium prausnitzii*, *Bacteroidetes*, *Methanobrevibacter smithii*, *Lactobacillus plantarum* and *Lactobacillus paracasei*, *L. rhamnosus*, and *Verrucomicrobia* (*Akkermansia muciniphila*) have been reported [16,65]. Depending on the microbiota alteration, dysbiosis can be produced by the loss of beneficial microbial organisms, overgrowth of potentially harmful microorganisms, or general microbial diversity loss [66]. Thus, obesity microbiota is characterised by a significant *Firmicutes* increase and a 50% decrease in Bacteroidetes at the terminal ileum [67]. It was also reported that *Lactobacillus reuteri* and *Lactobacillus sakei* are directly related to weight gain in adults, mainly in conjunction with a high-fat diet consumption [68], while on the other hand, microorganisms of the *Bifidobacterium* genus decrease the comorbidities associated with obesity, such as metabolic syndrome [69].

High-fat and high-carbohydrate diet consumption leads to *Bacteroides*, *Bifidobacterium*, *Lactobacillus*, and *Akkermansia* deficit with a considerable increase in *Clostridium* and *Prevotella* driving Toll-like receptor 4 (TLR4) activation via lipopolysaccharides pathway triggering to inflammation and claudin 1 and 3 expression decrease [70]. Claudin is a family of 18 proteins that play essential structural and functional roles in determining tight junction structure and permeability. Therefore, a reduction in these protein's expression via SCFA levels decrease alters the integrity gut epithelial barrier, causing bacterial translocation and expression of inflammatory cytokines [71] such as TNFα and interleukin-1 [72], increasing Gram-negative bacteria adherence to the intestinal epithelium [73], leading to a chronic pro-inflammatory state that triggers obesity and cardiometabolic comorbidities [74].

Furthermore, it has been recognised that high-glucose or fructose rich-foods produce microbiota dysbiosis, also affecting intestinal permeability and inducing hepatic steatosis [75], while on the other hand, glutamine, vitamin A, vitamin D, and dietary fibre preserve intestinal permeability by increasing the production of butyrate and propionate [76].

6. Are Probiotics Effective in Endocrine-Metabolic Disease Treatment? Are These Supplements Effective in Intestinal Dysbiosis?

According to The World Health Organization, probiotics are *"Live microorganisms which when administered in adequate amounts confer a health benefit on the host"* [77]. In this area of intense development, scientific evidence has been accumulated, influencing the appearance of new, rich, and sophisticated terminology. Since it has been shown that inactivated, non-viable, or broken probiotics have beneficial effects on health, the term paraprobiotics has been incorporated, including the true probiotics (functional), pseudoprobiotics (inactive), and phantom probiotics (non-viable or broken) [78]. Thus, a true probiotic, for instance, *Lactobacillus plantarum* improves IL-10 in the colon [79] by adhering to the gut epithelium. *Lactobacillus rhamnousus*, adhering to the epithelium and, in this case, also producing lactic acid [80]; Lactobacillus acidophilus is found at the intestinal level and whose mechanism of action is by lactacin production and further cholesterol adherence [81]. *Bifidobacterium animalis* increase intestinal motility and bile salts hydrolysis [82]. Furthermore, *Saccharomyces boullardii* redistributes T cells in vitro (Table 1) [83].

Table 1. The major species used as probiotics for the gastrointestinal tract in humans and their main locations and mechanisms of action [78].

Microorganism	Location	Mechanism of Action
Lactobacillus plantarum	Gastrointestinal tract	Adhesion to epithelial cells. Improves IL-10 production in the colon
Lactobacillus rhamnosus	Gastrointestinal tract and brain	Adhesion to epithelial cells, lactic acid production, Regeneration of epithelial cells, increases GABA receptors in cortical regions and decreases in the amygdala, hypothalamus, and *Locus ceruleus*
Lactobacillus salivarius	Gastrointestinal tract	Secretion of low molecular weight bacteriocins.
Lactobacillus reuteri	Gastrointestinal tract	Reuterin (3-hydroxypropionaldehyde) production
Lactobacillus acidophilus	Intestine	Cholesterol adherence
Lactobacillus casei	Intestine	Inhibits bacterial translocation, increases MUC gene expression, inhibits cholesterol mycelia formation, enhances NK cell activity, inhibits bacterial translocation, increases MUC gene expression, inhibits cholesterol mycelia formation, and enhances NK cell activity
Lactobacillus bulgaricus	Intestine	Adherence to cholesterol, inhibits the formation of cholesterol mycelia.
Bifidobacterium longum	Intestine	Binding to aflatoxin B1
Bifidobacterium adolescentis	Intestine	Binding to aflatoxin B1
Bifidobacterium animalis	Intestine	Increases intestinal motility and bile salts hydrolysis.
Saccharomyces boullardii	Intestine	T-cell redistribution
Lactobacillus plantarum	Intestine	Decreased translocation and adherence of pathogens
Lactobacillus paracasei	Intestine	Enhances cancer cell apoptosis
Saccharomyces boulardii	Intestine	Improves intestinal barrier function
Bifidobacterium sp.	Intestine	Secretes superoxide dismutase
Lactobacillus helveticus	Intestine	Secretes vitamin E

There is a growing body of evidence that probiotics improve, maintain, or restore the intestinal microbiota, a critical action because obesity has been linked to dysbiosis [84], thus opening the door to innovative manoeuvres directed to microbiota architecture and diversity.

7. Efficacy of Probiotics in Obesity and Its Comorbidities: Fiction or Reality?

The benefit of probiotics in overweight and obese patients has long been controversial. However, most research suggests limited health benefits, so they are only recommended as adjuvant therapy for cardiovascular disease biomarkers reduction [85].

In this regard, a meta-analysis by Koutnikova et al. on 105 trials assessing the probiotic's efficacy in obese patients concluded that while probiotics improved BMI and weight by 3–5%, there was no statistically significant effect on HbA1c, cholesterol, triglycerides, HOMA-IR, or liver function [86]. Conversely, a recent meta-analysis of randomised controlled trials (RCTs) by Tabrizi et al., assessing probiotic effectiveness on clinical symptoms, weight loss, glycemic control, blood lipids, endocrine profiles, inflammation biomarkers, and oxidative stress tests in women with polycystic ovary syndrome, found improvements in women consuming probiotics related to weight, BMI, FPG, insulin, HOMA-IR, triglycerides, VLDL-cholesterol, C reactive protein, malondialdehyde, hirsutism, total testosterone, QUICKI, nitric oxide, total antioxidant capacity, reduced glutathione, and sexual hormones binding globulin. However, it did not find changes in dehydroepiandrosterone sulfate levels and total cholesterol, LDL, and HDL cholesterol levels in patients with PCOS [87].

Similarly, a meta-analysis by Lau et al. evaluated the probiotic effect on obesity, type 2 diabetes, hypertension, and dyslipidemia in 38,802 adults from the National Health and Nutrition Examination Survey (NHANES) data between 1999 and 2014. In this research, Probiotic ingestion was considered when a subject reported yoghurt consumption or when a commercial probiotic supplemented it during the 24-h dietary recall or the Dietary Supplement use 30-Day questionnaire. This study found a 13.1% reported probiotic ingestion in the participants. The prevalence of obesity and hypertension was lower in the probiotic group (obesity-adjusted Odds Ratio (OR): 0.84, 95% CI 0.76–0.92, $p < 0.001$; hypertension-adjusted OR: 0.79, 95% CI 0.71–0.88, $p < 0.001$). Accordingly, even after analytic adjustments, body mass index (BMI) was significantly lower in the probiotic group, as were systolic and diastolic blood pressure and triglycerides; high-density lipoprotein (HDL) was significantly higher in the probiotic group for the adjusted model [88].

In an interesting meta-analysis conducted by Kim et al. with data from 1953 and 2018, including 246 obese cases and 198 normal controls, the primary goal was to determine whether SCFA levels differ between obese and non-obese individuals and determine their faecal microbiota structure. This study found differences in the levels of SCFAs in faeces between obese cases and non-obese controls. The findings show that individuals with obesity had higher acetate, propionate, and butyrate faecal levels. In addition, this study found that obese individuals had low bacterial abundance in faeces regarding microbiota architecture, but the differences were not statistically significant. The meta-regression analysis demonstrated that the abundance of the phylum *Firmicutes* was positively associated with obesity for individuals 37 years or younger, while the Bacteroidetes abundance was negatively associated with obesity for 47 or younger participants.

8. Prebiotics, the Cornerstone of Gut Microbiota

Since the prebiotic concept has experienced a continuous evolution over decades, the classic definition proposed by Gibson et al. is *"a non-digestible food ingredient that beneficially affects the host by selectively stimulating the growth and/or activity of one or a limited number of bacteria in the colon, thereby improving host's health"* [89] still being useful to understand the fundamental properties of this substances. This concept has become more sophisticated to include noncarbohydrate substances affecting the colonisation of beneficial bacteria within our microbiota. Prebiotics are non-digestible oligosaccharides with diverse chemical structures and functions, differing in molecular weight, monosaccharide type, origin (vegetables, fruits, among others), and branching degree. Prebiotics are currently a new and flourishing research area with a profound impact as modulators of gut microbiota and their effects on cancer, ulcerative colitis, irritable bowel syndrome, type 2 diabetes, response to chemotherapy, immune modulation, and obesity, among others. Prebiotics exert beneficial effects based on stimulating the growth of colon probiotics and beneficial taxons with many anti-inflammatory capacities and in their catabolic products, especially butyrate, which can carry out a diverse and complex cell cycle regulation in colonic cell tumour, leading towards their apoptosis [90].

Prebiotics has demonstrated their usefulness in regulating satiety by increasing GLP-1 and PYY [91], as well as decreasing ghrelin secretion [92], which results in a reduction in food intake and consequent weight loss [93]. Nutritionally, AX are the main component of dietary fiber, and their enzymatic hydrolysis produces AXOS and XOS; which, when cereal-based foods, such as bread and beer, are consumed, exhibit all of the characteristics of prebiotics, including resistance to gastric acidity, fermentation by the intestinal microbiota, and selective stimulation of the growth or activity of beneficial bacteria [55]. As a result, AXOS and XOS selectively stimulate *Bifidobacterium*, which stops the increase in cholesterol, triglycerides, postprandial glucose, and insulin levels [94].

9. Concluding Remarks

Humans have not escaped from the co-evolution with the vast microbial community residing in our bodies. As a superorganism, the mammalian gut is an excellent niche for microbes because of its constant temperature, predictable humidity, pH, and steady food supply. In return, the microbes perform a pleiad of functions ranging from vitamin production to immune system regulation and appetite control.

Until now, we had never had enough knowledge to modify this interaction to our benefit since 10,000 years ago, when the most significant change in the host-microbiota symbiosis occurred during the Neolithic revolution, a transition from hunting and gathering to agriculture and permanent settlement. In this period, agriculture and animal husbandry began to shape the genomes within us in an accelerated and non-stop fashion. The second giant leap in this relationship occurred during the industrialisation process and, most recently, during the Cocacolonization [95] and McDonalization [96] era, at least in the last five decades, driving dramatic changes in the human gut microbiota structure as we see in people with obesity, diabetes and other chronic diseases in the 20th and 21st century.

While we cannot entirely deny that the rationale for probiotics administration seems solid, it is also clear that we have a long way to go in understanding both the microbiota complexity and probiotics' effects on many diseases, including obesity. Each of us has a unique gut microbiome, and thus, the effects of the different bacteria in commercial probiotics can be highly variable; therefore, we believe their use should be tailored within a framework of personalised medicine that takes into account the disease to be treated and the microbiota affected by that particular patient for optimal benefits. Thus, it is almost certain that current commercial products contain neither the correct strains nor the correct amounts of bacteria to provide benefits for most of the diseases to be treated. Therefore, while taking a supplement to improve health is undoubtedly an attractive prospect, there are no robust controlled clinical trials aimed at assessing the efficacy of probiotics as individual agents for treating obesity, as we have seen in dozens of anti-obesity drugs that have been developed over the decades. Until now, those patients seeking to improve chronic diseases such as obesity by helping their gut microbiota with probiotics pursue a mirage under a promise from the manufacturing companies that take advantage of not having to substantiate their claims with randomised controlled trials. Faced with this knowledge gap, it should consider consuming a healthy diet rich in soluble fibre from fruits and vegetables. In the meantime, rigorous clinical trials with very high-resolution genomic analysis are needed to corroborate the potential health benefits and confirm whether all the effects attributed to probiotics from the supplement industry are simply a myth or a new health revolution helping us stop the ominous obesity epidemic.

Author Contributions: Conceptualisation: X.E.L.A. and V.B.; Investigation: X.E.L.A. and V.B.; Writing—original draft: X.E.L.A., A.M., D.P. and V.B.; Writing—review and editing: X.E.L.A., A.M., D.P. and V.B.; Funding acquisition: V.B. All authors have reviewed and approved the final version of the work. All authors have read and agreed to the published version of the manuscript.

Funding: Ministerio de Ciencia, Tecnología e Innovación-Colombia and La Universidad Simón Bolívar-Colombia Joint Grant for strengthening health science, technology, and innovation for ongoing projects with young talent and regional impact. Call # 874-2020; Grant number (Contrato): No. 462, 2021; Internal funds for research strengthening from Universidad Simon Bolivar, Vicerrectoría de Investigación, Extensión e Innovación, Barranquilla, Colombia.

Institutional Review Board Statement: Not applicable.

Informed Consent Statement: Not applicable.

Data Availability Statement: Not applicable.

Conflicts of Interest: The authors declare no conflict of interest.

References

1. CarrGómez, J.C.; Ena, J.; Lorido, J.A.; Ripoll, J.S.; Carrasco-Sánchez, F.J.; Gómez-Huelgas, R.; Soto, M.P.; Lista, J.D.; Martínez, P.P. Obesity Is a Chronic Disease. Positioning Statement of the Diabetes, Obesity and Nutrition Workgroup of the Spanish Society of internal Medicine (SEMI) for An Approach Centred on individuals with Obesity. *Rev. Clín. Esp.* **2021**, *221*, 509–516.
2. Hales, C.M.; Carroll, M.D.; Fryar, C.D.; Ogden, C.L. Prevalence of Obesity and Severe Obesity Among Adults: United States, 2017–2018. *NCHS Data Brief.* **2020**, *360*, 1–8.
3. Safaei, M.; Sundararajan, E.A.; Driss, M.; Boulila, W.; Shapi'I, A. A Systematic Literature Review on Obesity: Understanding the Causes & Consequences of Obesity and Reviewing Various Machine Learning Approaches Used to Predict obesity. *Comput. Biol. Med.* **2021**, *136*, 104754.
4. Zhang, X.; Zhang, M.; Zhao, Z.; Huang, Z.; Deng, Q.; Li, Y. Obesogenic Environmental Factors of Adult Obesity in China: A Nationally Representative Cross-Sectional Study. *Environ. Res. Lett.* **2020**, *15*, 4. [CrossRef]
5. Prakash, K.; Munyanyi, M.E. Energy Poverty and Obesity. *Energy Econ.* **2021**, *101*, 105428. [CrossRef]
6. Pérez-Rodrigo, C.; Hervás Bárbara, G.; Gianzo Citores, M.; Aranceta-Bartrina, J. Prevalence of Obesity and Associated Cardiovascular Risk Factors in the Spanish Population: The ENPE Study. *Rev. Esp. Cardiol. Engl.* **2021**, *3*, 232–241. [CrossRef]
7. Corazzini, R.; Morgado, F.; Gascón, T.M.; Affonso Fonseca, F.L. Evaluation of Obesity Associated with Health Risk Factors in Brazilian Public School. *Obes. Med.* **2020**, *19*, 100223. [CrossRef]
8. Cornejo-Pareja, I.; Muñoz-Garach, A.; Clemente-Postigo, M.; Tinahones, F.J. Importance of Gut Microbiota in Obesity. *Eur. J. Clin. Nutr.* **2019**, *72*, 26–37. [CrossRef]
9. Wu, H.; Tremaroli, V.; Schmidt, C.; Lundqvist, A.; Olsson, L.M.; Krämer, M. The Gut Microbiota in Prediabetes and Diabetes: A Population-Based Cross-Sectional Study. *Cell Metab.* **2020**, *32*, 379–390. [CrossRef]
10. Pittayanon, R.; Lau, J.T.; Yuan, Y.; Leontiadis, G.I.; Tse, F.; Surette, M. Gut Microbiota in Patients with Irritable Bowel Syndrome—A Systematic Review. *Gastroenterology* **2019**, *157*, 97–108. [CrossRef]
11. Nielsen, S.D.; Pearson, N.M.; Seidler, K. The Link between the Gut Microbiota and Parkinson's Disease: A Systematic Mechanism Review with Focus on α-Synuclein Transport. *Brain Res.* **2021**, *1769*, 147609. [CrossRef]
12. Lukacs, N.W.; Huang, Y.J. Microbiota–Immune interactions in Asthma Pathogenesis and Phenotype. *Curr. Opin. Immunol.* **2020**, *66*, 22–26. [CrossRef]
13. Guo, L.; Yang, K.; Zhou, P.; Yong, W. Gut Microbiota in Obesity and Nonalcoholic Fatty *Liver. Disease. Surg. Pract. Sci.* **2021**, *5*, 100030. [CrossRef]
14. Mills, S.; Stanton, C.; Lane, J.; Smith, G.; Ross, R. Precision Nutrition and the Microbiome, Part I: Current State of the Science. *Nutrients* **2019**, *11*, 923. [CrossRef]
15. Gomaa, E.Z. Human Gut Microbiota/Microbiome in Health and Diseases: A Review. *Antonie Van Leeuwenhoek* **2020**, *113*, 2019–2040. [CrossRef]
16. Crovesy, L.; Masterson, D.; Rosado, E.L. Profile of the Gut Microbiota of Adults with Obesity: A Systematic Review. *Eur. J. Clin. Nutr.* **2020**, *74*, 1251–1262. [CrossRef]
17. Lilly, D.M.; Stillwell, R.H. Probiotics: Growth-Promoting Factors Produced by Microorganisms. *Science* **1965**, *147*, 747–748. [CrossRef]
18. Afrc, R.F. Probiotics in Man and Animals. *J. Appl. Bacteriol.* **1989**, *66*, 365–378. [CrossRef]
19. Gilliland, S.E. Health and Nutritional Benefits from Lactic Acid Bacteria. *FEMS Microbiol. Lett.* **1990**, *87*, 175–1788. [CrossRef]
20. Goldin, B.R.; Gorbach, S.L. The Effect of Milk and Lactobacillus Feeding on Human intestinal Bacterial Enzyme Activity. *Am. J. Clin. Nutr.* **1984**, *39*, 756–761. [CrossRef]
21. Perdigón, G.; Fuller, R.; Raya, R. Lactic Acid Bacteria and their Effect-on the Immune System. *Curr. Issues Intest. Microbiol.* **2001**, *2*, 27–42. [PubMed]

22. Vedamuthu, E.R. Starter Cultures for Yogurt and Fer-mented Milks. In *RC Chandan Manufacturing Yogurt and Fermented Milks*; Blackwell Publishing: Ames, IA, USA, 2006; pp. 88–115.
23. Siciliano, R.A.; Mazzeo, M.F. Molecular Mechanisms of Probiotic Action: A Perspective. *Curr. Opin. Microbiol.* **2012**, *15*, 390–396. [CrossRef] [PubMed]
24. Abdoli, M.; Mohammadi, G.; Mansouri, K.; Khaledian, S.; Taran, M.; Martinez, F. A Review on Anticancer, Antibacterial and Photo Catalytic Activity of Various Nanoparticles Synthesised by Probiotics. *J. Biotechnol.* **2022**, *354*, 63–71. [CrossRef] [PubMed]
25. Tian, P.; Zou, R.; Wang, L.; Chen, Y.; Qian, X.; Zhao, J. Multi-Probiotics Ameliorate Major Depressive Disorder and Accompanying Gastrointestinal Syndromes via Serotonergic System Regulation. *J. Adv. Res.* 2022, in press. [CrossRef]
26. Wang, C.; Li, S.; Xue, P.; Yu, L.; Tian, F.; Zhao, J. The Effect of Probiotic Supplementation on Lipid Profiles in Adults with Overweight or Obesity: A Meta-Analysis of Randomised Controlled Trials. *J. Funct. Foods* **2021**, *86*, 104711. [CrossRef]
27. Woźniak, D.; Cichy, W.; Przysławski, J.; Drzymała-Czyż, S. The Role of Microbiota and Enteroendocrine Cells in Maintaining Homeostasis in the Human Digestive Tract. *Adv. Med. Sci.* **2021**, *66*, 284–292. [CrossRef]
28. Specter, M. Germs are Us. *New Yorker*, 15 October 2012; Volume 88, 32–39.
29. Li, J.; Jia, H.; Cai, X.; Zhong, H.; Feng, Q. An integrated Catalog of Reference Genes in the Human Gut Microbiome. *Nat. Biotechnol.* **2014**, *32*, 834–841. [CrossRef]
30. Arumugam, M.; Raes, J.; Pelletier, E.; Le Paslier, D.; Yamada, T. Enterotypes of the Human Gut Microbiome. *Nature* **2011**, *473*, 174–180. [CrossRef]
31. Watanabe, M.; Kojima, H.; Fukui, M. Complete Genome Sequence and Cell Structure of Limnochorda Pilosa, a Gram-Negative Spore-former within the Phylum Firmicutes. *Int. J. Syst. Evol. Microbiol.* **2016**, *66*, 1330–1339. [CrossRef]
32. Qin, J.; Li, R.; Raes, J. A Human Gut Microbial Gene Catalogue Established by Metagenomic Sequencing. *Nature* **2010**, *464*, 59–65. [CrossRef]
33. Rinninella, E.; Raoul, P.; Cintoni, M.; Franceschi, F.; Miggiano, G.; Gasbarrini, A. What Is the Healthy Gut Microbiota Composition? A Changing Ecosystem Across Age, Environment, Diet, and Diseases. *Microorganisms* **2019**, *7*, 14. [CrossRef]
34. Binda, C.; Lopetuso, L.R.; Rizzatti, G.; Gibiino, G.; Cennamo, V.; Gasbarrini, A. Actinobacteria: A Relevant Minority for the Maintenance of Gut Homeostasis. *Dig. Liver. Dis.* **2018**, *50*, 421–428. [CrossRef]
35. Lapébie, P.; Lombard, V.; Drula, E.; Terrapon, N.; Henrissat, B. Bacteroidetes Use Thousands of Enzyme Combinations to Break Down Glycans. *Nat. Commun.* **2019**, *10*, 2043. [CrossRef]
36. Ivanov, I.I.; de Llanos Frutos, R.; Manel, N.; Yoshinaga, K.; Rifkin, D.B.; Sartor, R.B.; Finlay, B.B.; Littman, D.R. Specific Microbiota Direct the Differentiation of Th17 Cells in the Mucosa of the Small intestine. *Cell Host Microbe* **2008**, *4*, 337–349. [CrossRef]
37. Chassaing, B.; Koren, O.; Goodrich, J.K.; Poole, A.C.; Srinivasan, S.; Ley, R.E.; Gewirtz, A.T. Dietary Emulsifiers Impact the Mouse Gut Microbiota Promoting Colitis and Metabolic Syndrome. *Nature* **2015**, *519*, 92–96. [CrossRef]
38. Gibiino, G.; Lopetuso, L.R.; Scaldaferri, F.; Rizzatti, G.; Binda, C.; Gasbarrini, A. Exploring Bacteroidetes: Metabolic Key Points and Immunological Tricks of Our Gut Commensals. *Dig. Liver. Dis.* **2018**, *50*, 635–639. [CrossRef]
39. Quigley, E.M.M. Microbiota-Brain-Gut Axis and Neurodegenerative Diseases. *Curr. Neurol. Neurosci. Rep.* **2017**, *17*, 94. [CrossRef]
40. Lukiw, W.J. Bacteroides Fragilis Lipopolysaccharide and inflammatory Signaling in Alzheimer's Disease. *Front. Microbiol.* **2016**, *7*, 1544. [CrossRef]
41. Stilling, R.M.; Van de Wouw, M.; Clarke, G.; Stanton, C.; Dinan, T.G.; Cryan, J.F. The Neuropharmacology of Butyrate: The Bread and Butter of the Microbiota-Gut-Brain Axis? *Neurochem. Int.* **2016**, *99*, 110–132. [CrossRef]
42. Morrison, D.J.; Preston, T. Formation of Short Chain Fatty Acids by the Gut Microbiota and their Impact on Human Metabolism. *Gut Microbes* **2016**, *7*, 189–200. [CrossRef]
43. Thorburn, A.N.; Macia, L.; Mackay, C.R. Diet, Metabolites, and "Western-Lifestyle" inflammatory Diseases. *Immunity* **2014**, *40*, 833–842. [CrossRef]
44. Macfarlane, G.T.; Macfarlane, S. Bacteria, Colonic Fermentation, and Gastrointestinal Health. *J. AOAC Int.* **2012**, *95*, 50–60. [CrossRef]
45. Jung, T.-H.; Park, J.H.; Jeon, W.-M.; Han, K.-S. Butyrate Modulates Bacterial Adherence on LS174T Human Colorectal Cells by Stimulating Mucin Secretion and MAPK Signaling Pathway. *Nutr. Res. Pract.* **2015**, *9*, 343. [CrossRef]
46. Fukuda, S.; Toh, H.; Hase, K.; Oshima, K.; Nakanishi, Y.; Yoshimura, K.; Tobe, T.; Clarke, J.M.; Topping, D.L.; Suzuki, T.; et al. Bifidobacteria Can Protect from Enteropathogenic infection Through Production of Acetate. *Nature* **2011**, *469*, 543–547. [CrossRef]
47. Wrzosek, L.; Miquel, S.; Noordine, M.-L.; Bouet, S.; Chevalier-Curt, M.J.; Robert, V.; Philippe, C.; Bridonneau, C.; Cherbuy, C.; Robbe-Masselot, C.; et al. Bacteroides thetaiotaomicron and Faecalibacterium Prausnitziiinfluence the Production of Mucus Glycans and the Development of Goblet Cells in the Colonic Epithelium of a Gnotobiotic Model Rodent. *BMC Biol.* **2013**, *11*, 61. [CrossRef]
48. Miyauchi, S.; Gopal, E.; Fei, Y.J.; Ganapathy, V. Functional Identification of SLC5A8, A Tumor Suppressor Down-Regulated in Colon Cancer, as a Na+-coupled Transporter for Short-chain Fatty Acids. *J. Biol. Chem.* **2004**, *279*, 13293–13296. [CrossRef]
49. Chassard, C.; Lacroix, C. Carbohydrates and the Human Gut Microbiota. *Curr. Opin. Clin. Nutr. Metab. Care* **2013**, *16*, 453–460. [CrossRef]
50. Ríos-Covián, D.; Ruas-Madiedo, P.; Margolles, A.; Gueimonde, M.; de los Reyes-Gavilán, C.G.; Salazar, N. Intestinal Short Chain Fatty Acids and their Link with Diet and Human Health. *Front. Microbiol.* **2016**, *7*, 185. [CrossRef] [PubMed]

51. Parada Venegas, D.; De la Fuente, M.K.; Landskron, G.; González, M.J.; Quera, R.; Dijkstra, G.; Harmsen, H.J.; Faber, K.N.; Hermoso, M.A. Short Chain Fatty Acids (SCFAs)-Mediated Gut Epithelial and Immune Regulation and Its Relevance for inflammatory Bowel Diseases. *Front. Immunol.* **2019**, *10*, 277. [CrossRef] [PubMed]
52. Kim, C.H.; Park, J.; Kim, M. Gut Microbiota-Derived Short-Chain Fatty Acids, T Cells, and inflammation. *Immune Netw.* **2014**, *14*, 277–288. [CrossRef] [PubMed]
53. Zhao, Y.; Chen, F.; Wu, W.; Sun, M.; Bilotta, A.J.; Yao, S.; Xiao, Y.; Huang, X.; Eaves-Pyles, T.D.; Golovko, G.; et al. GPR43 Mediates Microbiota Metabolite SCFA Regulation of Antimicrobial Peptide Expression in intestinal Epithelial Cells via Activation of mTOR and STAT3. *Mucosal Immunol.* **2018**, *11*, 752–762. [CrossRef]
54. Park, J.; Kim, M.; Kang, S.G.; Jannasch, A.H.; Cooper, B.; Patterson, J.; Kim, C.H. Short-Chain Fatty Acids induce Both Effector and Regulatory T Cells by Suppression of Histone Deacetylases and Regulation of the mTOR–S6K Pathway. *Mucosal Immunol.* **2015**, *8*, 80–93. [CrossRef]
55. Kim, K.N.; Yao, Y.; Ju, S.Y. Short Chain Fatty Acids and Fecal Microbiota Abundance in Humans with Obesity: A Systematic Review and Meta-Analysis. *Nutrients* **2019**, *11*, 2512. [CrossRef]
56. Byrne, C.S.; Chambers, E.S.; Morrison, D.J.; Frost, G. The Role of Short Chain Fatty Acids in Appetite Regulation and Energy Homeostasis. *Int. J. Obes.* **2015**, *39*, 1331–1338. [CrossRef]
57. Larraufie, P. SCFas Strongly Stimulate PYY Production in Human Enteroendocrine Cells. *Sci. Rep.* **2018**, *74*, 1–8. [CrossRef]
58. Tolhurst, G.; Heffron, H.; Lam, Y.S.; Parker, H.E.; Habib, A.M.; Diakogiannaki, E.; Cameron, J.; Grosse, J.; Reimann, F.; Gribble, F.M. Short-Chain Fatty Acids Stimulate Glucagon-like Peptide-1 Secretion via the G-Protein–Coupled Receptor FFAR2. *Diabetes* **2012**, *61*, 364–371. [CrossRef]
59. Chambers, E.S.; Byrne, C.S.; Aspey, K.; Chen, Y.; Khan, S.; Morrison, D.J.; Frost, G. Acute Oral Sodium Propionate Supplementation Raises Resting Energy Expenditure and Lipid Oxidation in Fasted Humans. *Diabetes Obes. Metab.* **2018**, *20*, 1034–1039. [CrossRef]
60. Chambers, E.S.; Viardot, A.; Psichas, A.; Morrison, D.J.; Murphy, K.G.; Zac-Varghese, S.E.K.; MacDougall, K.; Preston, T.; Tedford, C.; Finlayson, G.S.; et al. Effects of Targeted Delivery of Propionate to the Human Colon on Appetite Regulation, Body Weight Maintenance and Adiposity in Overweight Adults. *Gut* **2015**, *64*, 1744–1754. [CrossRef]
61. Byrne, C.; Chambers, E.S.; Alhabeeb, H.; Chhina, N.; Morrison, D.J.; Preston, T.; Tedford, C.; Fitzpatrick, J.; Irani, C.; Busza, A.; et al. Increased Colonic Propionate Reduces Anticipatory Reward Responses in the Human Striatum to High-Energy Foods. *Am. J. Clin. Nutr.* **2016**, *104*, 5–14. [CrossRef]
62. Pluznick, J.L.; Protzko, R.J.; Gevorgyan, H.; Peterlin, Z.; Sipos, A.; Han, J.; Brunet, I.; Wan, L.X.; Rey, F.; Wang, T.; et al. Olfactory Receptor Responding to Gut Microbiota-Derived Signals Plays a Role in Renin Secretion and Blood Pressure Regulation. *Proc. Natl. Acad. Sci. USA* **2013**, *110*, 4410–4415. [CrossRef]
63. Natarajan, N.; Hori, D.; Flavahan, S.; Steppan, J.; Flavahan, N.A.; Berkowitz, D.E.; Pluznick, J.L. Microbial Short Chain Fatty Acid Metabolites Lower Blood Pressure via Endothelial G Protein-Coupled Receptor 41. *Physiol. Genom.* **2016**, *48*, 826–834. [CrossRef]
64. Benítez-Páez, A.; Del Pulgar, E.M.G.; Kjølbæk, L.; Brahe, L.K.; Astrup, A.; Larsen, L.; Sanz, Y. Impact of Dietary Fiber and Fat on Gut Microbiota Re-Modeling and Metabolic Health. *Trends Food Sci. Technol.* **2016**, *57*, 201–212. [CrossRef]
65. Broekaert, W.F.; Courtin, C.M.; Verbeke, K.; Van de Wiele, T.; Verstraete, W.; Delcour, J.A. Prebiotic and Other Health-Related Effects of Cereal-Derived Arabinoxylans, Arabinoxylan-Oligosaccharides, and Xylooligosaccharides. *Crit. Rev. Food Sci. Nutr.* **2011**, *51*, 178–194. [CrossRef]
66. McCleary, B.V. Dietary Fiber Analysis. *Proc. Nutr. Soc.* **2003**, *62*, 3–9. [CrossRef] [PubMed]
67. Garrido, D.; Ruiz-Moyano, S.; Jimenez-Espinoza, R.; Eom, H.-J.; Block, D.E.; Mills, D.A. Utilization of Galactooligosaccharides by Bifidobacterium Longum Subsp. Infantis Isolates. *Food Microbiol.* **2013**, *33*, 262–270. [CrossRef] [PubMed]
68. Rivière, A.; Moens, F.; Selak, M.; Maes, D.; Weckx, S.; De Vuyst, L. The Ability of Bifidobacteria to Degrade Arabinoxylan Oligosaccharide Constituents and Derived Oligosaccharides Is Strain Dependent. *Appl. Environ. Microbiol.* **2014**, *80*, 204–217. [CrossRef] [PubMed]
69. Sanchez, J.I.; Marzorati, M.; Grootaert, C.; Baran, M.; Van Craeyveld, V.; Courtin, C.M.; Broekaert, W.F.; Delcour, J.A.; Verstraete, W.; Van de Wiele, T. Arabinoxylan-oligosaccharides (AXOS) Affect the Protein/Carbohydrate Fermentation Balance and Microbial Population Dynamics of the Simulator of Human intestinal Microbial Ecosystem: AXOS Effect on Protein/Carbohydrate Fermentation Balance. *Microb. Biotechnol.* **2009**, *2*, 101–113. [CrossRef] [PubMed]
70. Chassard, C.; Goumy, V.; Leclerc, M.; Del'homme, C.; Bernalier-Donadille, A. Characterization of the Xylan-degrading Microbial Community from Human Faeces: Xylanolytic Microbiota from Human Faeces. *FEMS Microbiol. Ecol.* **2007**, *61*, 121–131. [CrossRef]
71. Martinez-Guryn, K.; Hubert, N.; Frazier, K.; Urlass, S.; Musch, M.W.; Ojeda, P.; Pierre, J.; Miyoshi, J.; Sontag, T.J.; Cham, C.M.; et al. Small intestine Microbiota Regulate Host Digestive and Absorptive Adaptive Responses to Dietary Lipids. *Cell Host Microbe* **2018**, *23*, 458–469. [CrossRef]
72. Maharshak, N.; Packey, C.D.; Ellermann, M.; Manick, S.; Siddle, J.P.; Huh, E.Y.; Plevy, S.; Sartor, R.B.; Carroll, I.M. Altered Enteric Microbiota Ecology in interleukin 10-Deficient Mice During Development and Progression of intestinal inflammation. *Gut Microbes* **2013**, *4*, 316–324. [CrossRef]
73. Tseng, C.H.; Wu, C.Y. The Gut Microbiome in Obesity. *J. Formos. Med. Assoc.* **2019**, *118*, 3–9. [CrossRef]
74. Gomes, A.C.; Hoffmann, C.; Mota, J.F. The Human Gut Microbiota: Metabolism and Perspective in Obesity. *Gut Microbes* **2018**, *18*, 308–325. [CrossRef]

75. Jáquez, J.L.; Lascurain, L.; Falcon, A.C.; Montoya, J.R. Obesidad, Disbiosis Y Trastornos Gastrointestinales Funcionales En Edades Pediátricas. *Neurogastrol. LATAM Rev.* **2020**, *4*, 4268. [CrossRef]
76. Petersen, C.; Round, J.L. Defining Dysbiosis and Its influence on Host Immunity and Disease. *Cell Microbiol.* **2014**, *16*, 1024–1033. [CrossRef]
77. Musso, G.; Gambino, R.; Cassader, M. Interactions between Gut Microbiota and Host Metabolism Predisposing to Obesity and Diabetes. *Annu. Rev. Med.* **2011**, *62*, 361–380. [CrossRef]
78. Million, M.; Thuny, F.; Angelakis, E.; Casalta, J.-P.; Giorgi, R.; Habib, G.; Raoult, D. Lactobacillus Reuteri and *Escherichia coli* in the Human Gut Microbiota May Predict Weight Gain Associated with Vancomycin Treatment. *Nutr. Diabetes* **2013**, *3*, 87. [CrossRef]
79. Wang, J.; Tang, H.; Zhang, C.; Zhao, Y.; Derrien, M.; Rocher, E.; van-Hylckama Vlieg, J.E.; Strissel, K.; Zhao, L.; Obin, M.; et al. Modulation of Ggut Microbiota During Probiotic-Mediated Attenuation of Metabolic Syndrome in High Fat Diet-Fed Mice. *ISME J.* **2015**, *9*, 1–15. [CrossRef]
80. de La Serre, C.B.; Ellis, C.L.; Lee, J.; Hartman, A.L.; Rutledge, J.C.; Raybould, H.E. Propensity to High-Fat Diet-induced Obesity in Rats Is Associated with Changes in the Gut Microbiota and Gut inflammation. *Am. J. Physiol.-Gastrointest. Liver. Physiol.* **2010**, *299*, 440–448. [CrossRef]
81. Krautkramer, K.A.; Kreznar, J.H.; Romano, K.A.; Vivas, E.I.; Barrett-Wilt, G.A.; Rabaglia, M.E.; Keller, M.P.; Attie, A.D.; Rey, F.E.; Denu, J.M. Diet-Microbiota interactions Mediate Global Epigenetic Programming in Multiple Host Tissues. *Mol. Cell* **2016**, *64*, 982–992. [CrossRef]
82. Farhadi, A.; Banan, A.; Fields, J.; Keshavarzian, A. Intestinal Barrier: An interface between Health and Disease. *J. Gastroenterol. Hepatol.* **2003**, *18*, 479–497. [CrossRef]
83. Rosenbaum, M.; Knight, R.; Leibel, R.L. The Gut Microbiota in Human Energy Homeostasis and Obesity. *Trends Endocrinol. Metab.* **2015**, *26*, 493–501. [CrossRef] [PubMed]
84. Amabebe, E.; Robert, F.O.; Agbalalah, T.; Orubu, E.S.F. Microbial Dysbiosis-induced Obesity: Role of Gut Microbiota in Homoeostasis of Energy Metabolism. *Br. J. Nutr.* **2020**, *123*, 1127–1137. [CrossRef] [PubMed]
85. Do, M.; Lee, E.; Oh, M.J.; Kim, Y.; Park, H.Y. High-Glucose or -Fructose Diet Cause Changes of the Gut Microbiota and Metabolic Disorders in Mice without Body Weight Change. *Nutrients* **2018**, *10*, 761. [CrossRef] [PubMed]
86. Suzuki, T. Regulation of the intestinal Barrier by Nutrients: The Role of Tight Junctions. *Anim. Sci. J.* **2020**, *91*, 13357. [CrossRef] [PubMed]
87. FAO/WHO Working Group. *Guidelines for the Evaluation of Probiotics in Food*; FAO/WHO Working Group: Geneva, Switzerland, 2002.
88. Zendeboodi, F.; Khorshidian, N.; Mortazavian, A.M.; da Cruz, A.G. Probiotic: Conceptualisation from a New Approach. *Curr. Opin. Food Sci.* **2020**, *32*, 103–123. [CrossRef]
89. Allen, A.P.; Hutch, W.; Borre, Y.E.; Kennedy, P.J.; Temko, A.; Boylan, G.; Murphy, E.; Cryan, J.F.; Dinan, T.G.; Clarke, G. Bifidobacterium Longum 1714 as a Translational Psychobiotic: Modulation of Sstress, Electrophysiology and Neurocognition in Healthy Volunteers. *Transl. Psychiatry* **2016**, *6*, 939. [CrossRef] [PubMed]
90. Lopez, M.; Li, N.; Kataria, J.; Russell, M.; Neu, J. Live and Ultraviolet-inactivated Lactobacillus Rhamnosus GG Decrease Flagellin-induced interleukin-8 Production in Caco-2 Cells. *J. Nutr.* **2008**, *138*, 2264–2268. [CrossRef]
91. Ajmal, S.; Ahmed, N. Probiotic Potential of Lactobacillus Strains in Human infections. *Afr. J. Microbiol. Res.* **2009**, *3*, 851–855.
92. Wegh, C.A.; Geerlings, S.Y.; Knol, J.; Roeselers, G.; Belzer, C. Postbiotics and their Potential Applications in Early Life Nutrition and Beyond. *Int. J. Mol. Sci.* **2019**, *20*, 4673. [CrossRef]
93. Sánchez, M.T.; Ruiz, M.A.; Morales, M.E. Microorganismos Probióticos Y Salud. *Ars Pharm.* **2015**, *56*, 45–59. [CrossRef]
94. Debédat, J.; Clément, K.; Aron-Wisnewsky, J. Gut Microbiota Dysbiosis in Human Obesity: Impact of Bariatric Surgery. *Curr. Obes. Rep.* **2019**, *8*, 229–242. [CrossRef]
95. da Silva Pontes, K.S.; Guedes, M.R.; da Cunha, M.R.; de Souza Mattos, S.; Silva, M.I.B.; Neves, M.F.; Marques, B.C.A.A.; Klein, M.R.S.T. Effects of Probiotics on Body Adiposity and Cardiovascular Risk Markers in individuals with Overweight and Obesity: A Systematic Review and Meta-Analysis of Randomised Controlled Trials. *Clin. Nutr.* **2021**, *40*, 4915–4931. [CrossRef]
96. Koutnikova, H.; Genser, B.; Monteiro-Sepulveda, M.; Faurie, J.M.; Rizkalla, S.; Schrezenmeir, J.; Clément, K. Impact of Bacterial Probiotics on Obesity Diabetes and Non-Alcoholic Fatty Liver Disease Related Variables: A Systematic Review and Meta-Analysis of Randomised Controlled Trials. *BMJ Open* **2019**, *9*, e017995. [CrossRef]

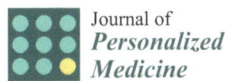

Article

Machine Learning Models for Nocturnal Hypoglycemia Prediction in Hospitalized Patients with Type 1 Diabetes

Vladimir B. Berikov [1,2], Olga A. Kutnenko [2], Julia F. Semenova [1] and Vadim V. Klimontov [1,*]

1. Laboratory of Endocrinology, Research Institute of Clinical and Experimental Lymphology—Branch of the Institute of Cytology and Genetics, Siberian Branch of Russian Academy of Sciences (RICEL—Branch of IC&G SB RAS), 630060 Novosibirsk, Russia; berikov@math.nsc.ru (V.B.B.); eekmxtyjr@yandex.ru (J.F.S.)
2. Laboratory of Data Analysis, Sobolev Institute of Mathematics, Siberian Branch of Russian Academy of Sciences, 630090 Novosibirsk, Russia; olga@math.nsc.ru
* Correspondence: klimontov@mail.ru; Tel.: +7-913-956-82-99

Abstract: Nocturnal hypoglycemia (NH) is a dangerous complication of insulin therapy that often goes undetected. In this study, we aimed to generate machine learning (ML)-based models for short-term NH prediction in hospitalized patients with type 1 diabetes (T1D). The models were trained on continuous glucose monitoring (CGM) data obtained from 406 adult patients admitted to a tertiary referral hospital. Eight CGM-derived metrics of glycemic control and glucose variability were included in the models. Combinations of CGM and clinical data (23 parameters) were also assessed. Random Forest (RF), Logistic Linear Regression with Lasso regularization, and Artificial Neuron Networks algorithms were applied. In our models, RF provided the best prediction accuracy with 15 min and 30 min prediction horizons. The addition of clinical parameters slightly improved the prediction accuracy of most models, whereas oversampling and undersampling procedures did not have significant effects. The areas under the curve of the best models based on CGM and clinical data with 15 min and 30 min prediction horizons were 0.97 and 0.942, respectively. Basal insulin dose, diabetes duration, proteinuria, and HbA1c were the most important clinical predictors of NH assessed by RF. In conclusion, ML is a promising approach to personalized prediction of NH in hospitalized patients with T1D.

Keywords: type 1 diabetes; hypoglycemia; continuous glucose monitoring; machine learning; random forest; artificial neuron networks; prediction

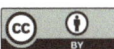

1. Introduction

Nocturnal hypoglycemia (NH) is a wide-spread and potentially dangerous complication of insulin therapy which often goes undetected. In subjects with diabetes, almost 50% of all episodes of severe hypoglycemia occur at night. A growing body of evidence indicates that NH can cause sleep disturbances, morning headache, chronic fatigue, and mood changes; it is also associated with cardiac arrhythmias resulting in "death-in-bed syndrome" [1,2]. Hypoglycemia induces a wide range of changes in gene expression in the cardiovascular and nervous systems and may be a trigger for the damage of target organs [3]. Repeated episodes of hypoglycemia cause defective glucose counterregulation and contribute to the development of an impaired awareness of hypoglycemia [4].

Patients with type 1 diabetes (T1D) on basal bolus insulin therapy are particularly prone to NH [5]. In healthy subjects, hypoglycemia triggers awakening, but patients with T1D are often unable to wake up when their blood glucose drops [6]. Therefore, reliable and personalized predictive methods are urgently needed to reduce the risk of NH in T1D subjects.

For a long time, the measurement of pre-bedtime glucose level was used for the NH risk assessment [7]. However, the value of the bedtime glucose in predicting NH is limited due to inter-individual and intra-individual differences in nocturnal glucose dynamics. A number of models based on clinical parameters, continuous glucose monitoring (CGM) data, indices of glycemic control, and glucose variability were proposed in recent years to identify patients at high risk of NH [8–11].

Machine learning (ML) technologies opened up new possibilities for personalized hypoglycemia forecasting. A comprehensive review [12] and meta-analysis [13] of research in this area were recently published. Currently, various ML algorithms have been tested for short-term NH prediction in subjects with T1D including Random Forest (RF) [14–16], Repeated Measures RF [17], Artificial Neural Networks (ANNs) [18], Support Vector Machine [14,19], Long Short-Term Memory [14], Linear Discriminant Analysis [9], and Multilayer Perceptron [19]. To be of practical use, a ML algorithm must provide enough time to take action to avoid hypoglycemia. In most of the above-mentioned studies, the prediction horizons (PHs) ranged from 15 to 60 min; in one study [15], it was extended to 6 h.

Improving the predictive accuracy of ML models and assessing their applicability in various clinical situations remains an important challenge. The complimenting of glucose time series data with insulin doses, carbohydrate intake, and other clinical parameters, as well as combinations of different ML algorithms, is used to improve the predictive accuracy of the models [12]. In previous studies, ML algorithms were trained on CGM data obtained under normal living conditions. Another urgent task is the prediction of hypoglycemia in a hospital setting. It was demonstrated that in hospitalized patients hypoglycemia occurs with greater frequency between 0 and 6 a.m. [20]. Inpatient hypoglycemia in people with diabetes is associated with increased mortality and a longer hospital stay [21]. Previously, Fralik M et al. applied supervised ML for prediction of severe hypoglycemia in patients hospitalized under general internal medicine and cardiovascular surgery [22].

In this study, we aimed to develop ML-based models for short-term prediction of NH in hospitalized patients with T1D. We have also tested whether the inclusion of a broad set of clinical data and CGM-derived glucose variability parameters in the ML model, as well as the application of an oversampling or undersampling technique, can improve the accuracy of NH prediction.

2. Materials and Methods

The process of ML model generation in our study included the following steps: (1) CGM data cleaning and preprocessing; (2) extracting metrics from CGM recordings; (3) data sampling; (4) combination of CGM data with clinical and laboratory parameters; (5) ML algorithm training; (6) evaluation of the model and NH predictors.

2.1. Databases

A database of CGM data obtained from 406 subjects with T1D was used to generate ML models for NH prediction. Data were collected from men and women aged from 18 to 70 years, on basal bolus insulin therapy. The treatment with sensor-augmented pumps with predictive low glucose suspend technology, current diabetic ketoacidosis or hyperglycemic hyperosmolar state, end-stage renal disease, congestive heart failure (class IV according to NYHA), malignant neoplasms, and acute infectious diseases were considered as exclusion criteria. Patients were observed at the clinic of RICEL—Branch of IC&G SB RAS, a tertiary referral hospital. All patients were admitted for a routine in-depth examination, screening for complications and correction of therapy.

Blinded CGM was performed with an iPro™2, MMT-7741 (iPro2) CGM system and CareLink iPro™ (CareLink iPro, MMT-7340) software (Medtronic, Minneapolis, MN, USA). This system measures interstitial glucose values ranging from 2.2 to 22.2 mmol/L every 5 min. At least 4 capillary blood glucose measurements per day were performed with a One Touch Verio Pro+ glucose meter (Johnson & Johnson, New Brunswick, NJ, USA) to calibrate the CGM system. Mean CGM duration was 6.7 days; the range was from 3 to 11 days.

The CGM database was matched to a clinical database containing demographic and anthropometric characteristics of the included subjects, information about diabetes, complications and associated diseases, data from laboratory tests, and instrumental examinations.

2.2. Model Building

For the modeling, CGM records representing nocturnal intervals (from 00:00 to 05:59 a.m.) were used. The NH was defined as an episode of interstitial glucose level <3.9 mmol/L for at least 15 min [23].

2.2.1. CGM Data Cleaning and Preprocessing

At the first step, we cleaned the data, looking for outliers and record defects. The CGM records with data gaps of 30 min or more were excluded. Shorter intervals of missed values were linearly extrapolated based on surrounding observations. At the preprocessing stage, we cut intervals of length T from the suitable CGM records and divided these intervals depending on the presence of an episode of NH at the selected PH value. Since the number of intervals without hypoglycemia (NH- intervals) was much higher than those with the episode (NH+ intervals) and their behavior for adjacent intervals looks quite similar, we considered a sample of NH- intervals with starting moments $t_1, t_{1+s}, t_{1+2s}, \ldots$ where $s \geq 1$ is a gap parameter. The number of obtained intervals depended on T and s; for example, for T = 45 min and s = 4 we had 216 NH+ intervals and 36684 NH- ones.

2.2.2. Extraction of CGM Metrics

Since CGM data had a significant stochastic component and the amount of available data was not very large, feature-based procedures were used. Each record was represented as a series $\{G_1, \ldots, G_n\}$, where n = T/(5 min). From the appropriate sets of CGM records we derived parameters of glucose dynamics. These parameters included indices of glucose variability and glycemic control that are used in diabetology: coefficient of variation (CV), lability index (LI), low blood glucose index (LBGI), and 1 h continuous overlapping net glycemic action (CONGA-1) [24,25]. In addition, we applied indices used in the time series analysis: minimal value, difference between the last two values (DLV), acceleration over the last values (ALV), and linear trend coefficient (LC). Ultimately, 8 metrics were chosen (Table 1).

Table 1. CGM-derived metrics used for the engineering of ML models.

Parameter	Formula
CV	$CV = \frac{SD}{\bar{G}} \times 100\%$, where $\bar{G} = \frac{\sum_{i=1}^{n} G_i}{n}$ and $SD = \sqrt{\frac{\sum_{i=1}^{n}(G_i - \bar{G})}{n-1}}$
LI	$LI = \sum_{i=1}^{n-1}(G_i - G_{i+1})^2 / 5$
LBGI	$LBGI = \frac{1}{n}\sum_{i=1}^{n} rl(G_i)$, where $rl(G_i) = r(G_i)$ if $f(G_i) < 0$ and 0 otherwise, $rh(G_i) = r(G_i)$ if $f(G_i) > 0$ and 0 otherwise, $r(G_i) = 10 \times f^2(G_i)$, $f(G_i) = 1.509 \times \left[(\log(18 \times G_i))^{1.084} - 5.381\right]$
CONGA-1	$CONGA(1) = \sqrt{\frac{\sum_{i=2}^{n}(D_i - \bar{D})}{n-1}}$ where $\bar{D} = \frac{\sum_{i=2}^{n} D_i}{n-1}$, $D_i = G_i - G_{i-1}$
Minimum value	$G_{min} = \min(G_1, \ldots, G_n)$
DLV	$G_{n-1} - G_n$
ALV	$(G_n - G_{n-1}) - (G_{n-1} - G_{n-2})$
LC	coefficient b_1 in a linear trend model $G_i = b_0 + b_1 t_i + \varepsilon_i$

Abbreviations: ALV, acceleration over the last values; CONGA-1, 1-h continuous overlapping net glycemic action; CV, coefficient of variation; DLV, difference between the last two values; LBGI, low blood glucose index; LC, linear trend coefficient; LI, lability index.

2.2.3. Data Sampling

As expected, the numbers of CGM intervals with a recorded NH episode were significantly less than that of the intervals without. To get a more balanced distribution of NH+ and NH- intervals in the training subset, we have applied oversampling and undersampling techniques. Oversampling consisted of perturbation with small Gaussian noise. For each feature, we used normal distribution $N(0,\sigma)$, where parameter σ equals 5% of the standard deviation of the sample. This technique was applied for generating artificial CGM records with a NH episode. Undersampling consisted of selecting the most representative records without NH. To determine the representative records, we clustered NH- intervals using a k-medoids algorithm with a number of clusters equal to the number of NH events. The obtained medoids representing the intervals without NH were used for the consequent analysis. The effects of oversampling and undersampling techniques on the prediction accuracy were estimated.

2.2.4. Input Clinical Parameters into the Models

At the next step, clinical characteristics of patients were entered into the models. In total, 23 clinical and laboratory parameters were assessed as potential contributors for NH risk. These parameters included age, sex, body mass index (BMI), diabetes duration, diabetic complications and associated diseases, insulin treatment characteristics, hypolipidemic and antihypertensive therapy, glycated hemoglobin A1c (HbA1c), renal function, and albuminuria (Table S1).

2.2.5. ML Algorithms

We conducted a number of preliminary experiments with different kinds of ML methods for constructing a prediction model. Finally, we decided to use RF, Logistic Linear Regression with Lasso regularization (LogRLasso), and ANN. RF is characterized by high generalization ability and robustness, especially in situations with redundant and possibly non-informative features [26]. LogRLasso is also a robust technique which provides an embedded opportunity to select the most important features [27]. The Levenberg–Marquardt algorithm, known for its fast convergence and robustness [28], was applied for ANN training. We used an ANN with a fully connected feed-forward network architecture with two hidden layers (5 neurons in each layer).

2.3. Model Evaluation

The quality of prediction was evaluated using 10-fold cross-validation. The model parameters were evaluated for the PHs of 15 and 30 min.

If a decision taken by a classifier depended on a certain threshold, ROC curve analysis was performed. Assessment of the quality of classifiers was carried out by the estimation of area under the curve (AUC). This metric is independent of the decision threshold and can be used in situations of significant differences in class frequencies. In addition, the numbers of true positive, false positive, false negative, and true negative forecast results were calculated. Based on these parameters, sensitivity (Se) and specificity (Sp) of the models were estimated.

2.4. Assessment of NH Predictors

We used RF as a standard tool for estimating the value of predictors in a model [26]. This method ranks all available features according to their usefulness in the prediction: the more frequently a feature is chosen in the ensemble of decision trees, and the more accurate predictions it yields, the higher the rank. There were 500 trees in the ensemble. In addition, we used LogRLasso to evaluate feature importance. Due to the embedded regularization, this method reveals non-significant features which are attributed with zero model coefficients. The method makes it possible to assess the direction of the influence of features on the outcome (in our case, whether the risk of NH increases or decreases with an increase in a feature value).

3. Results

3.1. Characteristics of Patients

The clinical characteristics of patients are shown in Table 2. We observed individuals aged from 18 to 70 years (median 36 years), with diabetes duration 0.5–55 years (median 16 years). The HbA1c level was 8.1% (range: 4.7–15.1%). All patients were on basal bolus therapy with insulin analogues. One hundred and fourteen patients (28.1%) had severe hypoglycemia in their medical history. An impaired awareness of hypoglycemia, assessed by the Clarke method [29], was revealed in 148 (36.5%) subjects.

Table 2. Clinical characteristics of T1D patients.

General Demographic and Clinical Parameters	
Sex, m/f, n (%)	147/259 (36.2/63.8)
Age, years	36 (28–48)
BMI, kg/m^2	23.6 (21.2–27.1)
Waist-to-hip ratio	0.84 (0.78–0.91)
Current smoking, n (%)	68 (16.7)
Diabetes-related parameters and associated diseases	
Diabetes duration, years	16 (10–25)
Daily insulin dose, IU	40 (29.1–53.6)
Daily insulin dose, IU/kg	0.59 (0.47–0.76)
Daily basal insulin dose, IU	19.0 (13.6–26)
Daily basal insulin dose, IU/kg	0.28 (0.21–0.38)
Diabetic retinopathy, n (%)	246 (60.6)
Chronic kidney disease, n (%)	274 (67.5)
Neuropathy, n (%)	301 (74.1)
Impaired awareness of hypoglycemia, n (%)	148 (36.5)
Arterial hypertension, n (%)	159 (39.2)
Coronary artery disease, n (%)	31 (7.6)
Laboratory parameters	
HbA1c, %	8.1 (7.1–9.2)
Total cholesterol, mmol/L	5.0 (4.2–5.9)
LDL cholesterol, mmol/L	3.0 (2.4–3.7)
HDL cholesterol, mmol/L	1.5 (1.3–1.7)
Triglycerides, mmol/L	1.0 (0.7–1.4)
Serum creatinine, µmol/L	81.9 (73.7–94.0)
eGFR, mL/min/1.73 m^2	88.0 (73.0–100.0)
UACR, mg/mmoL	2.1 (2.0–7.65)

Continuous data are presented as medians (25th–75th percentiles). Abbreviations: BMI, body mass index; eGFR, estimated glomerular filtration rate; HbA1c, glycated hemoglobin A1c; HDL, high-density lipoprotein; LDL, low-density lipoprotein; T1D, type 1 diabetes; UACR, urinary albumin-to-creatinine ratio.

3.2. Evaluation of ML Models

Three ML methods, including RF composed of 500 trees, LogRLasso, and ANN, were evaluated using baseline (no-sampling), oversampling, and undersampling procedures. We have also compared the models based on the CGM metrics only with those included combinations of CGM and clinical data (Table 3).

Table 3. Quality metrics (%) of the ML models for NH prediction.

PH	Sampling/Parameters		RF		LogRLasso		ANN	
			CGM	CGM + Clinical Data	CGM	CGM + Clinical Data	CGM	CGM + Clinical Data
15 min	OS	Se	93.6 (3.4)	90.9 (2.8)	93.6 (1.9)	93.0 (3.0)	90.5 (5.9)	90.8 (2.5)
		Sp	90.1 (2.4)	91.8 (2.3)	91.9 (2.2)	93.0 (2.0)	91.4 (1.6)	89.1 (4.5)
		AUC	0.958 (0.011)	0.953 (0.012)	**0.962 (0.010)**	**0.968 (0.014)**	0.946 (0.032)	0.935 (0.029)
	NS	Se	91.8 (1.2)	94.5 (2.6)	93.6 (3.4)	92.4 (2.5)	88.6 (3.6)	90.3 (3.1)
		Sp	91.1 (3.9)	91.4 (3.3)	91.2 (2.5)	92.3 (3.7)	92.6 (3.1)	91.0 (1.6)
		AUC	**0.959 (0.020)**	**0.97 (0.017)**	0.957 (0.021)	0.958 (0.025)	0.934 (0.032)	0.935 (0.027)
	US	Se	88.2 (5.2)	92.3 (3.4)	90.5 (6.7)	90.8 (4.7)	90.0 (4.7)	91.9 (3.7)
		Sp	92.7 (2.1)	90.6 (1.3)	91.4 (1.4)	91.2 (2.4)	90.2 (2.8)	88.9 (3.6)
		AUC	0.953 (0.023)	0.956 (0.009)	0.947 (0.036)	0.947 (0.018)	**0.947 (0.033)**	**0.945 (0.017)**
30 min	OS	Se	87.6 (1.9)	86.6 (3.6)	90.4 (1.7)	91.0 (3.5)	87.6 (3.9)	84.6 (5.2)
		Sp	88.9 (3.1)	87.0 (2.6)	87.5 (2.2)	87.7 (3.7)	88.0 (4.0)	87.2 (5.5)
		AUC	**0.927 (0.03)**	0.911 (0.019)	**0.932 (0.06)**	0.94 (0.012)	0.918 (0.031)	0.881 (0.034)
	NS	Se	87.1 (4.6)	90.4 (4.7)	87.1 (4.0)	86.9 (4.0)	86.6 (3.2)	83.3 (4.2)
		Sp	87.1 (6.0)	87.4 (1.6)	90.8 (1.9)	90.3 (1.9)	88.7 (2.2)	86.3 (2.8)
		AUC	0.92 (0.036)	**0.942 (0.028)**	0.928 (0.012)	**0.933 (0.012)**	**0.924 (0.018)**	0.881 (0.049)
	US	Se	89.5 (3.6)	92.4 (3.1)	85.1 (5.6)	90.3 (3.2)	85.1 (5.3)	85.2 (3.6)
		Sp	86.5 (2.8)	85.3 (1.2)	89.5 (1.8)	86.7 (1.9)	87.5 (2.7)	84.8 (2.2)
		AUC	0.912 (0.031)	0.923 (0.021)	0.913 (0.027)	0.92 (0.03)	0.908 (0.028)	**0.901 (0.023)**

The SD values of the estimates obtained with cross-validation process are shown in the parentheses. The highest AUC values for each PH and ML algorithm are highlighted in bold. Abbreviations: ANN, Artificial Neural Networks; AUC, area under the curve; CGM, continuous glucose monitoring; LogRLasso, Logistic Linear Regression with Lasso regularization; NP, nocturnal hypoglycemia; PH, prediction horizon; RF, Random Forest; OS, oversampling; NS, no sampling; US, undersampling; Se, sensitivity; Sp, specificity.

The models based on the LogRlasso algorithm and operating only with CGM data were characterized by the highest AUC values (0.962 in a model with oversampling and 15 min PH; 0.932 in a model with oversampling and 30 min PH). At the same time, RF provided the best prediction accuracy when CGM and clinical data were combined (AUC: 0.97 in a model without sampling and 15 min PH; 0.942 in a model without sampling and 30 min PH). ANN provided slightly worse results in the models trained on CGM only and CGM and clinical data.

The sampling effect was quite modest and depended on the ML algorithm and PH. In a one-way ANOVA, the effect of sampling on AUC was insignificant ($p = 0.8$ for all algorithms). An application of a no-sampling approach provided the highest AUC values in the RF model trained on the CGM and clinical data.

3.3. Evaluation of NH Predictors

Lower minimal glucose and LC, and higher LBGI, DLV, CONGA-1, proteinuria, basal insulin dose, diabetes duration, and HbA1c, as well as the presence of autonomic neuropathy, formed the list of the 10 most reliable NH predictors assessed by RF with a 15 min PH (Table 4). At a 30 min PH, lower minimal glucose and HbA1c, higher LBGI, DVL, daily and basal insulin doses, diabetes duration, proteinuria, eGFR, and BMI demonstrated the highest importance. Among the clinical factors, insulin dose, diabetes duration, and proteinuria were associated with the risk of hypoglycemia positively; meanwhile, HbA1c, eGFR, and BMI demonstrated negative associations.

Table 4. The most important NH predictors revealed by RF in patients with T1D.

PH	Parameters	Importance	Effect
15 min	Minimal glucose	1.000	−
	LBGI	0.786	+
	DLV	0.723	+
	CONGA-1	0.625	+

Table 4. Cont.

PH	Parameters	Importance	Effect
	LC	0.542	−
	Proteinuria	0.494	+
	Basal insulin dose, IU/kg	0.488	+
	Diabetes duration	0.457	+
	Autonomic neuropathy	0.383	+
	HbA1c	0.379	−
30 min	Minimal glucose	1.000	−
	LBGI	0.845	+
	Daily insulin dose, IU/kg	0.770	+
	HbA1c	0.698	−
	Diabetes duration	0.693	+
	Basal insulin dose, IU/kg	0.666	+
	Proteinuria	0.653	+
	eGFR	0.652	+
	DLV	0.589	+
	BMI	0.577	−

Effect: the risk of NH increases as the parameter value increases (+); the risk of NH decreases as the parameter value increases (−). Abbreviations: BMI, body mass index; CONGA-1, 1 h continuous overlapping net glycemic action; DLV, difference between the last two values; eGFR, estimated glomerular filtration rate; HbA1c, glycated hemoglobin A1c; LBGI, Low Blood Glucose Index; LC, linear trend coefficient; NH, nocturnal hypoglycemia; RF, Random Forest; T1D, type 1 diabetes.

4. Discussion

The prevention of hypoglycemia, a frequent and potentially life-threatening complication of insulin therapy, remains a priority in diabetes care. Recent progress in the field is related to the implementation of sensor-augmented pumps with predictive low glucose suspend technology and closed-loop systems [30,31]. However, a significant proportion of patients with diabetes remain on multiple daily insulin injections. Therefore, it is important to develop reliable methods of hypoglycemia prediction for these patients also. In this study, we engineered ML models for real-time NH prediction in patients with T1D in a hospital setting. We assessed the predictive accuracy of the models based on CGM data and three ML algorithms: RF, LogRLasso, and ANN. We also evaluated the effectiveness of the use of clinical data as additional parameters, as well as oversampling and undersampling techniques, in the NH prediction.

In our models, RF provided the best prediction accuracy (in terms of AUC crossvalidated estimates) at 15 min and 30 min PHs. LogRLasso was ranked as the second and ANN as the third algorithm. The more modest result of ANN can be explained by the relatively small sample size and the inherent stochastic nature of the data.

The choice of PH is an important step in the building of predictive models. In a recent review, Mujahid et al. indicated a 30 min PH as the most commonly used in ML-based models for NH prediction [12]. However, the optimal PH duration is still debatable, since the rate of development and severity of hypoglycemia, as well as the response to carbohydrates, can vary. Obviously, in the case of NH, the PH should not be too long; otherwise, the duration and quality of sleep can be reduced significantly. However, the PH should be long enough to enable patient or medical staff to take preventive actions. The American Diabetes Association advises patients to follow the "15:15" rule for the treatment of hypoglycemia: "have 15 g of carbohydrate to raise your blood sugar and check it after 15 min. If it's still below 70 mg/dL, have another serving" [32]. Therefore, we believe that 15 min or 30 min PHs are acceptable in most cases.

An uneven distribution of observations between the classes, or the problem of imbalanced data, is a challenge in the building of ML models. In our sample, the number of CGM intervals with at least one episode of NH was much less than that of the intervals without an episode: depending on the PH, we have analyzed 209-256 intervals with NH and about 40,000 intervals without. In data analysis, oversampling and undersampling techniques are used to adjust the class distribution of a data set. These methods involve the generation of artificial observations of the minority class (oversampling, or augmentation technique) or the partial exclusion of observations from the majority class (undersampling) [33,34]. In this work, we have tried both oversampling and undersampling techniques and estimated the effects of these techniques on the prediction quality. The effect of the sampling depended on the ML method and the PH. The use of the oversampling provided slightly better results (in terms of AUC metric) compared to other techniques. At the same time, in the models generated by RF, the application of a no-sampling approach provided the highest quality of forecasting.

First, we trained ML models on CGM data only. The minimal glucose, LBGI, and DVL were the most reliable NH predictors at 15 min and 30 min PHs. Besides, CONGA-1 and LC were important in 15 min forecasting. At a 15 min PH, the highest AUC levels were 0.959% for RF, 0.962% for LogRLasso, and 0.947% for the ANN algorithm. In the models with a 30 min PH, the highest AUC values: 0.927%, 0.932%, and 0.924% were obtained by RF, LogRLasso, and ANN, respectively. Thus, parameters characterizing the concentration of glucose and the dynamics of glucose levels before the episode of hypoglycemia had the greatest prognostic value, as expected.

We have also investigated whether the inclusion of a set of clinical and laboratory data could improve the quality of CGM-based prediction. For this purpose, we input 23 parameters in the models, including demographic characteristics, information about diabetes, its complications and associated diseases, and laboratory test results. We did not include carbohydrate data, having taken into account frequent inconsistence of these data and the fact that most patients do not eat at night. Incorporating the clinical data in the models increased the sensitivity and specificity of the forecast up to 2% at a 30 min PH. Proteinuria, basal insulin dose, diabetes duration, and HbA1c turned out to be the most important clinical predictors of NH at 15 min and 30 min PHs. Besides, daily insulin dose, eGFR, and BMI were important for 30 min forecasting.

In general, all the models we had built showed good prediction quality assessed by the sensitivity, specificity, and AUC. In particular, sensitivity and specificity varied from 94.5% and 91.4%, respectively, at a 15 min PH to 90.4% and 87.4% at a 30 min PH.

Our study has some evident limitations. The duration of CGM was quite short. The datasets used were not very large and the number of observations with NH was limited. At the same time, as far as we know, this is the first study aimed to develop ML-based methods for short-term NH prediction in hospitalized patients with T1D. The resulting models can be used to develop a decision support system for the prevention of NH in hospitalized patients with T1D.

5. Conclusions

In this study, we have developed a ML-based approach for predicting NH in patients with T1D in a hospital setting. The models trained on CGM data and operating RF, LogRLasso, and ANN algorithms showed acceptable prediction accuracy in terms of specificity, sensitivity, and AUC with PH lengths of 15 and 30 min. The incorporation of clinical data into the models improved the sensitivity and specificity of forecast up to 2%. Among the clinical parameters, basal insulin dose, diabetes duration, proteinuria, and HbA1c turned out to be the most reliable NH predictors.

The development and implementation of decision support systems based on ML algorithms seems to be a promising approach to reduce the burden of NH in patients with T1D on multiple daily insulin injections.

Supplementary Materials: The following supporting information can be downloaded at: https://www.mdpi.com/article/10.3390/jpm12081262/s1, Table S1: Clinical and laboratory parameters of T1D patients that were included in the models for NH prediction.

Author Contributions: Conceptualization, V.B.B. and V.V.K.; methodology, V.B.B.; software, validation, and formal analysis, V.B.B. and O.A.K.; investigation, V.B.B., J.F.S. and V.V.K.; data curation, V.B.B. and J.F.S.; writing—original draft preparation, V.B.B. and V.V.K.; writing—review and editing, V.V.K.; supervision, project administration, and funding acquisition, V.V.K. All authors have read and agreed to the published version of the manuscript.

Funding: This research was funded by the Russian Science Foundation, grant number 20-15-00057.

Institutional Review Board Statement: The study was conducted in accordance with the Declaration of Helsinki, and approved by the Ethics Committee of RICEL–branch of IC & G SB RAS (protocol N. 158, date of approval 1 June 2020).

Informed Consent Statement: Written informed consent was obtained from all subjects involved in the study.

Data Availability Statement: The data supporting reported results are available in Supplementary Materials. The source data are available from the corresponding authors upon request.

Conflicts of Interest: The authors declare no conflict of interest. The funder had no role in the design of the study; in the collection, analyses, or interpretation of data; in the writing of the manuscript; or in the decision to publish the results.

Abbreviations

ANN	Artificial Neural Networks
AUC	area under the curve
AVL	acceleration over the last values
BMI	body mass index
CGM	continuous glucose monitoring
CONGA-1	1 h continuous overlapping net glycemic action
CV	coefficient of variation
DVL	difference between the last two values
eGFR	estimated glomerular filtration rate
HbA1c	glycated hemoglobin A1c
LBGI	Low Blood Glucose Index
LC	linear trend coefficient
LI	Lability Index
LogRLasso	Logistic Linear Regression with Lasso regularization
ML	machine learning
NH	nocturnal hypoglycemia
PH	prediction horizon
RF	Random Forest
Se	sensitivity
Sp	specificity
T1D	type 1 diabetes
t-SNE	t-distributed Stochastic Neighbor Embedding
UACR	urinary albumin-to-creatinine ratio

References

1. Allen, K.V.; Frier, B.M. Nocturnal hypoglycemia: Clinical manifestations and therapeutic strategies toward prevention. *Endocr. Pract.* **2003**, *9*, 530–543. [CrossRef] [PubMed]
2. Graveling, A.J.; Frier, B.M. The risks of nocturnal hypoglycaemia in insulin-treated diabetes. *Diabetes Res. Clin. Pract.* **2017**, *133*, 30–39. [CrossRef] [PubMed]
3. Saik, O.V.; Klimontov, V.V. Hypoglycemia, Vascular Disease and Cognitive Dysfunction in Diabetes: Insights from Text Mining-Based Reconstruction and Bioinformatics Analysis of the Gene Networks. *Int. J. Mol. Sci.* **2021**, *22*, 12419. [CrossRef] [PubMed]

4. Seaquist, E.R.; Anderson, J.; Childs, B.; Cryer, P.; Dagogo-Jack, S.; Fish, L.; Heller, S.R.; Rodriguez, H.; Rosenzweig, J.; Vigersky, R. Hypoglycemia and diabetes: A report of a workgroup of the American Diabetes Association and the Endocrine Society. *Diabetes Care* **2013**, *36*, 1384–1395. [CrossRef]
5. Siamashvili, M.; Davis, H.A.; Davis, S.N. Nocturnal hypoglycemia in type 1 and type 2 diabetes: An update on prevalence, prevention, pathophysiology and patient awareness. *Expert Rev. Endocrinol. Metab.* **2021**, *16*, 281–293. [CrossRef] [PubMed]
6. Schultes, B.; Jauch-Chara, K.; Gais, S.; Hallschmid, M.; Reiprich, E.; Kern, W.; Oltmanns, K.M.; Peters, A.; Fehm, H.L.; Born, J. Defective awakening response to nocturnal hypoglycemia in patients with type 1 diabetes mellitus. *PLoS Med.* **2007**, *4*, e69. [CrossRef] [PubMed]
7. Whincup, G.; Milner, R.D. Prediction and management of nocturnal hypoglycaemia in diabetes. *Arch. Dis. Child.* **1987**, *62*, 333–337. [CrossRef]
8. Ling, Q.; Lu, J.; Li, X.; Qiao, C.; Zhu, D.; Bi, Y. Value of Capillary Glucose Profiles in Assessing Risk of Nocturnal Hypoglycemia in Type 1 Diabetes Based on Continuous Glucose Monitoring. *Diabetes Ther.* **2020**, *11*, 915–925. [CrossRef]
9. Jensen, M.H.; Dethlefsen, C.; Vestergaard, P.; Hejlesen, O. Prediction of Nocturnal Hypoglycemia from Continuous Glucose Monitoring Data in People with Type 1 Diabetes: A Proof-of-Concept Study. *J. Diabetes Sci. Technol.* **2020**, *14*, 250–256. [CrossRef] [PubMed]
10. Sampath, S.; Tkachenko, P.; Renard, E.; Pereverzev, S.V. Glycemic Control Indices and Their Aggregation in the Prediction of Nocturnal Hypoglycemia from Intermittent Blood Glucose Measurements. *J. Diabetes Sci. Technol.* **2016**, *10*, 1245–1250. [CrossRef]
11. Klimontov, V.V.; Myakina, N.E. Glucose variability indices predict the episodes of nocturnal hypoglycemia in elderly type 2 diabetic patients treated with insulin. *Diabetes Metab. Syndr.* **2017**, *11*, 119–124. [CrossRef] [PubMed]
12. Mujahid, O.; Contreras, I.; Vehi, J. Machine learning techniques for hypoglycemia prediction: Trends and challenges. *Sensors* **2021**, *21*, 546. [CrossRef] [PubMed]
13. Kodama, S.; Fujihara, K.; Shiozaki, H.; Horikawa, C.; Yamada, M.H.; Sato, T.; Yaguchi, Y.; Yamamoto, M.; Kitazawa, M.; Iwanaga, M.; et al. Ability of Current Machine Learning Algorithms to Predict and Detect Hypoglycemia in Patients with Diabetes Mellitus: Meta-analysis. *JMIR Diabetes* **2021**, *6*, e22458. [CrossRef] [PubMed]
14. Li, J.; Ma, X.; Tobore, I.; Liu, Y.; Kandwal, A.; Wang, L.; Lu, J.; Lu, W.; Bao, Y.; Zhou, J.; et al. A Novel CGM Metric-Gradient and Combining Mean Sensor Glucose Enable to Improve the Prediction of Nocturnal Hypoglycemic Events in Patients with Diabetes. *J. Diabetes Res.* **2020**, *2020*, 8830774. [CrossRef]
15. Vu, L.; Kefayati, S.; Idé, T.; Pavuluri, V.; Jackson, G.; Latts, L.; Zhong, Y.; Agrawal, P.; Chang, Y.C. Predicting Nocturnal Hypoglycemia from Continuous Glucose Monitoring Data with Extended Prediction Horizon. *AMIA Annu. Symp. Proc.* **2020**, *2019*, 874–882.
16. Dave, D.; DeSalvo, D.J.; Haridas, B.; McKay, S.; Shenoy, A.; Koh, C.J.; Lawley, M.; Erraguntla, M. Feature-Based Machine Learning Model for Real-Time Hypoglycemia Prediction. *J. Diabetes Sci. Technol.* **2021**, *15*, 842–855. [CrossRef]
17. Calhoun, P.; Levine, R.A.; Fan, J. Repeated measures random forests (RMRF): Identifying factors associated with nocturnal hypoglycemia. *Biometrics* **2021**, *77*, 343–351. [CrossRef]
18. Vehí, J.; Contreras, I.; Oviedo, S.; Biagi, L.; Bertachi, A. Prediction and prevention of hypoglycaemic events in type-1 diabetic patients using machine learning. *Health Inform. J.* **2020**, *26*, 703–718. [CrossRef]
19. Bertachi, A.; Viñals, C.; Biagi, L.; Contreras, I.; Vehí, J.; Conget, I.; Giménez, M. Prediction of Nocturnal Hypoglycemia in Adults with Type 1 Diabetes under Multiple Daily Injections Using Continuous Glucose Monitoring and Physical Activity Monitor. *Sensors* **2020**, *20*, 1705. [CrossRef]
20. Ulmer, B.J.; Kara, A.; Mariash, C.N. Temporal occurrences and recurrence patterns of hypoglycemia during hospitalization. *Endocr. Pract.* **2015**, *21*, 501–507. [CrossRef]
21. Pratiwi, C.; Mokoagow, M.I.; Made Kshanti, I.A.; Soewondo, P. The risk factors of inpatient hypoglycemia: A systematic review. *Heliyon* **2020**, *6*, e03913. [CrossRef] [PubMed]
22. Fralick, M.; Dai, D.; Pou-Prom, C.; Verma, A.A.; Mamdani, M. Using machine learning to predict severe hypoglycaemia in hospital. *Diabetes Obes. Metab.* **2021**, *23*, 2311–2319. [CrossRef] [PubMed]
23. Danne, T.; Nimri, R.; Battelino, T.; Bergenstal, R.M.; Close, K.L.; DeVries, J.H.; Garg, S.; Heinemann, L.; Hirsch, I.; Amiel, S.A.; et al. International Consensus on Use of Continuous Glucose Monitoring. *Diabetes Care* **2017**, *40*, 1631–1640. [CrossRef] [PubMed]
24. Rodbard, D. Glucose Variability: A Review of Clinical Applications and Research Developments. *Diabetes Technol. Ther.* **2018**, *20*, S25–S215. [CrossRef]
25. Kovatchev, B. Glycemic Variability: Risk Factors, Assessment, and Control. *J. Diabetes Sci. Technol.* **2019**, *13*, 627–635. [CrossRef]
26. Breiman, L. Random Forests. *Mach. Learn.* **2001**, *45*, 5–32. [CrossRef]
27. Friedman, J.; Hastie, T.; Tibshirani, R. Regularization Paths for Generalized Linear Models via Coordinate Descent. *J. Stat. Softw.* **2010**, *33*, 1–22. [CrossRef]
28. Kanzow, C.; Yamashita, N.; Fukushima, M. Levenberg–Marquardt methods with strong local convergence properties for solving nonlinear equations with convex constraints. *J. Comp. Appl. Math.* **2005**, *173*, 321–343. [CrossRef]
29. Clarke, W.L.; Cox, D.J.; Gonder-Frederick, L.A.; Julian, D.; Schlundt, D.; Polonsky, W. Reduced awareness of hypoglycemia in adults with IDDM. A prospective study of hypoglycemic frequency and associated symptoms. *Diabetes Care* **1995**, *18*, 517–522. [CrossRef]

30. Steineck, I.; Ranjan, A.; Nørgaard, K.; Schmidt, S. Sensor-Augmented Insulin Pumps and Hypoglycemia Prevention in Type 1 Diabetes. *J. Diabetes Sci. Technol.* **2017**, *11*, 50–58. [CrossRef] [PubMed]
31. Chen, E.; King, F.; Kohn, M.A.; Spanakis, E.K.; Breton, M.; Klonoff, D.C. A Review of Predictive Low Glucose Suspend and Its Effectiveness in Preventing Nocturnal Hypoglycemia. *Diabetes Technol. Ther.* **2019**, *21*, 602–609. [CrossRef] [PubMed]
32. American Diabetes Association. Healthy Living. Hypoglycemia (Low Blood Glucose). Available online: https://www.diabetes.org/healthy-living/medication-treatments/blood-glucose-testing-and-control/hypoglycemia (accessed on 8 February 2022).
33. Provost, F. Machine learning from imbalanced data sets 101. In *AAAI Technical Report WS-00-05, Proceedings of the AAAI'2000 Workshop on Imbalanced Data Sets, Austin, TX, USA, 31 July 2000*; AAAI Press: Palo Alto, CA, USA, 2000; Volume 68, p. 2000.
34. Chawla, N.V. Data mining for imbalanced datasets: An overview. In *Data Mining and Knowledge Discovery Handbook*; Springer: Berlin/Heidelberg, Germany, 2009; pp. 875–886.

MDPI AG
Grosspeteranlage 5
4052 Basel
Switzerland
Tel.: +41 61 683 77 34

Journal of Personalized Medicine Editorial Office
E-mail: jpm@mdpi.com
www.mdpi.com/journal/jpm

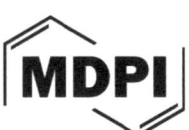

Disclaimer/Publisher's Note: The title and front matter of this reprint are at the discretion of the Guest Editors. The publisher is not responsible for their content or any associated concerns. The statements, opinions and data contained in all individual articles are solely those of the individual Editors and contributors and not of MDPI. MDPI disclaims responsibility for any injury to people or property resulting from any ideas, methods, instructions or products referred to in the content.

www.ingramcontent.com/pod-product-compliance
Lightning Source LLC
LaVergne TN
LVHW070000100526
838202LV00019B/2589